Management of the Difficult Pediatric Airway

Management of the Difficult Pediatric Airway

Edited by

Narasimhan Jagannathan
Ann & Robert H. Lurie Children's Hospital of Chicago
Northwestern University Feinberg School of Medicine

John E. Fiadjoe
Perelman School of Medicine, University of Pennsylvania
Children's Hospital of Philadelphia

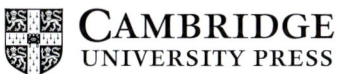

CAMBRIDGE
UNIVERSITY PRESS

University Printing House, Cambridge CB2 8BS, United Kingdom

One Liberty Plaza, 20th Floor, New York, NY 10006, USA

477 Williamstown Road, Port Melbourne, VIC 3207, Australia

314–321, 3rd Floor, Plot 3, Splendor Forum, Jasola District Centre, New Delhi – 110025, India

79 Anson Road, #06-04/06, Singapore 079906

Cambridge University Press is part of the University of Cambridge.

It furthers the University's mission by disseminating knowledge in the pursuit of education, learning, and research at the highest international levels of excellence.

www.cambridge.org
Information on this title: www.cambridge.org/9781108492584
DOI: 10.1017/9781316658680

© Cambridge University Press 2020

This publication is in copyright. Subject to statutory exception and to the provisions of relevant collective licensing agreements, no reproduction of any part may take place without the written permission of Cambridge University Press.

First published 2020

Printed in Singapore by Markono Print Media Pte Ltd

A catalogue record for this publication is available from the British Library.

Library of Congress Cataloging-in-Publication Data

Names: Jagannathan, Narasimhan, 1975– editor. | Fiadjoe, John E., 1972– editor.
Title: Management of the difficult pediatric airway / edited by Narasimhan Jagannathan, John E. Fiadjoe.
Description: Cambridge, United Kingdom ; New York, NY : Cambridge University Press, 2019. | Includes bibliographical references and index.
Identifiers: LCCN 2019012183 | ISBN 9781108492584 (hardback : alk. paper)
Subjects: | MESH: Airway Obstruction–surgery | Airway Management–methods | Child | Infant
Classification: LCC RF51 | NLM WF 145 | DDC 617.5/40083–dc23
LC record available at https://lccn.loc.gov/2019012183

ISBN 978-1-108-49258-4 Hardback

Cambridge University Press has no responsibility for the persistence or accuracy of URLs for external or third-party internet websites referred to in this publication and does not guarantee that any content on such websites is, or will remain, accurate or appropriate.

••

Every effort has been made in preparing this book to provide accurate and up-to-date information that is in accord with accepted standards and practice at the time of publication. Although case histories are drawn from actual cases, every effort has been made to disguise the identities of the individuals involved. Nevertheless, the authors, editors, and publishers can make no warranties that the information contained herein is totally free from error, not least because clinical standards are constantly changing through research and regulation. The authors, editors, and publishers therefore disclaim all liability for direct or consequential damages resulting from the use of material contained in this book. Readers are strongly advised to pay careful attention to information provided by the manufacturer of any drugs or equipment that they plan to use.

Contents

List of Contributors   vii

Section 1 Basic Principles, Assessment, and Planning of Airway Management

1. **Developmental Anatomy of the Airway**   1
   Rebecca S. Isserman and Ronald S. Litman

2. **The Difficult Pediatric Airway: Predictors, Incidence, and Complications**   8
   Nicholas E. Burjek

3. **Universal Algorithms and Approaches to Airway Management**   20
   Thomas Engelhardt and Andreas Machotta

Section 2 Devices and Techniques to Manage the Abnormal Airway

4. **Direct Laryngoscopy Equipment and Techniques**   27
   Maria Matuszczak and Cheryl K. Gooden

5. **Supraglottic Airway Equipment and Techniques**   38
   Andrea S. Huang, Lisa E. Sohn, Suman Rao, and Narasimhan Jagannathan

6. **Oxygenation Techniques for Children with Difficult Airways**   55
   Paul A. Baker

7. **Video Laryngoscopy Equipment and Techniques**   69
   Agnes I. Hunyady, James Peyton, Sarah Lee, and Raymond Park

8. **Flexible Bronchoscopy Techniques: Nasal and Oral Approaches**   90
   Paul Stricker and Pete G. Kovatsis

9. **Optical Stylet and Light-Guided Equipment and Techniques**   103
   Rajeev Subramanyam and Mohamed Mahmoud

10. **Rigid Bronchoscopy Equipment and Techniques**   112
    Jessica M. Van Beek-King and Jeffrey C. Rastatter

11. **Hybrid Approaches to the Difficult Pediatric Airway**   118
    Patrick N. Olomu, Grace Hsu, and Justin L. Lockman

12. **Muscle Relaxants**   129
    Annery Garcia-Marcinkiewicz and John E. Fiadjoe

13. **Management of the "Can't Intubate, Can't Oxygenate" Scenario**   132
    Vivian Man-ying Yuen, Stefano Sabato, and Birgitta Wong

14. **Ultrasonography for Airway Management**   143
    Michael S. Kristensen, Wendy H. Teoh, and Thomas Engelhardt

15. **Difficult Airway Cart**   155
    Alyson Walker and Britta S. von Ungern-Sternberg

Section 3 Special Topics

16. **Extubation in Children with Difficult Airways**   161
    Luis Sequera-Ramos, Alec Zhu, Benjamin Kiesel, and Narasimhan Jagannathan

17. **Airway Management in the Child with an Airway Injury**   169
    Somaletha T. Bhattacharya

18. **Airway Management Outside of the Operating Room: the Emergency Department**   177
    Aaron Donoghue

Contents

19 **Airway Management of the Neonate and Infant: the Difficult and Critical Airway in the Intensive Care Unit Setting** 185
Janet Lioy, Erin Tkach, and Luv Javia

20 **Airway Management in EXIT Procedures** 204
Debnath Chatterjee and Timothy M. Crombleholme

21 **One-Lung Ventilation** 212
T. Wesley Templeton and Eduardo Goenaga-Diaz

Appendix Airway Management Videos 229
Michelle Tsao, Anthony Tantoco, and Narasimhan Jagannathan
Index 230

Contributors

Paul A. Baker, MBChB MD FANZCA
Department of Anaesthesiology, Faculty of Medical and Health Science, University of Auckland, and Department of Paediatric Anaesthesia, Starship Children's Hospital, Auckland, New Zealand

Jessica M. Van Beek-King, MD
Pediatric Otolaryngology, Clinical Science Center, Madison, WI, USA

Somaletha T. Bhattacharya, MD, FFARCSI
Department of Anesthesia, Critical Care, and Pain Medicine, Massachusetts General Hospital, Boston, MA, USA

Nicholas E. Burjek, MD
Department of Pediatric Anesthesiology, Ann & Robert H. Lurie Children's Hospital of Chicago, and Northwestern University Feinberg School of Medicine, Chicago, IL, USA

Debnath Chatterjee, MD, FAAP
Children's Hospital Colorado and Colorado Fetal Care Center, University of Colorado School of Medicine, Aurora, CO, USA

Timothy M. Crombleholme, MD
Children's Hospital Colorado and Colorado Fetal Care Center, University of Colorado School of Medicine, Aurora, CO, USA

Aaron Donoghue, MD, MSCE
Critical Care Medicine and Pediatrics, Perelman School of Medicine, University of Pennsylvania, and Critical Care Medicine and Emergency Medicine, Children's Hospital of Philadelphia, Philadelphia, PA, USA

Thomas Engelhardt, MD, PhD FRCA
Department of Anaesthesia, Royal Aberdeen Children's Hospital, Aberdeen, Scotland, UK

John E. Fiadjoe, MD
Department of Anesthesiology and Critical Care at the University of Pennsylvania, Perelman School of Medicine in Philadelphia, PA, USA

Annery Garcia-Marcinkiewicz, MD
Department of Anesthesiology and Critical Care, Children's Hospital of Philadelphia and Perelman School of Medicine, University of Pennsylvania Philadelphia, PA, USA

Eduardo Goenaga-Diaz, MD
Department of Anesthesiology, Wake Forest School of Medicine, NC, USA

Cheryl K. Gooden, MD, FAAP, FASA
Yale New Haven Children's Hospital, and Yale University School of Medicine
New Haven, CT, USA

Grace Hsu, MD
Department of Anesthesiology and Critical Care, Children's Hospital of Philadelphia and Perelman School of Medicine, University of Pennsylvania Philadelphia, PA, USA

Andrea S. Huang, MD
Department of Pediatric Anesthesiology, Ann & Robert H. Lurie Children's Hospital of Chicago, and Northwestern University Feinberg School of Medicine, Chicago, IL, USA

Agnes I. Hunyady, MD
Seattle Children's Hospital, and University of Washington School of Medicine, Seattle, WA, USA

Rebecca S. Isserman, MD
Department of Anesthesiology and Critical Care, Children's Hospital of Philadelphia and Perelman School of Medicine, University of Pennsylvania Philadelphia, PA, USA

List of Contributors

Narasimhan Jagannathan, MD, MBA
Department of Pediatric Anesthesiology, Ann & Robert H. Lurie Children's Hospital of Chicago, and Northwestern University Feinberg School of Medicine, Chicago, IL, USA

Luv Javia, MD
Cochlear Implant Program, Center for Pediatric Airway Disorders, Pediatric Otolaryngology, Children's Hospital of Philadelphia and Department of Clinical Otorhinolaryngology / Head and Neck Surgery, University of Pennsylvania Perelman School of Medicine, PA, USA

Benjamin Kiesel, MD
Department of Emergency Medicine, Northwestern Medicine, Chicago, IL, USA

Pete G. Kovatsis, MD, FAAP
Department of Anesthesiology, Critical Care, and Pain Medicine, Boston Children's Hospital, and Department of Anaesthesiology, Harvard Medical School, Boston, MA, USA

Michael S. Kristensen, MD
Rigshospitalet, University Hospital of Copenhagen, Denmark

Sarah Lee, MD
Harborview Medical Center, and University of Washington School of Medicine, Seattle, WA, USA

Janet Lioy, MD, FAAP
Children's Hospital of Philadelphia, PA, USA

Ronald S. Litman, DO, ML
Department of Anesthesiology and Critical Care, Children's Hospital of Philadelphia, and Perelman School of Medicine, University of Pennsylvania Philadelphia, PA, USA

Justin L. Lockman, MD, MSEd
Department of Anesthesiology and Critical Care, Children's Hospital of Philadelphia and Perelman School of Medicine, University of Pennsylvania Philadelphia, PA, USA

Andreas Machotta, MD, DEAA
Department of Anesthesiology, Sophia Children's Hospital, Erasmus MC, Rotterdam, Netherlands

Mohamed Mahmoud, MD
Cincinnati Children's Hospital Medical Center, University of Cincinnati, Cincinnati, OH, USA

Maria Matuszczak, MD
Department of Anesthesiology, McGovern Medical School, UTHealth, Houston, TX, USA

Patrick N. Olomu, MD, FRCA
Department of Anesthesiology and Pain Medicine, University of Texas Southwestern Medical Center and Children's Health System of Texas, Dallas, TX, USA

Raymond Park, MD
Department of Anesthesiology, Critical Care, and Pain Medicine, Boston Children's Hospital, and Department of Anaesthesiology, Harvard Medical School, Boston, MA, USA

James Peyton, MBChB MRCP FRCA
Department of Anesthesiology, Critical Care, and Pain Medicine, Boston Children's Hospital, and Department of Anaesthesiology, Harvard Medical School, Boston, MA, USA

Suman Rao, MD
Northwestern University Feinberg School of Medicine, Chicago, IL, USA

Jeffrey C. Rastatter, MD
Pediatric Otolaryngology, Ann & Robert H. Lurie Children's Hospital of Chicago, Northwestern University Feinberg School of Medicine, Chicago, IL, USA

Luis Sequera-Ramos, MD
Department of Anesthesiology and Critical Care, Children's Hospital of Philadelphia and Perelman School of Medicine, University of Pennsylvania Philadelphia, PA, USA

Stefano Sabato, MBBS, FANZCA
Department of Anaesthesia and Pain Management, Royal Children's Hospital Melbourne, Victoria, Australia; Murdoch Children's Research Institute, Parkville, Victoria, Australia

Lisa E. Sohn, MD
Department of Pediatric Anesthesiology, Ann & Robert H. Lurie Children's Hospital of Chicago, and Northwestern University Feinberg School of Medicine, Chicago, IL, USA

List of Contributors

Paul Stricker, MD
Department of Anesthesiology and Critical Care, Children's Hospital of Philadelphia and Perelman School of Medicine, University of Pennsylvania Philadelphia, PA, USA

Rajeev Subramanyam, MBBS, MD, MS
Department of Anesthesiology and Critical Care Medicine, Children's Hospital of Philadelphia, Philadelphia, PA, USA

Anthony Tantoco, MD
Department of Pediatric Anesthesiology, Ann & Robert H. Lurie Children's Hospital of Chicago, and Northwestern University Feinberg School of Medicine, Chicago, IL, USA

Erin Tkach, MD, FAAP
Desert Neonatal Associates, an Envision Physician Services Provider, AZ, USA

Michelle Tsao, MD
Department of Pediatric Anesthesiology, Ann & Robert H. Lurie Children's Hospital of Chicago, and Northwestern University Feinberg School of Medicine, Chicago, IL, USA

T. Wesley Templeton, MD
Department of Anesthesiology, Wake Forest School of Medicine, NC, USA

Wendy H. Teoh, MBBS, FANZCA
Wendy Teoh Pte. Ltd, Private Anaesthesia Practice, Singapore

Britta S. von Ungern-Sternberg, MD, PhD, DEAA, FANZCA
Department of Anaesthesia and Pain Management, Perth Children's Hospital, and
Medical School, The University of Western Australia, and Telethon Kids Institute, Perth, Australia

Alyson Walker, MBChB BSc MRCP FRCA
Department of Anaesthesia and Pain Management, Royal Hospital for Children, Glasgow, Scotland, UK

Birgitta Wong, MBBS
Department of Surgery, Li Ka Shing Faculty of Medicine, The University of Hong Kong, Hong Kong

Vivian Man-ying Yuen, MBBS
Department of Anaesthesiology, The University of Hong Kong, Hong Kong

Alec Zhu, BS
Department of Urology, Northwestern University Feinberg School of Medicine, Chicago, IL, USA

Section 1 Basic Principles, Assessment, and Planning of Airway Management

Chapter 1

Developmental Anatomy of the Airway

Rebecca S. Isserman and Ronald S. Litman

Expertise in airway management in infants and young children requires a comprehensive knowledge and understanding of the developmental anatomy of the human upper airway from birth through adolescence. This chapter will review these topics as well as the anatomical and developmental causes for common syndromes that are associated with difficult mask ventilation or difficult tracheal intubation.

Embryonic Development[1–5]

The upper airway consists of the air-conducting passages from the nose to the carina.[3] The structures of the upper airway continue to change their shape and properties until late into the first decade of life. Less is known about their developmental course during fetal life as compared with other organ systems because much of this understanding is gained from postmortem studies.

Upper airway structures develop with the cranium and the most cephalad boundaries of the digestive and respiratory systems. The lateral surface of a 5-week-old 4.0 mm embryo contains five or six pairs of narrow masses called *branchial (pharyngeal) arches*. Each branchial arch contains characteristic types of ectoderm and mesoderm, the primordial precursors of epithelial (e.g., skin) and mesothelial structures (e.g., muscle, bone), respectively. The structures of each branchial arch receive motor or sensory innervation from an adjacent cranial nerve. When the primordial muscle cell migrates, it retains its original embryonic innervation. The structures between the branchial arches are the *branchial (pharyngeal) clefts*, which, with the exception of the first cleft, disappear during the course of development. The tissue underlying the branchial clefts contains outpouchings of the foregut region called pharyngeal pouches. The pharyngeal pouches will develop into the corresponding endothelial structures of the upper digestive and respiratory organ systems.

The first branchial arch develops into the mandible, maxilla, and the muscles of mastication. It contributes to development of the bones of the middle ear and the muscles between the ear and mandible, such as the tensor tympani, tensor veli palatini, and the anterior belly of the digastric muscle. Motor and sensory innervation to the structures derived from the first arch are supplied by the trigeminal nerve (cranial nerve V).

The second branchial arch forms bony and muscular structures from the ear (proximally) to the hyoid bone (distally), including the muscles of the face and inner ear that are innervated by the facial nerve (cranial nerve VII). Skeletal contribution from the second branchial arch includes the styloid process and the lesser cornu of the hyoid bone.

The third branchial arch develops into the body and greater cornu of the hyoid bone and the stylopharyngeus muscle, which aids in elevating the pharynx during swallowing, and is innervated by the glossopharyngeal nerve (cranial nerve IX).

The fourth through sixth branchial arches contribute to the formation of the thyroid, cricoid, arytenoid, corniculate, and cuneiform laryngeal cartilages, as well as the muscles that form the pharynx, larynx, and upper half of the esophagus. These structures are innervated by the vagus (cranial nerve X) and accessory (cranial nerve XI) nerves. The earliest appearance of the future larynx is seen as a bud growing out from the ventral part of the foregut at approximately 4 weeks' gestation. The laryngeal and esophageal tracts are initially seen as one common tube, which eventually separates into two adjacent and functionally different conduits. By 16 weeks' gestation, the larynx contains all its definitive elements in their proper proportions. During fetal and postnatal growth, the development of the size of the larynx closely parallels the size of the surrounding bony and cartilaginous structures.[6]

The first branchial cleft becomes part of the external auditory canal, while the remaining clefts do not correspond to recognizable human structures. Nevertheless, abnormal formation here can lead to cysts or more significant malformations.

The first pharyngeal pouch becomes incorporated into the future temporal bone and forms the epithelial lining of the middle ear and the tympanic membrane. The second pharyngeal pouch develops into the tonsil. The superior portion of the third pharyngeal pouch differentiates into the inferior parathyroid, and the inferior portion migrates caudally to become the thymus. The fourth pharyngeal pouch forms the superior parathyroid gland; the area roughly corresponding to the fifth and sixth pharyngeal pouches is incorporated into the thyroid gland.

Postnatal Development

Airway management of infants and young children will be influenced by developmental differences in head and neck anatomy. These differences are influenced by two major growth spurts during childhood that contribute to the vertical growth of the facial structures: the first at the time of the acquisition of permanent dentition (i.e., 7–10 years of age), and the second during puberty in the teenage years.

When compared to the older child, the infant's skull (especially the occipital region) is relatively larger, such that neck flexion may not be required to attain the classic sniffing position that optimizes visualization of the glottic structures during laryngoscopy. At birth, the neurocranium-to-face size ratio is 8:1, and declines to 6:1 at 2 years of age, 4:1 at 5 years of age, and approximately 2:1 by adulthood.[7,8] The growth of the lower facial bones is proportionately linear from 1 to 11 years of age.[6]

The mandibular arch of the infant is U-shaped and becomes more V-shaped during childhood until it is completely developed during adolescence. The angle between the ramus and the body of the mandible is more obtuse in infants than in adults. This largely accounts for the relatively low incidence of difficult intubations in children compared with adults.

Overall, the most important difference in nasal anatomy between young children and adults is merely the smaller size. Small nasal passages are more likely to become obstructed with blood or secretions as a result of instrumentations during airway management. Children are less likely to have occult nasal polyps or septal deviations when compared with adults.[9] The anatomical dimensions of the nasopharynx increase linearly between 1 and 11 years of age.[6]

Early literature indicated that small infants were obligate nasal breathers, which predisposed them to breathing difficulties during periods of nasal obstruction. However, this has largely been disproven,[10] although infants with choanal atresia will often develop upper airway obstruction, which results in varying degrees of hypoxemia.[11]

The infant tongue is relatively larger in proportion to the oral cavity when compared with the adult. Tongue volume increases linearly between ages 1 and 11 years.[6] Magnetic resonance imaging (MRI) studies of the upper airway during general anesthesia have demonstrated that, as in adults,[12] upper airway obstruction occurs primarily at the levels of the soft palate and epiglottis, and not at the base of the tongue.[13]

The 20 primary teeth, identified by a lettering system, begin to erupt during the first year of life, and are shed between 6 and 12 years of age. The 32 permanent teeth begin to appear at the same time as the primary teeth are shed and are identified by a numbering system.

In newborns, the uvula and epiglottis are in close proximity within the oropharynx, which facilitates nasal breathing and oral ingestion of liquids simultaneously. This anatomical relationship is maintained throughout most of the first year of life, but during the second year, the larynx begins to descend as it adapts to its greater role in phonation.

Although the mechanisms have not been elucidated, the pharynx of premature newborns is susceptible to passive collapse, especially during apnea, but may also collapse as a result of cervical flexion or nasal obstruction.[14] These effects are exacerbated by the administration of general anesthesia or sedatives, which decrease pharyngeal muscle tone. Furthermore, pharyngeal collapse often occurs in premature infants during application of cricoid pressure.

Of interest, the upper airway of a normal infant is smaller in both inspiration and expiration at 6 weeks of age compared with the neonatal period. This relative narrowing may be caused by postnatal growth of adenoid tissue or thickening of the mucous membrane lining in response to infection or second-hand smoke exposure. The linear dimensions of the soft palate and oropharynx increase linearly between 1 and 11 years of age.[6,15]

Adenoidal and tonsillar tissue is minimal at birth, and then grows rapidly between 4 and 7 years of age. The growth of airway lymphoid tissue parallels the growth of the facial and cervical bony structures.[6] Hypertrophied tonsil and adenoid tissue is likely the most common cause of upper airway obstruction after administration of general anesthesia in children in this age group.

The epiglottis of infants is relatively narrow and short, and angled into the lumen of the airway. The lower portion of the oropharynx at the level of the epiglottis is particularly compliant and prone to collapse during anesthetic or sedative-induced loss of consciousness. Obstruction at the level of the epiglottis can be significantly decreased by placing the child in the lateral position.[16]

The effect of sex on oropharyngeal length has been studied, with particular reference to an association between relatively longer airway length and the predisposition to obstructive sleep apnea.[17] Prior to the onset of puberty, boys and girls have relatively similar oropharyngeal length, but after the onset of puberty, the oropharyngeal lengths in boys are greater than those of girls, even after correcting for height and weight. The relatively longer upper airway length in males has been implicated as a possible etiologic factor in the greater disposition in males toward obstructive sleep apnea.[18] Thus, postpubertal males may have a greater disposition toward upper airway collapse in response to administration of pharmacological agents that depress consciousness.

During infancy, the relative position of the larynx is slightly higher in the neck than in older children and adults. Although its position relative to the cervical spine is complete by 3 years of age (it descends from C2–C3 to C4–C5), it continues to descend relative to other facial structures such as the mandible.[19] The tip of the epiglottis proceeds in a gradual and linear descent from C2 to C3 from birth to 18 years of age.[20] This relative movement is unique to humans because of the shifting functionality from sucking and swallowing while breathing to the development of speech later in life. Early in life, a relatively high larynx facilitates simultaneous sucking and respiration due to the apposition of the epiglottis (as high as C1) and the soft palate. Additional differences in early life that protect against aspiration during feeding include relatively thicker aryepiglottic folds and larger arytenoids.

The chest wall of neonates and small infants is highly compliant and tends to collapse inward, thus reducing functional residual capacity (FRC) and promoting atelectasis. To preserve FRC, the adductor muscles of the larynx act as an expiratory "valve," and restrict exhalation in order to maintain positive end-expiratory pressure (PEEP). This is referred to as "laryngeal braking."[21,22]

The higher position of the larynx during infancy influences airway management to the extent that the glottic opening is more easily visualized using a straight, rather than a curved, laryngoscope. In infants of less than 1 year of age, elevation of the base of the skull during direct laryngoscopy is usually not necessary.[23]

In children who have received neuromuscular blockade, the fixed-diameter cricoid cartilage is the narrowest structure of the upper airway because of its inability to distend in a similar manner to the vocal cords.[24–26] A tracheal tube that easily passes through the relatively compliant vocal cords may compress surface mucosa at the subglottic level or the cricoid cartilage and predispose to inflammation, edema, and subsequent scarring and stenosis.[27–29] Tracheal edema is more likely to increase airway resistance in smaller diameter airways since the resistance to flow through a tube is related to the fifth power of the radius of the tube (since this flow is largely turbulent). In non-intubated, sedated children without neuromuscular blockade, the adductor muscles of the vocal cords are tonically active, and are the basis for the narrowest portion of the upper airway to occur at this level.[30–32] The relationship between the sizes of the structures along the upper airway remains relatively stable throughout growth and development.[32] There is no specific age during childhood at which the use of an uncuffed tracheal tube would be beneficial.

Tracheal lengths (distance between glottis and carina) increase linearly during childhood.[25,33] A familiarity with these distances in infants will facilitate proper placement of the tracheal tube midway between the glottis and carina to minimize the risk of displacement (either too high out of the larynx or too low into the main bronchus) with changes in head or neck position.

Anatomical Basis for Syndromes Associated with Difficult Airways

Up to 3% of children have congenital or acquired upper airway abnormalities, frequently associated with a craniofacial anomaly, which may result in difficulty in mask ventilation or tracheal intubation.[1] Successful airway management requires an understanding of the anatomical basis of these abnormalities and the relationship to normal development. To organize these craniofacial anomalies, the Committee on Nomenclature and Classification of Craniofacial Anomalies of the American Cleft Palate Association has organized them into five distinct categories: *hypoplasia*, *clefts*, *synostosis*, *hyperplasia*, and *unclassified*.[34,35] The first three of these are often implicated in difficult airways.

Anomalies within the *hypoplasia* category are characterized by hypoplasia or atrophy of a portion of the craniofacial skeleton. Micrognathia, or mandibular hypoplasia, is a common cause of difficulty with either ventilation or intubation in the neonatal period and beyond.[36] The finding of micrognathia along with glossoptosis and resultant airway obstruction defines Pierre Robin sequence, which occurs in up to 1:8500 live births. PRS can occur in isolation, associated with additional congenital malformations, or as part of a clinical syndrome with a specific chromosomal anomaly (in approximately 60% of cases).[37] The wide range of clinical conditions demonstrating PRS suggests a diverse developmental pathogenesis of the sequence, with a few leading hypotheses elucidated.[38]

Intrauterine constraint, leading to compression of the chin and limitation of jaw growth prenatally has been implicated in both asymmetric and symmetric micrognathia. Support for this theory includes findings of pressure indentations on the chest at birth, associated with muscular torticollis on the same side as unilateral micrognathia, and an increased incidence of PRS in twin gestations.[39] The hypothesis that PRS develops as a primary failure of mandibular outgrowth traces development of the mandible back to its origin in the first branchial arch. Unlike the maxilla, which forms as bone in close association with the developing facial bones, the mandible forms in relative isolation, initially as cartilage, called Meckel's cartilage. Micrognathia, in this theory, is due to defective generation and/or growth of this cartilage.[38] In either case, mandibular hypoplasia prevents fusion of the palatal shelf, which normally occurs between the eighth and tenth weeks of gestation.[37] This causes the retrognathia, glossoptosis, and airway obstruction that characterizes PRS, and explains the frequent occurrence of cleft palate with PRS.[38]

Aberrant development of the first and second branchial arches is implicated in the etiology of *oculoauriculovertebral spectrum* (OAVS; hemifacial microsomia, Goldenhar syndrome), which involves unilateral hypoplasia of the craniofacial skeleton. As the names imply, there is a wide clinical spectrum associated with this disorder. There is also no consensus on minimum diagnostic criteria; however, the majority of patients have asymmetric microsomia and external ear abnormalities.[40] The reported prevalence varies from as common as 1 in 5600 to 1 in 45 000.[41] While most cases of OAVS are sporadic, there is evidence that genetic, epigenetic, and environmental factors all contribute to the complex etiology of this disorder, likely also involving the neural crest cells in the first and second branchial arches.[40]

Clefting most frequently involves the lip and/or palate, typically not associated with a difficult airway, but also may involve the midface, as in Treacher Collins syndrome (Figure 1.1). This is an autosomal dominant inherited disorder associated with severe airway obstruction, and inability to provide mask ventilation or tracheal intubation. It is associated with a genetic mutation on chromosome 5 and occurs in

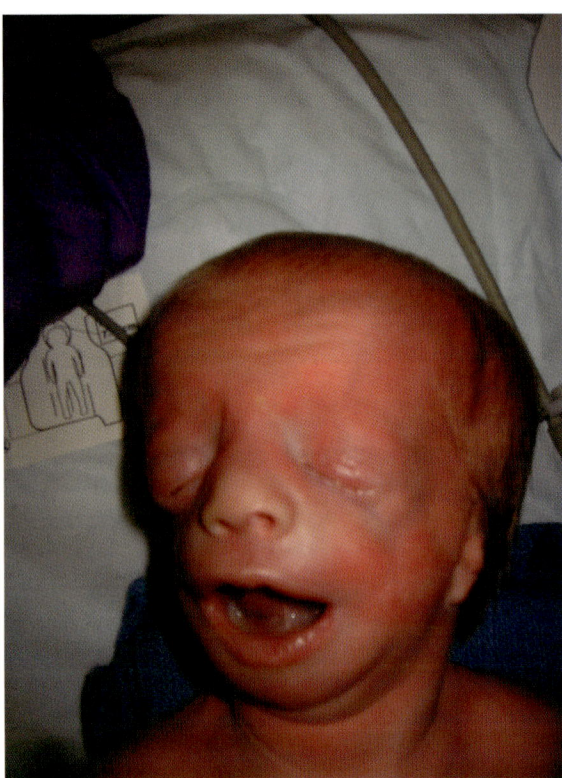

Figure 1.1 Treacher Collins syndrome. (From *Basics of Pediatric Anesthesia*, Litman, RS, ed., 2016, with permission.)

approximately 1:50 000 live births.[42] Specific findings include symmetric maxillary and zygomatic hypoplasia, a high arched and/or cleft palate, downward sloping palpebral fissures, and microtia often associated with hearing loss.[38,42] Most of these findings occur in tissues that arise from the first and second branchial arches and are due to mutations (in the *treacle ribosome biogenesis factor 1 [TCOF1]* gene) associated with a decreased number of cranial neural crest cells in these regions.[42]

Craniosynostosis refers to the abnormal closure of one or more of the cranial sutures, and is commonly associated with midface hypoplasia in syndromes that also have difficult airways. Airway issues are usually related to mask ventilation, with poor mask fit, combined with choanal stenosis and excessive nasopharyngeal soft tissue leading to multilevel airway obstruction. Intubation may also prove difficult and may be worsened by fibrosis or mechanical limitations following midface advancement surgery.[37,43]

Apert syndrome is inherited in an autosomal dominant fashion and is associated with mutations in the *fibroblast growth factor receptor 2 (FGFR-2)* gene on chromosome 10, causing abnormalities in suture closure and bone formation of structures originating from the first branchial arch.[44] Mutations in *FGFR* genes also cause additional craniosynostosis syndromes associated with midface hypoplasia and potential difficult airways, such as Pfeiffer syndrome (Figure 1.2) and Crouzon syndrome.[45] Evaluation of the hands of these patients will help distinguish between these otherwise similarly appearing syndromes. Patients with Apert syndrome have syndactyly, while Pfeiffer syndrome is associated with a broad thumb, and patients with Crouzon syndrome have completely normal hands.[35]

Understanding the changing airway anatomy as children grow, as well as the anatomical causes of difficult airway syndromes is the first step in developing safe and effective airway management plans in the difficult pediatric airway.

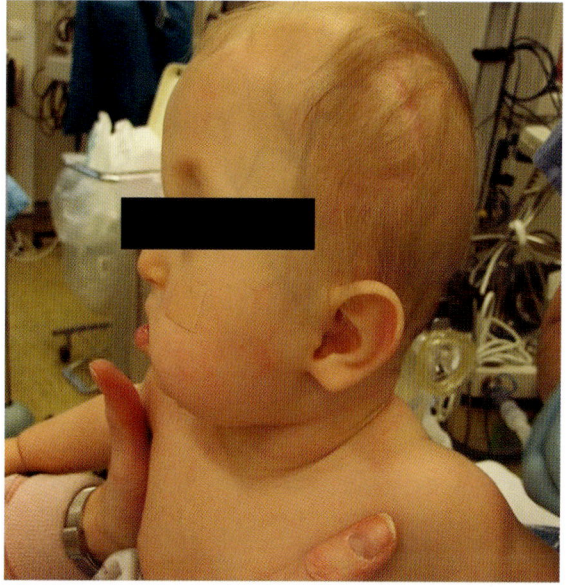

Figure 1.2 Pfeiffer syndrome. (From *Basics of Pediatric Anesthesia*, Litman, RS, ed., 2016, with permission.)

References

1. Pohunek P. Development, Structure and Function of the Upper Airways. *Paediatric Respiratory Reviews* 2004; **5**(1): 2–8.

2. Hast MH. The Developmental Anatomy of the Larynx. *Otolaryngologic Clinics of North America* 1970; **3**: 413–38.

3. Marcus CL, Smith RJH, Mankarious LA, Arens R, Mitchell GS, Elluru RG, et al. Developmental Aspects of the Upper Airway: Report from an NHLBI Workshop, March 5–6, 2009. *Proceedings of the American Thoracic Society* 2009; **6**(6): 513–20.

4. Zaw-Tun HA, Burdi AR. Reexamination of the Origin and Early Development of the Human Larynx. *Cells Tissues Organs* 2016; **122**(3): 163–84.

5. Moore KL, Persaud TVN, Torchia MG. Pharyngeal Apparatus, Face, and Neck. In *The Developing Human*. Elsevier Health Sciences; 2016: 155–93.

6. Arens R, McDonough JM, Corbin AM, Hernandez ME, Maislin G, Schwab RJ, et al. Linear Dimensions of the Upper Airway Structure during Development. *American Journal of Respiratory and Critical Care Medicine* 2012; **165**(1): 117–22.

7. Dorst JP. Changes of the Skull during Childhood. In Newton TH, Potts DG, eds. *Radiology of the Skull and Brain*. St. Louis: Mosby; 1971: 118–31.

8. Sullivan PG. Skull, Jaw, and Teeth Growth Patterns. In Falkner F, Tanner JM, eds. *Human Growth: a Comprehensive Treatise*. New York: Springer; 1986: 243–65.

9. Smith JE, Reid AP. Asymptomatic Intranasal Abnormalities Influencing the Choice of Nostril for Nasotracheal Intubation. *British Journal of Anaesthesia* 1999; **83**(6): 882–6.

10. Miller MJ, Martin RJ, Carlo WA, Fouke JM, Strohl KP, Fanaroff

Section 1: Basic Principles, Assessment, and Planning of Airway Management

AA. Oral Breathing in Newborn Infants. *The Journal of Pediatrics* 1985; **107**(3): 465–9.

11. Cozzi F, Steiner M, Rosati D, Madonna L, Colarossi G. Clinical Manifestations of Choanal Atresia in Infancy. *Journal of Pediatric Surgery* 1988; **23**(3): 203–6.

12. Mathru M, Esch O, Lang J, Herbert ME, Chaljub G, Goodacre B, et al. Magnetic Resonance Imaging of the Upper Airway. Effects of Propofol Anesthesia and Nasal Continuous Positive Airway Pressure in Humans. *Anesthesiology* 1996; **84**(2): 273–9.

13. Litman RS, Weissend EE, Shrier DA, Ward DS. Morphologic Changes in the Upper Airway of Children during Awakening from Propofol Administration. *Anesthesiology* 2002; **96**(3): 607–11.

14. Praud J-P, Reix P. Upper Airways and Neonatal Respiration. *Respiratory Physiology & Neurobiology* 2005; **149**(1–3): 131–41.

15. Jeans WD, Fernando DCJ, Maw AR, Leighton BC. A Longitudinal Study of the Growth of the Nasopharynx and its Contents in Normal Children. *British Journal of Radiology* 2014; **54**(638): 117–21.

16. Litman RS, Wake N, Chan L-ML, McDonough JM, Sin S, Mahboubi S, et al. Effect of Lateral Positioning on Upper Airway Size and Morphology in Sedated Children. *Anesthesiology* 2005; **103**(3): 484–8.

17. Ronen O, Malhotra A, Pillar G. Influence of Gender and Age on Upper-Airway Length during Development. *Pediatrics* 2007; **120**(4): e1028–34.

18. Malhotra A, Huang Y, Fogel RB, Pillar G, Edwards JK, Kikinis R, et al. The Male Predisposition to Pharyngeal Collapse. *American Journal of Respiratory and Critical Care Medicine* 2012; **166**(10): 1388–95.

19. Sasaki CT, Levine PA, Laitman JT, Crelin ES. Postnatal Descent of the Epiglottis in Man: a Preliminary Report. *Archives of Otolaryngology* 1977; **103**(3): 169–71.

20. Schwartz DS, Keller MS. Maturational Descent of the Epiglottis. Archives of Otolaryngology – Head & Neck Surgery. 1997 Jun; **123**(6): 627–8.

21. Radvanyi-Bouvet MF, Monset-Couchard M, Morel-Kahn F, Vicente G, Dreyfus-Brisac C. Expiratory Patterns during Sleep in Normal Full-Term and Premature Neonates. *Neonatology* 1982; **41**(1–2): 74–84.

22. Mortola JP, Milic-Emili J, Noworaj A, Smith B, Fox G, Weeks S. Muscle Pressure and Flow during Expiration in Infants. *American Review of Respiratory Disease* 1984; **129**(1): 49–53.

23. Westhorpe RN. The Position of the Larynx in Children and its Relationship to the Ease of Intubation. *Anaesthesia and Intensive Care* 1987; **15**(4): 384–8.

24. Eckenhoff JE. Some Anatomic Considerations of the Infant Larynx Influencing Endotracheal Anesthesia. *Anesthesiology* 1951; **12**(4): 401–10.

25. Butz RO. Length and Cross-Section Growth Patterns in the Human Trachea. *Pediatrics* 1968; **42**(2): 336–41.

26. Wailoo MP, Emery JL. Normal Growth and Development of the Trachea. *Thorax* 1982; **37**(8): 584–7.

27. Benjamin B. Prolonged Intubation Injuries of the Larynx: Endoscopic Diagnosis, Classification, and Treatment. *Annals of Otology, Rhinology & Laryngology Supplement* 1993; **160**: 1–15.

28. Gould SJ, Howard S. The Histopathology of the Larynx in the Neonate Following Endotracheal Intubation. *The Journal of Pathology* 1985; **146**(4): 301–11.

29. Joshi VV, Mandavia SG, Stern L, Wiglesworth FW. Acute Lesions Induced by Endotracheal Intubation: Occurrence in the Upper Respiratory Tract of Newborn Infants with Respiratory Distress Syndrome. *American Journal of Diseases in Children* 1972; **124**(5): 646–9.

30. Dalal PG, Murray D, Messner AH, Feng A, McAllister J, Molter D. Pediatric Laryngeal Dimensions: an Age-Based Analysis. *Anesthesia & Analgesia* 2009; **108**(5): 1475–9.

31. Dalal PG, Murray D, Feng A, Molter D, McAllister J. Upper Airway Dimensions in Children Using Rigid Video-Bronchoscopy and a Computer Software: Description of a Measurement Technique. *Pediatric Anesthesia* 2008; **18**(7): 645–53.

32. Litman RS, Weissend EE, Shibata D, Westesson P-L. Developmental Changes of Laryngeal Dimensions in Unparalyzed, Sedated Children. *Anesthesiology* 2003; **98**(1): 41–5.

33. Griscom NT, Wohl ME. Dimensions of the Growing Trachea Related to Age and Gender. *American Journal of Roentgenology* 2012; **146**(2): 233–7.

34. Whitaker LA, Pashayan H, Reichman J. A Proposed New Classification of Craniofacial Anomalies for The American Cleft Palate Association Committee on Nomenclature and Classification of Craniofacial Anomalies. *Cleft Palate Journal* 1981; **18**(3): 161–75.

35. Cladis FP, Grunwaldt L, Losee J. Anesthesia for Plastic Surgery. In Davis PJ, Cladis FP, eds. *Smith's Anesthesia for Infants and Children*. 8th ed. Philadelphia, PA: Elsevier; 2017: 821–41.

36. Evans KN, Sie KC, Hopper RA, Glass RP, Hing AV, Cunningham ML. Robin Sequence: From Diagnosis to Development of an Effective Management Plan. *Pediatrics* 2011; **127**(5): 936–48.

37 Raj D, Luginbuehl I. Managing the Difficult Airway in the Syndromic Child. *Continuing Education in Anaesthesia Critical Care & Pain* 2015; **15**(1): 7–13.

38 Tan TY, Kilpatrick N, Farlie PG. Developmental and Genetic Perspectives on Pierre Robin Sequence. *Seminars in Medical Genetics, Part C of American Journal of Medical Genetics* 2013; **163**(4): 295–305.

39 Graham JM Jr., Sanchez-Lara PA. *Smith's Recognizable Patterns of Human Deformation*. 4th ed. Philadelphia: Elsevier; 2016.

40 Beleza-Meireles A, Clayton-Smith J, Saraiva JM, Tassabehji M. Oculo-Auriculo-Vertebral Spectrum: a Review of the Literature and Genetic Update. *Journal of Medical Genetics* 2014; **51**(10): 635–45.

41 Barisic I, Odak L, Loane M, Garne E, Wellesley D, Calzolari E, et al. Prevalence, Prenatal Diagnosis and Clinical Features of Oculo-Auriculo-Vertebral Spectrum: a Registry-Based Study in Europe. *European Journal of Human Genetics* 2014; **22**(8): 1026–33.

42 van Gijn DR, Tucker AS, Cobourne MT. Craniofacial Development: Current Concepts in the Molecular Basis of Treacher Collins Syndrome. *British Journal of Oral & Maxillofacial Surgery* 2013; **51**(5): 384–8.

43 Gripp K, Escobar LF. Facial Bones. In Stevenson RE, Hall JG, eds. *Human Malformations and Related Anomalies*. Oxford: Oxford University Press; 2005: 267–95.

44 Lomri A, Lemonnier J, Hott M, de Parseval N, Lajeunie E, Munnich A, et al. Increased Calvaria Cell Differentiation and Bone Matrix Formation Induced by Fibroblast Growth Factor Receptor 2 Mutations in Apert Syndrome. *The Journal of Clinical Investigation* 1998; **101**(6): 1310–17.

45 Buchanan EP, Xue AS, Hollier LH Jr. Craniofacial Syndromes. *Plastic and Reconstructive Surgery* 2014; **134**(1): 128e–53e.

Section 1 Basic Principles, Assessment, and Planning of Airway Management

Chapter 2

The Difficult Pediatric Airway: Predictors, Incidence, and Complications

Nicholas E. Burjek

Airway and respiratory complications are frequent causes of anesthetic-related morbidity in the pediatric patient.[1,2] Often, these complications occur in patients who are difficult to mask-ventilate, intubate, or manage with a supraglottic airway (SGA) device. While not all challenging airways can be identified preoperatively, recognizing anatomical features predictive of difficult intubation will facilitate preparation and enhance safety. When faced with the anticipated difficult airway, the anesthesiologist may change his or her plan for induction and ventilation, prepare additional airway equipment and emergency medications, and have extra help available for the airway management. This likely explains the lower complication rates seen with the management of anticipated versus unanticipated difficult airways.[3] In addition to identifying the potentially difficult airway, understanding the most common airway complications, their risk factors, and strategies for prevention and treatment are vital components of safe pediatric airway management.

Unique Features of the Pediatric Airway

General Pediatric Population

Even the "normal" pediatric airway has anatomical features that may make airway management difficult for the anesthesiologist accustomed to caring for adults, and may predispose patients to airway-related complications. A large occiput results in neck flexion when the patient is in the supine position. This leads to compression of the pharyngeal soft tissues and upper airway during mask ventilation, along with poor alignment of the oral, pharyngeal, and laryngeal axes during laryngoscopy. The tongue and tonsils are large compared to the rest of the oral cavity, leading to anatomical obstruction during mask ventilation. Additionally, bleeding from tonsillar trauma can obstruct the laryngoscopist's view and lead to airway irritation. The larynx sits in a more cranial position in the neck, making visualization of the glottic opening more difficult. The epiglottis is long and floppy, can be difficult to lift, and may obstruct the view of the glottic opening. The smaller size of the pharynx and larynx complicates maneuvering of airway equipment, and may predispose to tissue damage. The glottic opening and lower airways have a small diameter, and any further narrowing due to edema or bronchospasm can rapidly lead to serious airway obstruction.

Aspects of pediatric respiratory physiology may also predispose to complications. The chest wall is compliant and prone to collapse during anesthesia, leading to atelectasis and loss of functional reserve capacity. Along with a faster rate of oxygen consumption, this leads to rapid oxygen desaturation during apneic episodes. The predominance of parasympathetic tone in small children results in bradycardia and cardiovascular collapse in response to hypoxemia. Increased airway reactivity predisposes children to laryngospasm and bronchospasm. Increased reactivity is particularly important among patients with disease states such as asthma, bronchopulmonary dysplasia (BPD), and upper respiratory tract infections: all of which occur more frequently in children.

Despite these challenges, anesthesiologists accustomed to mask ventilating and intubating children can safely and easily manage the majority of pediatric patients.

Airway Anomalies

A small number of pediatric patients have additional features that can make mask ventilation and intubation very difficult or impossible with conventional techniques. These conditions can be categorized as congenital and acquired abnormalities of the face, mouth, neck, or trachea[4] (Table 2.1).

Chapter 2: The Difficult Pediatric Airway: Predictors, Incidence, and Complications

Table 2.1 Classification of Conditions That Affect Airway Management

Functional classification	Condition
Supraglottic abnormalities:	
Maxillary hypoplasia	Apert syndrome Crouzon syndrome Pfeiffer syndrome Saethre–Chotzen syndrome DiGeorge syndrome Achondroplasia
Mandibular hypoplasia	Pierre Robin sequence Treacher Collins syndrome Goldenhar syndrome Stickler syndrome Moebius syndrome Micrognathia CHARGE syndrome (coloboma, heart defects, atresia choanae, restricted growth, genital anomalies, ear anomalies) Cri du chat syndrome
Large obstructive tongue	Beckwith–Wiedemann syndrome Down syndrome Hypothyroidism Lingual tumor

Abnormalities of the entire airway, including glottis	Mucopolysaccharidoses:
	  Hurler syndrome
	  Hunter syndrome
	  Sanfilippo syndrome
	  Morquio syndrome
	  Maroteaux–Lamy syndrome
	Vascular/lymphatic malformation syndromes
	Epidermolysis bullosa

Subglottic abnormalities	Subglottic stenosis Laryngeal stenosis Tracheal stenosis Laryngomalacia Tracheomalacia Airway masses/tumors
Limited mouth opening	Freeman–Sheldon syndrome
Limited neck mobility	Klippel–Feil syndrome Noonan syndrome Arthrogryposis Spinal fusion Cervical stenosis Cervical instability Achondroplasia

Other abnormalities	Infections:
	  Epiglottitis
	  Croup
	Burns
	Anaphylaxis
	Presence of foreign body
	Airway trauma

Conditions such as Treacher Collins syndrome, Apert syndrome, Goldenhar syndrome, and Pierre Robin sequence result from abnormalities in embryologic development of the face and skull. Other syndromes, such as Klippel–Feil, achondroplasia, and the mucopolysaccharidoses result from genetic abnormalities of the soft tissues and skeleton. These disorders may be associated with features such as micrognathia, limited mouth opening, mandibular hypoplasia, midface hypoplasia, macroglossia, microstomia, cleft lip or palate, cervical spine immobility or instability, facial asymmetry, and masses involving the airway: all of which complicate airway management. While these conditions are rare, many of these patients will require multiple anesthetics for diagnostic and therapeutic procedures in their lifetimes. These procedures are often elective, allowing time for optimization and review of prior anesthetic records. These patients are usually cared for at tertiary pediatric hospitals, with anesthesiologists accustomed to dealing with these difficult airways.

Acquired conditions of the airway include infection (croup or epiglottitis), foreign-body aspiration, trauma, anaphylaxis, and burns. These may occur in otherwise healthy children, and often progress rapidly, requiring emergent intubation for ventilatory support, airway protection, or surgical intervention. These patients are more likely to present to non-specialty care centers. Therefore, all anesthesiologists must be prepared to employ the advanced airway maneuvers described in this book, and all hospitals should have the equipment needed to treat the child with the compromised and difficult airway.

Table 2.2 Patient Factors Associated with Difficult Airway Management

Difficult mask ventilation	Age: < 1 year
	Presentation for ENT surgery
Difficult intubation	Age: < 1 year
	Presence of craniofacial syndrome
	American Society of Anesthesiologists (ASA) Physical Status III or IV
	Intensive care unit (ICU) status
	Low body mass index (BMI)
	Mallampati score 3 or 4 (if patient cooperative)
Difficult SGA device placement	Age: < 2 years
	Presentation for ENT surgery
	Presence of craniofacial syndrome
	Inpatient status

Predictors and Incidence of the Difficult Airway

Difficult Mask Ventilation

Valois-Gomez studied the incidence and risk factors for difficult mask ventilation among 484 patients 0–8 years of age undergoing elective surgery at a single tertiary-care children's hospital. Patients who were anticipated to be difficult to mask-ventilate (such as those with congenital craniofacial malformations, cervical instability, or history of difficult airways) were excluded from the study. Difficult mask ventilation was defined as the requirement for at least two of the following maneuvers during mask ventilation: two-person mask ventilation, use of an oral or nasal airway, application of $\geq 5\,cmH_2O$ continuous positive airway pressure (CPAP), or unanticipated need for increased FiO_2. The incidence of unexpected difficult mask ventilation was 6.6%, which is higher than the incidence found in adults, typically cited as 1.5%.[5,6] Younger age and presentation for ear, nose, and throat (ENT) surgery were identified as patient risk factors for difficult mask ventilation. Difficult intubation by direct laryngoscopy was not associated with difficult mask ventilation (Table 2.2). This study may overestimate the true incidence of difficult mask ventilation because many anesthesiologists do not consider placing an oral airway or applying $\geq 5\,cmH_2O$ of CPAP as indicative of a difficult mask ventilation.

Difficult Intubation

Rates of difficult intubation will vary depending on the population examined; however, most studies have found an incidence of 1–3% among pediatric patients presenting for anesthesia. The previously mentioned study by Valois-Gomez found a 1.2% incidence of difficult intubation (Cormack–Lehane laryngoscopic view grade III or IV, intubation time > 5 min, or desaturation to < 95% SpO_2) among patients who were not anticipated to be challenging.[6] Another study of direct laryngoscopy in 11 219 patients undergoing general anesthesia at a tertiary-care pediatrics hospital found a Cormack–Lehane laryngoscopic view of grade III or IV in 1.35% of the patients. This study did not differentiate between anticipated and unanticipated difficulty. The rate was highest among patients younger than 1 year of age (4.7% versus 0.7% in older patients).[7] A study of 511 pediatric patients aged 0–14 years found difficult laryngoscopy in 16% of neonates less than 1 month old, 2.6% of patients aged 1 month to 5 years of age, and no cases of difficult intubation in patients over 5 years of age.[8] In a study of pediatric cardiac surgery patients, the incidence of difficult intubation was 1.25%. Fifty percent of the difficult-to-intubate patients were diagnosed with a craniofacial syndrome, and 81% were younger than 1 year of age.[9] Critically ill patients requiring intubation in the ICU are more likely to be difficult to intubate, with a reported incidence of 9%.[10]

Clearly, the most important predictor of difficult intubation is age of less than 1 year. Other patient factors include ASA Physical Status Classification III and IV, low BMI, presentation for oromaxillofacial surgery, and presence of a craniofacial syndrome.[7,9] While the airway exam is difficult in young patients who are unable to cooperate, two features require mention. The Mallampati score, an important part of evaluation of the adult airway, has been shown to correlate with the Cormack–Lehane laryngoscopic view in patients over 4 years of age who cooperate with the exam. In this population, a Mallampati score of 3 or 4 had a 43% positive predictive value for poor laryngoscopic view, while a Mallampati score of 1 or 2 had a negative predictive value of 99%.[11] The Mallampati score is not useful in younger patients, who are unable to cooperate. In this age group, the most important physical exam finding is micrognathia, or short thyromental distance (Figure 2.1). Micrognathia, while easily missed if not specifically looked for, is the most common physical exam finding in difficult-to-intubate infants, and its presence is associated with intubation- and airway-related complications.[3,8]

Difficult SGA Device Placement

Traditionally, patients were considered to have difficult airways if they were difficult to mask-ventilate or intubate. However, in recent decades, there has been an increased use of SGA devices for elective airway management and airway rescue, including in patients with challenging airways.[12–17] Placement of an SGA device is now an early step in all difficult airway algorithms, including ones specifically designed for pediatric patients.[18,19] As such, identification of

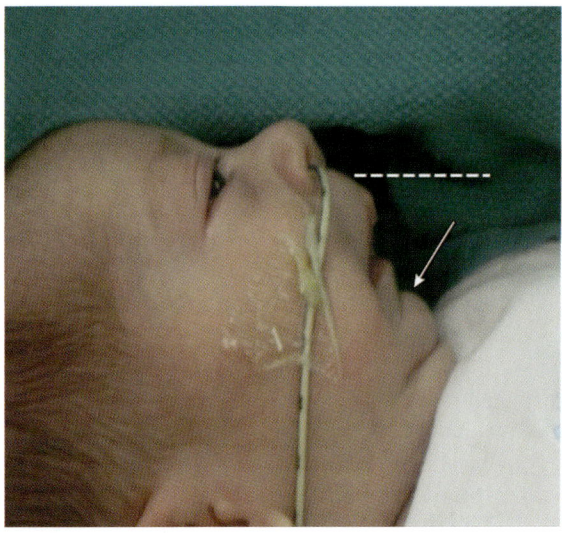

Figure 2.1 Micrognathia is a common and easily missed anatomical feature, which is associated with difficult airway management and airway-related complications, especially in infants.

patients who may be at risk for SGA device failure is an important part of the airway evaluation.

SGA devices, when used for elective airway management, have a failure rate of 0.86% in children.[20] This compares favorably with a reported failure rate of 1.1% in adults.[21] Pediatric risk factors for SGA device failure include patient presentation for ENT surgery, inpatient admission status, known airway abnormality, age less than 2 years, and use for prolonged surgery or during transport. Adequate ventilation through an SGA device may be lost at any point during a procedure, with the majority of failures occurring at induction and device insertion. While the overall failure rate for elective SGA device use is low, the risk factors overlap with those identified for difficult mask ventilation and intubation. Therefore, while SGA device placement should be an early step in the management of unanticipated difficult intubation and mask ventilation, there may be a higher rate of failure in this scenario.

Unanticipated Difficult Airways

While the majority of difficult-to-intubate patients can be identified by history and physical exam, some are not recognized preoperatively. The Pediatric Difficult Intubation (PeDI) Registry prospectively collected data from 13 pediatric centers following all episodes where intubation was difficult. Difficult intubation was defined as a Cormack–Lehane view of grade III or IV on direct laryngoscopy by an attending pediatric anesthesiologist, impossible direct laryngoscopy due to anatomical reasons, failed direct laryngoscopy in the prior six months, or instances where the attending felt direct laryngoscopy was unsafe due to an unfavorable physical exam. Among 1018 difficult intubation encounters, 20% were unanticipated. Compared to patients with anticipated difficult airways, the unanticipated group was three times as likely to experience severe complications, including cardiac arrest.[3] A separate study of ICU patients found that emergency intubation was associated with a higher rate of severe adverse events compared to elective intubation.[22] These data highlight the importance of proper preparation for the difficult airway as a way to prevent complications.

Complications of Airway Management

Incidence of Complications

The majority of anesthesia complications in children are airway related. The 2017 APRICOT study was a prospective observational study of children under 15 years of age undergoing anesthesia for all elective and urgent diagnostic and surgical procedures at 261 centers across 33 European countries. Among 31 127 anesthetics, 5.2% of all cases involved severe critical events. Sixty percent of these critical events were respiratory, with 3.1% of all patients experiencing a respiratory complication. The most common respiratory events were severe laryngospasm and bronchospasm; each occurring in 1.2% of anesthetics. Postoperative stridor and bronchial aspiration had respective incidences of 0.7% and 0.1%. Bradycardia occurred in 0.2% of all anesthetics. While the cause of bradycardia was not reported for these cases, this arrhythmia frequently follows hypoxemia. Of ten total cardiac arrests, four were directly related to hypoxemia.[1]

The APRICOT study examined an undifferentiated pediatric population, and the incidence of anticipated or unanticipated difficult airways among the cohort was unreported. The PeDI Registry specifically examined patients who were difficult to intubate, and found even higher rates of complications. Twenty percent of all children in the PeDI cohort experienced at least one complication, with 3% having a severe complication. The most common complication was hypoxemia, with 9% of all patients experiencing a drop in SpO_2 of at least 10% during the intubation attempt. Other common non-severe airway complications included minor airway trauma or bleeding (6%), esophageal intubation (3%), laryngospasm (3%), and bronchospasm (1%). The most common severe complications were severe airway trauma (1%) and cardiac arrest (1%). All types of complications occurred more frequently when the challenging airway was unanticipated, with a 3% incidence of cardiac arrest among unanticipated difficult airway patients. Compared to the incidence of cardiac arrest in the APRICOT study (0.03% of all anesthetics), the PeDI rates of cardiac arrest suggest at least a 33–100-fold increase in the risk of this very serious complication among patients with difficult airways.[3]

Further highlighting the risk of cardiac arrest as a direct consequence of airway management are data from the Pediatric Perioperative Cardiac Arrest (POCA) Registry. This registry includes data submitted from nearly 80 North American centers following perioperative cardiac arrest in children under 18 years of age. An analysis of 193 anesthetic-related arrests from 1998 to 2004 found respiratory causes in 53 (27%) cases. The most common direct cause was laryngospasm, which accounted for 6% of all perioperative arrests. Other respiratory causes included inadequate oxygenation, inadvertent extubation, airway obstruction, esophageal or endobronchial intubation, bronchospasm, aspiration, and difficult intubation.[23]

An analysis of closed malpractice claims found that respiratory events were more common in pediatric claims (43% versus 30% of adult claims). Again, hypoxemia leading to bradycardia and cardiac arrest was a common source of death and ischemic brain injury among children.[24]

Predictors of Airway Complications

In addition to providing data regarding the incidence of airway-related complications, the previously mentioned studies also identify risk factors that may predispose patients to these events. The most important risk factors are patient age and need for multiple intubation attempts (Table 2.3).

Table 2.3 Patient and Procedural Factors Associated with Complications During Airway Management

Weight < 10 kg

Presence of micrognathia

> 2 intubation attempts

≥ 3 attempts at direct laryngoscopy

While the age cutoff for elevated risk has varied among studies, an increased incidence of complications has consistently been found among younger patients. Morray and colleagues found the highest rate of closed claims among patients aged less than 6 months.[24] The PeDI study found a higher rate of airway-related complications among children less than 10 kg; most of whom were less than 1 year of age. This study also showed that complications occurred more frequently in patients with micrognathia: a physical exam finding that can be easily missed in infants.[3] Graciano and colleagues confirmed that, among an ICU population, adverse events during intubation were more common in children less than 1 year old.[10] The APRICOT authors found a significantly higher rate of complications in children aged less than 3 years of age, and went so far as to recommend that patients in this age range be cared for by anesthesiologists with special pediatric training or experience.[1]

The second major risk factor for complications is repeated instrumentation of the airway. Patients with more than two intubation attempts, and especially those with three or more attempts at direct laryngoscopy, were more likely to experience adverse events in the PeDI dataset.[3] Complications were also more common in ICU patients who experienced more than two attempts at direct laryngoscopy before successful intubation.[10] Another study of ICU patients found more frequent and serious airway injuries occurred when patients were intubated for the second time in the same hospital stay.[25]

Important lessons can be taken from these studies of adverse events. First, any attempt to manage the airway of a neonate or infant must be considered high risk. While the preoperative physical exam is an important step in any anesthetic, special attention should be paid to the airway exam of the infant; in particular looking for micrognathia. Anesthesiologists should have a lower threshold for preparation of advanced airway equipment or the use of apneic oxygenation techniques in this group. The second lesson is to avoid fixation on unsuccessful airway management techniques. If direct laryngoscopy is unsuccessful, but ventilation with a mask or SGA device is possible, additional help should be sought and advanced equipment used for subsequent attempts. Repeated attempts at direct laryngoscopy frequently leads to airway trauma, bleeding, and edema: all of which can complicate further intubation attempts. Even worse, they may make mask ventilation more difficult, leading to a dangerous "can't intubate, can't oxygenate" scenario. Finally, as many complications are caused by trauma and airway reactivity, use of less invasive airway management techniques can decrease morbidity. Multiple studies of patients of all ages undergoing appropriate procedures have shown decreased rates of complications when an SGA device is used instead of an endotracheal tube (ETT).[26,27] This is particularly true in patients with increased airway reactivity due to upper respiratory tract infections or asthma.[5,28]

Prevention and Management of Complications

Hypoxemia

The most important principle in airway management for patients of any age is the primacy of oxygenation over any other goal, including tracheal intubation. Due to previously described physiologic features, such as increased oxygen consumption and loss of FRC, hypoxemia occurs rapidly in the apneic, anesthetized child. While a drop in SpO_2 is often quickly reversible with effective mask ventilation, even brief periods of hypoxemia can have greater consequences, including bradycardia and cardiac arrest. The PeDI study found that 16% of all patients with difficult airways experienced a drop in SpO_2 of 10% or more, and 2% experienced cardiac arrest.[3]

With this in mind, apneic time should be minimized during pediatric airway management. If a difficult intubation is anticipated, induction techniques that maintain spontaneous ventilation should be considered, with supplemental oxygen supplied during intubation attempts. A downside to this technique is that intubation attempts place any spontaneously breathing patient at risk for laryngospasm, which can itself lead to rapid desaturation. Alternatively, if paralysis is used, apneic oxygenation should be considered.[29] Multiple techniques can be used to supply oxygen to the posterior pharynx during intubation attempts and prolong the time to desaturation.[30,31] These techniques are described in greater detail in a later chapter of this book. With either of these strategies, the time spent on any individual intubation attempt should be limited, and the anesthesiologist must be ready to quickly abandon the intubation attempt in order to reoxygenate through mask ventilation.

Finally, as bradycardia, hemodynamic collapse, and cardiac arrest are the most dangerous sequelae of hypoxemia, atropine (0.02 mg/kg) and epinephrine at an appropriate dilution should be immediately available during any intubation attempts when difficulty is anticipated.

Laryngospasm

One of the most common perioperative respiratory adverse events, laryngospasm is the involuntary, reflexive closure of the vocal cords in response to irritation of the larynx or trachea. It often occurs during light planes of anesthesia, and leads to rapid oxygen desaturation. Laryngospasm may be triggered by airway instrumentation, or by substances such as mucus, blood, or saliva. It may occur during airway instrumentation, maintenance of anesthesia if an ETT is not in place, or during emergence and extubation. Laryngospasm may be partial, in which there is increased upper airway resistance, making air movement by mask ventilation difficult, but not impossible, or complete, in which no air movement is possible.

Risk factors for laryngospasm include younger age, recent upper respiratory tract infection, passive smoke exposure, and surgical procedures involving the airway, such as tonsillectomy.[32-36] Prevention strategies include rescheduling elective procedures in patients with a recent upper respiratory tract infection, ensuring an appropriate depth of anesthesia prior to intubation attempts, avoidance of multiple intubation attempts, and suctioning of oral blood or secretions prior to intubation attempts or extubation.

Treatment of partial laryngospasm includes administration of 100% FiO_2, a tight mask seal with CPAP, and deepening the plane of anesthesia with

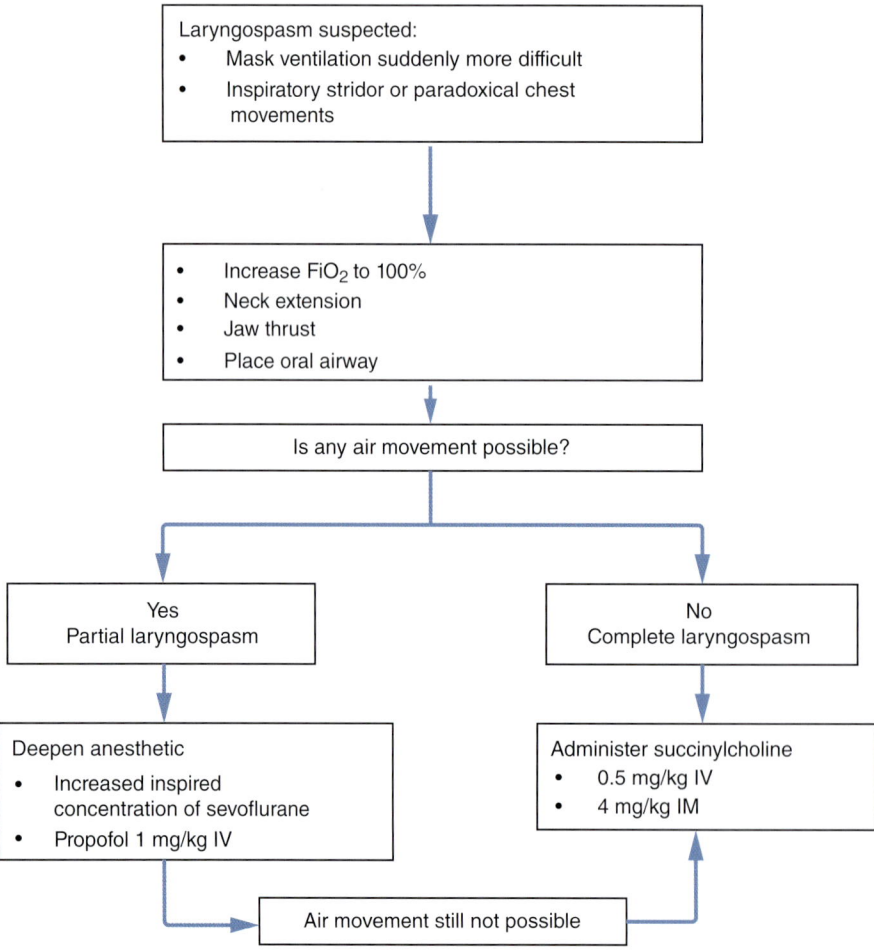

Figure 2.2 Algorithm for the management of laryngospasm.

propofol or volatile anesthetic. Complete laryngospasm requires administration of rapid-acting paralytics, such as succinylcholine, or rocuronium if succinylcholine is contraindicated. If mask ventilation becomes suddenly difficult or impossible in a previously easy to ventilate patient, laryngospasm is the most likely cause, and paralytics should be rapidly administered[37] (Figure 2.2).

Bronchospasm

Bronchospasm, the reversible reflex spasm of bronchial smooth muscle, is more common in children with asthma, recent upper respiratory tract infections, and passive smoke exposure. It is caused by stimulation and irritation of the airway, which may occur with ETT placement. Bronchospasm may cause severe airway obstruction, making air movement, oxygenation, and ventilation impossible. It can quickly lead to hypoxemia, and high airway pressures may cause a tension pneumothorax or cardiovascular deterioration. Intraoperative signs of bronchospasm include wheezing on chest auscultation, upsloping or decreased waveform on capnography, loss of tidal volume, increased airway pressures, and hypoxemia.

To prevent intraoperative bronchospasm, asthma control should be optimized preoperatively. Severe asthmatics should receive a course of glucocorticoids, and nebulized albuterol should be administered within 30 minutes of induction.[38,39] Postponement of surgery should be considered in patients with active or recent upper respiratory tract infections, depending on the severity of illness and urgency of surgery.[33] Airway instrumentation should only occur under deep planes of anesthesia in patients at risk of bronchospasm, and intravenous induction with propofol is preferred.[40] If appropriate, an SGA device, which is less stimulating to the airway, should be used instead of an ETT.[27,28,41,42] Management of bronchospasm includes administration of 100% oxygen, deepening the plane of anesthesia (with intravenous or inhaled anesthetics), albuterol administration through the ETT, intravenous magnesium sulfate, anticholinergics such as glycopyrrolate and atropine, and intravenous epinephrine. If severe bronchospasm occurs in an anesthetized patient without an ETT, a cuffed tube should be placed, as this allows the use of higher inspiratory pressures.

Postintubation Croup

Pressure of the ETT on glottic and subglottic structures can lead to acute narrowing and postintubation croup. Symptoms include a barking cough, subcostal retractions, respiratory distress, and hypoxemia following extubation. According to Poiseuille's law, resistance to laminar flow of a fluid through a pipe (such as air through the trachea) is inversely proportional to the pipe's radius to the fourth power. Therefore, even a small amount of airway narrowing due to edema can cause a rapid and profound increase in resistance; leading to the above symptoms.

Risk factors include young age, a history of infectious croup, multiple intubation attempts, lack of a leak around the ETT at 25 cmH_2O airway pressure, operations involving the neck, intubation for greater than one hour, and coughing with an ETT in place.[43] Prevention strategies include use of an appropriately sized ETT; switching to a smaller ETT if no leak is audible at 25 cmH_2O; use of ETTs with high-volume, low-pressure cuffs; and administration of dexamethasone 0.5–0.6 mg/kg in at-risk patients.[44–46] Postintubation croup can be managed with nebulized racemic epinephrine and observation for at least two hours. If symptoms do not reoccur in that time, the patient may be safely discharged home. If symptoms return, the patient should be admitted to the ward or ICU for monitoring, supplemental oxygen, and additional racemic epinephrine.[47–49]

Aspiration

Aspiration of gastric contents into the trachea is an infrequent anesthetic complication in children. It may occur during induction, airway management, maintenance, or emergence from anesthesia and extubation. Severity of complications varies widely, with some patients having no observable consequences. In other cases, aspiration may lead to laryngospasm or bronchospasm and subsequent rapid oxygen desaturation, mild respiratory insufficiency requiring supplemental oxygen for hours to days, severe acute respiratory distress syndrome, or even death.

Risk factors for pulmonary aspiration include emergency procedures, ASA Physical Status of III–IV, and light anesthesia or high abdominal pressures during airway management with a supraglottic device.[1,50–52] The risk of aspiration may be minimized (but not eliminated) by observing recommended fasting guidelines before elective procedures.[53] If aspiration occurs during an anesthetic, the patient should be placed in a head-down position, and the mouth and pharynx suctioned. Supplemental oxygen should be provided, and the anesthesiologist should be ready to treat secondary laryngospasm or bronchospasm. The decision to proceed with the planned procedure will depend on the urgency of the procedure and the severity of respiratory symptoms. Symptoms typically reach maximum severity within an hour following pulmonary aspiration; at which time disposition decisions may be made.[50,52]

Endotracheal Tube Misplacement

The distal end of an appropriately placed ETT should be positioned halfway between the vocal cords and carina. The average tracheal length in neonates less than 3 months old is 4 cm.[54] The trachea may be even shorter in premature infants. As a result, even small changes in tube depth may result in advancement into an endobronchial position or withdrawal into the pharynx. Endobronchial intubation leads to atelectasis of the contralateral lung and hypoxemia from pulmonary shunting, while all ability to ventilate is lost with inadvertent extubation. The visual appearance of the glottic and upper esophageal openings may also be more difficult to distinguish in small children, increasing the risk of esophageal intubation.

The increased risk of misplacement makes careful positioning of the ETT during intubation very important. The ETT should be advanced just past the vocal cords during laryngoscopy, and bilateral breath sounds confirmed following intubation. A stable end-tidal carbon dioxide tracing on capnography for several breaths confirms placement. The ETT should be securely taped above and below the mouth. As the tube may be advanced or withdrawn with small neck movements, breath sounds should be checked following any position change. A change in pulmonary compliance or end-tidal carbon dioxide along with oxygen desaturation, especially following position changes, suggests endobronchial intubation. In this case, the ETT must be carefully withdrawn in increments of less than a half cm until bilateral breath sounds are auscultated. Likewise, sudden loss of end-tidal carbon dioxide and a new airway leak suggests inadvertent extubation. If possible, laryngoscopy should be used to evaluate ETT placement and reintubate the trachea. If surgical positioning makes laryngoscopy impossible, the ETT should be removed and an SGA device placed until the patient can be repositioned, or equipment such as a fiberoptic bronchoscope can be obtained for replacement of the ETT.[55]

Airway Trauma

Trauma to the airway caused by the ETT or laryngoscope during intubation attempts can have short- and long-term consequences. Bleeding of the pharyngeal or tonsillar tissue can obscure the glottic view on laryngoscopy, trigger laryngospasm or bronchospasm, and lead to hypoxemia from aspiration. ETT trauma or barotrauma can cause a pneumothorax, with positive-pressure ventilation quickly leading to a tension pneumothorax and cardiac arrest if needle decompression and chest tube placement are not performed.[56,57]

Arytenoid dislocation causes vocal cord paralysis, hoarseness, and respiratory distress, and may require surgical reduction. Ulceration of the glottis and subglottis can lead to granulation tissue, fibrous nodules, arytenoid adhesion, and subglottic membranes.[25] These injuries, especially severe ones, are at risk for progression to subglottic stenosis.[58] Subglottic stenosis can cause chronic upper airway obstruction that worsens with upper respiratory tract infections, and requires balloon dilation, tracheostomy, or laryngotracheal reconstruction for treatment.

Conclusion

When managing the pediatric airway, the anesthesiologist's primary goals should always be to maintain oxygenation and avoid complications. The techniques described may be used to increase the likelihood of successful and safe airway management, but many require special equipment and advanced preparation. Preoperative identification of patients who are likely to pose a challenge allows the anesthesiologist to formulate a plan and proceed with airway management in a safe and controlled manner. Understanding the most common airway complications and their contributing factors allows one to be more effective at prevention, recognition, and treatment of these potentially life-threatening events.

References

1. Habre W, Disma N, Virag K, et al. Incidence of Severe critical Events in Paediatric Anaesthesia (APRICOT): a Prospective Multicentre Observational Study in 261 Hospitals in Europe. *The Lancet Respiratory Medicine* 2017; 5: 412–25.

2. Mir Ghassemi A, Neira V, Ufholz LA, et al. A Systematic Review and Meta-Analysis of Acute Severe Complications of Pediatric

Anesthesia. *Paediatric Anaesthesia* 2015; **25**: 1093–102.

3. Fiadjoe JE, Nishisaki A, Jagannathan N, et al. Airway Management Complications in Children with Difficult Tracheal Intubation from the Pediatric Difficult Intubation (PeDI) Registry: a Prospective Cohort Analysis. *The Lancet Respiratory Medicine* 2016; **4**: 37–48.

4. Hall SC. The Difficult Pediatric Airway – Recognition, Evaluation, and Management. *Canadian Journal of Anesthesia/Journal canadien d'anesthésie* 2001; **48**: R22–5.

5. Valois-Gomez T, Oofuvong M, Auer G, Coffin D, Loetwiriyakul W, Correa JA. Incidence of Difficult Bag-Mask Ventilation in Children: a Prospective Observational Study. *Paediatric Anaesthesia* 2013; **23**: 920–6.

6. Kheterpal S, Han R, Tremper KK, et al. Incidence and Predictors of Difficult and Impossible Mask Ventilation. *Anesthesiology* 2006; **105**: 885–91.

7. Heinrich S, Birkholz T, Ihmsen H, Irouschek A, Ackermann A, Schmidt J. Incidence and Predictors of Difficult Laryngoscopy in 11 219 Pediatric Anesthesia Procedures. *Paediatric Anaesthesia* 2012; **22**: 729–36.

8. Mirghassemi A, Soltani AE, Abtahi M. Evaluation of Laryngoscopic Views and Related Influencing Factors in a Pediatric Population. *Paediatric Anaesthesia* 2011; **21**: 663–7.

9. Akpek EA, Mutlu H, Kayhan Z. Difficult Intubation in Pediatric Cardiac Anesthesia. *Journal of Cardiothoracic and Vascular Anesthesia* 2004; **18**: 610–12.

10. Graciano AL, Tamburro R, Thompson AE, Fiadjoe J, Nadkarni VM, Nishisaki A. Incidence and Associated Factors of Difficult Tracheal intubations in Pediatric ICUs: a Report from National Emergency Airway Registry for Children: NEAR4KIDS. *Intensive Care Medicine* 2014; **40**: 1659–69.

11. Santos AP, Mathias LA, Gozzani JL, Watanabe M. Difficult Intubation in Children: Applicability of the Mallampati Index. *Revista Brasileira de Anestesiologia* 2011; **61**: 156–8, 9–62, 84–7.

12. Jagannathan N, Sequera-Ramos L, Sohn L, Wallis B, Shertzer A, Schaldenbrand K. Elective Use of Supraglottic Airway Devices for Primary Airway Management in Children with Difficult Airways. *British Journal of Anaesthesia* 2014; **112**: 742–8.

13. Asai T. Is it Safe to Use Supraglottic Airway in Children with Difficult Airways? *British Journal of Anaesthesia* 2014; **112**: 620–2.

14. Cox RG, Lardner DR. Supraglottic Airways in Children: Past Lessons, Future Directions. *Canadian Journal of Anesthesia/Journal canadien d'anesthésie* 2009; **56**: 636–42.

15. Lopez-Gil M, Brimacombe J, Alvarez M. Safety and Efficacy of the Laryngeal Mask Airway. A Prospective Survey of 1400 Children. *Anaesthesia* 1996; **51**: 969–72.

16. Jagannathan N, Ramsey MA, White MC, Sohn L. An Update on Newer Pediatric Supraglottic Airways with Recommendations for Clinical Use. *Paediatric Anaesthesia* 2015; **25**: 334–45.

17. Patel A, Clark SR, Schiffmiller M, Schoenberg C, Tewfik G. A Survey of Practice Patterns in the Use of Laryngeal Mask by Pediatric Anesthesiologists. *Paediatric Anaesthesia* 2015; **25**: 1127–31.

18. Black AE, Flynn PE, Smith HL, et al. Development of a Guideline for the Management of the Unanticipated Difficult Airway in Pediatric Practice. *Paediatric Anaesthesia* 2015; **25**: 346–62.

19. Apfelbaum JL, Hagberg CA, Caplan RA, et al. Practice Guidelines for Management of the Difficult Airway: an Updated Report by the American Society of Anesthesiologists Task Force on Management of the Difficult Airway. *Anesthesiology* 2013; **118**: 251–70.

20. Mathis MR, Haydar B, Taylor EL, et al. Failure of the Laryngeal Mask Airway Unique and Classic in the Pediatric Surgical Patient: a Study of Clinical Predictors and Outcomes. *Anesthesiology* 2013; **119**: 1284–95.

21. Ramachandran SK, Mathis MR, Tremper KK, Shanks AM, Kheterpal S. Predictors and Clinical Outcomes from Failed Laryngeal Mask Airway Unique: a Study of 15 795 Patients. *Anesthesiology* 2012; **116**: 1217–26.

22. Nishisaki A, Turner DA, Brown CA 3rd, et al. A National Emergency Airway Registry for Children: Landscape of Tracheal Intubation in 15 PICUs. *Critical Care Medicine* 2013; **41**: 874–85.

23. Bhananker SM, Ramamoorthy C, Geiduschek JM, et al. Anesthesia-Related Cardiac Arrest in Children: Update from the Pediatric Perioperative Cardiac Arrest Registry. *Anesthesia & Analgesia* 2007; **105**: 344–50.

24. Morray JP, Geiduschek JM, Caplan RA, Posner KL, Gild WM, Cheney FW. A Comparison of Pediatric and Adult Anesthesia Closed Malpractice Claims. *Anesthesiology* 1993; **78**: 461–7.

25. Gomes Cordeiro AM, Fernandes JC, Troster EJ. Possible Risk Factors Associated with Moderate or Severe Airway Injuries in Children who Underwent Endotracheal Intubation. *Pediatric Critical Care Medicine* 2004; **5**: 364–8.

26. Drake-Brockman TFE, Ramgolam A, Zhang G, Hall GL,

von Ungern-Sternberg BS. The Effect of Endotracheal Tubes versus Laryngeal Mask Airways on Perioperative Respiratory Adverse Events in Infants: a Randomised Controlled Trial. *The Lancet* 2017; **389**: 701–8.

27 Luce V, Harkouk H, Brasher C, et al. Supraglottic Airway Devices vs Tracheal Intubation in Children: a Quantitative Meta-Analysis of Respiratory Complications. *Paediatric Anaesthesia* 2014; **24**: 1088–98.

28 Parnis SJ, Barker DS, Van Der Walt JH. Clinical Predictors of Anaesthetic Complications in Children with Respiratory Tract Infections. *Paediatric Anaesthesia* 2001; **11**: 29–40.

29 Fiadjoe JE, Litman RS. Oxygen Supplementation during Prolonged Tracheal Intubation Should be the Standard of Care. *British Journal of Anaesthesia* 2016; **117**: 417–8.

30 Steiner JW, Sessler DI, Makarova N, et al. Use of Deep Laryngeal Oxygen Insufflation during Laryngoscopy in Children: a Randomized Clinical Trial. *British Journal of Anaesthesia* 2016; **117**: 350–7.

31 Windpassinger M, Plattner O, Gemeiner J, et al. Pharyngeal Oxygen Insufflation during AirTraq Laryngoscopy Slows Arterial Desaturation in Infants and Small Children. *Anesthesia & Analgesia* 2016; **122**: 1153–7.

32 Olsson GL, Hallen B. Laryngospasm during Anaesthesia. A Computer-Aided Incidence Study in 136 929 Patients. *Acta Anaesthesiologica Scandinavica* 1984; **28**: 567–75.

33 von Ungern-Sternberg BS, Boda K, Chambers NA, et al. Risk Assessment for Respiratory Complications in Paediatric Anaesthesia: a Prospective Cohort Study. *The Lancet* 2010; **376**: 773–83.

34 Flick RP, Wilder RT, Pieper SF, et al. Risk Factors for Laryngospasm in Children during General Anesthesia. *Paediatric Anaesthesia* 2008; **18**: 289–96.

35 Lakshmipathy N, Bokesch PM, Cowen DE, Lisman SR, Schmid CH. Environmental Tobacco Smoke: a Risk Factor for Pediatric Laryngospasm. *Anesthesia & Analgesia* 1996; **82**: 724–7.

36 Mamie C, Habre W, Delhumeau C, Argiroffo CB, Morabia A. Incidence and Risk Factors of Perioperative Respiratory Adverse Events in Children Undergoing Elective Surgery. *Paediatric Anaesthesia* 2004; **14**: 218–24.

37 Weiss M, Engelhardt T. Cannot Ventilate – Paralyze! *Paediatric Anaesthesia* 2012; **22**: 1147–9.

38 Kabalin CS, Yarnold PR, Grammer LC. Low Complication Rate of Corticosteroid-Treated Asthmatics Undergoing Surgical Procedures. *Archives of Internal Medicine* 1995; **155**: 1379–84.

39 von Ungern-Sternberg BS, Habre W, Erb TO, Heaney M. Salbutamol Premedication in Children with a Recent Respiratory Tract Infection. *Paediatric Anaesthesia* 2009; **19**: 1064–9.

40 Eames WO, Rooke GA, Wu RS, Bishop MJ. Comparison of the Effects of Etomidate, Propofol, and Thiopental on Respiratory Resistance after Tracheal Intubation. *Anesthesiology* 1996; **84**: 1307–11.

41 Drake-Brockman TF, Ramgolam A, Zhang G, Hall GL, von Ungern-Sternberg BS. The Effect of Endotracheal Tubes versus Laryngeal Mask Airways on Perioperative Respiratory Adverse Events in Infants: a Randomised Controlled Trial. *The Lancet* 2017; **389**: 701–8.

42 Tait AR, Pandit UA, Voepel-Lewis T, Munro HM, Malviya S. Use of the Laryngeal Mask Airway in Children with Upper Respiratory Tract Infections: a Comparison with Endotracheal Intubation. *Anesthesia & Analgesia* 1998; **86**: 706–11.

43 Koka BV, Jeon IS, Andre JM, MacKay I, Smith RM. Postintubation Croup in Children. *Anesthesia & Analgesia* 1977; **56**: 501–5.

44 Dullenkopf A, Gerber A, Weiss M. The Microcuff Tube Allows a Longer Time Interval until Unsafe Cuff Pressures are Reached in Children. *Canadian Journal of Anesthesia Journal/Journal canadien d'anesthésie* 2004; **51**: 997–1001.

45 Salgo B, Schmitz A, Henze G, et al. Evaluation of a New Recommendation for Improved Cuffed Tracheal Tube Size Selection in Infants and Small Children. *Acta Anaesthesiologica Scandinavica* 2006; **50**: 557–61.

46 Weiss M, Dullenkopf A, Fischer JE, Keller C, Gerber AC. Prospective Randomized Controlled Multi-Centre Trial of Cuffed or Uncuffed Endotracheal Tubes in Small Children. *British Journal of Anaesthesia* 2009; **103**: 867–73.

47 Bjornson C, Russell K, Vandermeer B, Klassen TP, Johnson DW. Nebulized Epinephrine for Croup in Children. *Cochrane Database Systematic Reviews* 2013: Cd006619.

48 Rizos JD, DiGravio BE, Sehl MJ, Tallon JM. The Disposition of Children with Croup Treated with Racemic Epinephrine and Dexamethasone in the Emergency Department. *Journal of Emergency Medicine* 1998; **16**: 535–9.

49 Kunkel NC, Baker MD. Use of Racemic Epinephrine, Dexamethasone, and Mist in the Outpatient Management of Croup. *Pediatric Emergency Care* 1996; **12**: 156–9.

50. Walker RW. Pulmonary Aspiration in Pediatric Anesthetic Practice in the UK: a Prospective Survey of Specialist Pediatric Centers Over a One-Year Period. *Paediatric Anaesthesia* 2013; **23**: 702–11.

51. Borland LM, Sereika SM, Woelfel SK, et al. Pulmonary Aspiration in Pediatric Patients during General Anesthesia: Incidence and Outcome. *Journal of Clinical Anesthesia* 1998; **10**: 95–102.

52. Warner MA, Warner ME, Warner DO, Warner LO, Warner EJ. Perioperative Pulmonary Aspiration in Infants and Children. *Anesthesiology* 1999; **90**: 66–71.

53. Practice Guidelines for Preoperative Fasting and the Use of Pharmacologic Agents to Reduce the Risk of Pulmonary Aspiration: Application to Healthy Patients Undergoing Elective Procedures: an Updated Report by the American Society of Anesthesiologists Task Force on Preoperative Fasting and the Use of Pharmacologic Agents to Reduce the Risk of Pulmonary Aspiration. *Anesthesiology* 2017; **126**: 376–93.

54. Lee KS, Yang CC. Tracheal Length of Infants under Three Months Old. *Annals of Otology, Rhinology & Laryngology* 2001; **110**: 268–70.

55. Sohn L, Sawardekar A, Jagannathan N. Airway Management Options in a Prone Achondroplastic Dwarf with a Difficult Airway after Unintentional Tracheal Extubation during a Wake-Up Test for Spinal Fusion: To Flip or Not to Flip? *Canadian Journal of Anesthesia/Journal canadien d'anesthésie* 2014; **61**: 741–4.

56. Chan IA, Gamble JJ. Tension Pneumothorax during Flexible Bronchoscopy in a Nonintubated Infant. *Paediatric Anaesthesia* 2016; **26**: 452–4.

57. Parekh UR, Maguire AM, Emery J, Martin PH. Pneumothorax in Neonates: Complication during Endotracheal Intubation, Diagnosis, and Management. *Journal of Anaesthesiology Clinical Pharmacology* 2016; **32**: 397–9.

58. Schweiger C, Manica D, Kuhl G, Sekine L, Marostica PJ. Post-Intubation Acute Laryngeal Injuries in Infants and Children: a New Classification System. *International Journal of Pediatric Otorhinolaryngology* 2016; **86**: 177–82.

Section 1 Basic Principles, Assessment, and Planning of Airway Management

Chapter 3

Universal Algorithms and Approaches to Airway Management

Thomas Engelhardt and Andreas Machotta

Introduction

Airway problems are a significant cause of perioperative morbidity and mortality in children. This is a direct consequence of a shorter apnea tolerance in children and the necessity to rectify airway obstructions in a timely manner. A simple, time critical, pediatric-specific airway algorithm in conjunction with dedicated teaching, training, and frequent practice is likely to reduce the airway-related pediatric morbidity and mortality.

This chapter outlines key aspects of a successful pediatric airway algorithm and its implementation into clinical practice. A simple, universal, and pragmatic approach to pediatric airway management is suggested. It is essential to establish a minimum standard of pediatric airway equipment and medication wherever children are treated.

Small Airways Create Big Problems

Airway Problems are a Significant Cause for Perioperative Cardiac Arrest

Airway obstruction rapidly leads to profound hypoxia and bradycardia as children have a decreased oxygen reserve and increased oxygen consumption when compared with adults.[1,2] In general, the smaller and younger the patient, the shorter the time to rectify the underlying problem. Therefore, neonates and young children are at particular high risk,[3,4] as are compromised children undergoing emergency procedures in the operating room or beyond.[5,6] The apnea tolerance is measured in seconds, leaving only a limited time window to respond. Perioperative cardiac arrest secondary to perioperative hypoxia is a consequence of prolonged airway obstruction frequently associated with a poor outcome. Transient short perioperative hypoxia, however, may not necessarily result in evident short-term postoperative morbidity. Long-term consequences of transient hypoxemia are only poorly understood in children, with the exception of preterm neonates. The latter have an increased risk of cognitive and motor impairment in later life with an increasing duration of hypoxia and bradycardia.[7]

Wake Up is Not an Option

A very low FRC and increased closing capacity develops rapidly into significant hypoxemia and profound bradycardia, compromising the well-being of the child. "Optimal" preoxygenation does not result in a sufficiently long "safety period," necessitating intermittent ventilation and oxygenation in all situations, including rapid-sequence inductions.[8] A severe airway obstruction and increased carbon dioxide retention leads to significant respiratory acidosis. This is an accelerating downward spiral, requiring swift and exact intervention. There are no reports suggesting a severely hypoxic, bradycardic, and acidotic child with a prolonged acute airway obstruction will resume spontaneous ventilation and airway patency with a good neurological outcome. Such faith is misplaced in pediatric anesthesia.

Current Solutions

Numerous published difficult airway algorithms are in existence. They are available in various formats and languages, and mostly have their primary origin in adult anesthesia. This is likely due to the occurrence of "mixed" anesthesia practices of adult and pediatric anesthesia. The resulting designed algorithms are, therefore, less suitable for pediatric-specific problems.

Various pediatric specialist anesthesia societies and groups have published their own expert-opinion-based pediatric airway management algorithms; not necessarily compatible with each other. In addition, different medical and surgical specialties have also devised their own recommendations, making it difficult for the individual practitioner to identify the optimal approach.

Routine pediatric airway management is easy for the experienced practitioner. However, even a previously healthy child without any signs or symptoms of airway anomalies can quickly deteriorate, requiring the correct sequence of steps to be carried out rapidly to avoid harm. The following section describes principles underlying such an approach.

Principle Approaches to a Universal Pediatric Difficult Airway Algorithm

Simplicity

The perioperative care of a child undergoing anesthesia can be a stressful situation for the less experienced practitioner. A rapid deterioration and the quick onset of hypoxia and bradycardia adds significantly to this stress,[9] and may lead to poor decision-making. Any suggested solution to resolve such a crisis requires a simple and intuitive approach. Box 3.1 shows six essential aspects to make such an approach effective.

A forward-only, "step-by-step," easy-to-memorize algorithm significantly reduces cognitive load in a situation of a clinical crisis. It enables the practitioner to focus on the essential step without distraction. The "open-box" principle allows the use of existing local expertise to become part of the crisis resolution. There is currently no consensus of which airway device is superior and applicable in all difficult pediatric airway situations.[10] Only a solution adapting these principles can build acceptance across various specialists, pediatric specialties, and pediatric anesthesia societies and groups.

Prevention of the Difficult Pediatric Airway

A short clinical examination must be performed before starting any procedure involving anesthesia and should be directed toward the respiratory system. In particular, symptoms and signs of airway obstruction, such as stridor, cyanosis, dyspnea, and suprasternal retractions are acute indicators of imminent difficulties. Apneic episodes and the use of auxiliary respiratory muscles may also indicate an acutely impaired airway. Subtle craniofacial anomalies are frequently overlooked and can be part of an underlying syndrome.

A clear airway management plan, including the knowledge of all possible complications and their management, are essential before embarking on anesthesia. This is best achieved through regular practice, continuing medical education, and training for all practitioners involved in pediatric airway management.

All equipment, such as tubes, laryngoscopes, blades, stylets, forceps, face masks, nasopharyngeal and oropharyngeal airways, suction devices, and all potentially necessary drugs, should be prepared in appropriate sizes and dosages. In case of a severe airway problem, a child can become hypoxic and bradycardic within seconds. All tools to establish a safe pediatric airway and to manage possible complications must, therefore, be ready for immediate use.

Clear Separation of Airway Problems

Oxygenation and (face-mask) ventilation saves lives.[11] Fortunately, difficult face-mask ventilation is easy to manage in experienced hands. According to the findings of a large cohort study, difficult face-mask ventilation could always be controlled by the recognition and treatment of airway obstruction.[10] Successful (face-mask) oxygenation and ventilation is the key to prevent harm in pediatric airway management.

In contrast, pediatric tracheal intubation can be more challenging and even be difficult in the younger child, neonate, or syndromic patient.[12,13] There is no universally accepted best equipment or technique for all tracheal intubation situations, but it is clear that repeated tracheal intubation attempts may render a difficult tracheal intubation into an impossible one.[10]

Recognize and Treat Airway Obstruction

Airway obstruction is the most common cause of anesthesia-related perioperative hypoxia in pediatric

---

Box 3.1 A Successful, Universally Adapted Approach to the Difficult Airway:

- simple and intuitive
- forward only
- easy to memorize
- easy to practice
- "open box" (use of existing expertise)
- applicable to all situations

Table 3.1 The Causes and Treatment of Airway Obstruction

Severe airway obstructions during anesthesia are generally divided into anatomical (mechanical) and functional airway obstructions. This distinction necessitates different treatments: anesthetic techniques for anatomical airway obstructions and pharmacological interventions for severe functional airway obstructions.

Anatomical/mechanical airway obstructions

Causes	Treatment
Poor face-mask technique	Two-hand/two-person technique
Inadequate head position	Repositioning, reopening
Large adenoids/tonsils/obesity/pharyngeal obstruction	Oropharyngeal/nasopharyngeal/SGA device
Blood/foreign bodies/secretions[1]	Suction, removal

Functional airway obstructions

Causes	Treatment
Inadequate anesthesia	Deepen anesthesia
Laryngospasm[2]	Propofol, muscle relaxants
Muscle rigidity	Muscle relaxants
Bronchospasm[3]	Epinephrine, bronchodilators (sevoflurane)

[1] Preexisting copious secretions (upper respiratory tract infection) may benefit from a preinduction antisialagogue.
[2] Minimal laryngospasm can initially be treated with jaw thrust and positive pressure.
[3] Use epinephrine (titrate) in the peri-arrest situation.

and adult patients, and may occur at any time in the perioperative period. To manage such a situation successfully, it is important to distinguish the two possible mechanisms of airway obstructions, which require two different strategies of treatment:[14]

The first is an *anatomical/mechanical airway obstruction*, which is a physical obstruction of the airway, requiring the intervention of the person who performs ventilation or the anesthesia practitioner. This is in contrast to the second possible mechanism: a *functional airway obstruction*, which is due to acute physiological changes. This is relieved through the administration of drugs. Table 3.1 shows the causes of these two different mechanisms of airway obstruction and their treatment.

Help

It is essential that help and assistance is sought at an early stage. This must be clearly identified on a locally adapted algorithm, including emergency contact details.

Anatomical/Mechanical Airway Obstructions

Anatomical and mechanical airway obstructions are, in most cases, caused by a poor anesthetic technique. This includes inadequate head position, incorrect selection and use of the face mask, and a failure to appreciate an airway obstruction secondary to large adenoids and tonsils in pre-school children.

Anatomical/mechanical airway obstruction must be recognized and treated by the clinician.

A "triple-airway maneuver" (head tilt, chin lift, jaw thrust), while maintaining a mouth opening, are simple treatments employed in daily practice. Alternatively, the use of an appropriately sized oropharyngeal or nasopharyngeal airway can be used when the airway is obstructed by large tonsils and adenoids. Forceful bag-mask ventilation frequently results in gastric distension and requires decompression by orogastric suctioning.

Saliva, blood, regurgitation, or supraglottic foreign bodies can also lead to a mechanical obstruction and necessitate suction and its removal under direct vision (*plan A*). Rarely, an unexpected subglottic or inhaled foreign body needs to be bypassed with a small tracheal tube. Careful lung recruitment maneuvers are required to prevent atelectasis and to restore optimal oxygenation and ventilation following prolonged tracheal intubation attempts.

If no anatomical or mechanical obstruction is apparent during direct laryngoscopy and the trachea cannot be intubated, a laryngeal mask airway (LMA) or an SGA device should be used to overcome any potentially overlooked anatomical supraglottic airway problems (*plan B*).[11]

Functional Airway Obstructions

Functional airway obstruction can occur above (upper) or below (lower) the glottis. Functional upper airway obstruction is commonly encountered, and are usually caused by insufficient depth of anesthesia, laryngospasm, or opioid-induced glottic closure.[15] Functional lower airway obstruction is induced by bronchospasm in children with recent respiratory tract infections, bronchial hyper-reactivity, or thoracic wall rigidity as a consequence of opioid use.

Severe functional airway obstructions are generally treated with drugs.

Hypnotics, such as propofol, are commonly used in otherwise healthy, non-compromised children to overcome acute functional airway problems such as insufficient depth of anesthesia and laryngospasm. Careful hemodynamic monitoring and intervention is essential. Muscle relaxants can be used as an alternative to overcome nearly all functional airway obstructions except for bronchospasm. Epinephrine is useful in this impending peri-arrest situation.[14] Moreover, muscle relaxants should always be used before any attempts to perform a surgical airway such as emergency cricothyroidotomy, needle insertion, or tracheostomy.[16]

Structured Algorithm

"Open Box" and Local Expertise

As previously discussed, a universally accepted and implemented approach to the difficult pediatric

Pediatric Oxygenation and Ventilation
(Please adapt according to local expertise and facilities)

Prevention, teaching, training, facilities
Careful assessment and planning

Recognize and treat
Anatomical/mechanical airway obstructions
Treatment (specify)
Positioning, mouth–opening, oral airway, supraglottic airway

Call for help
(Insert contact details)

Recognize and treat
Functional airway obstructions
Treatment (specify)
Hypnotic, muscle relaxant, epinephrine

Plan A
DL/VL
(specify local choice)

Plan B
LMA/SGA
(specify local choice)

Figure 3.1 Simple, universal, locally adaptable ("open box") difficult pediatric airway algorithm. (DL: direct laryngoscopy; VL: video laryngoscopy; LMA: laryngeal mask airway; SGA: supraglottic airway device)

airway requires the recognition and use of local expertise, resources, and facilities. The following adapted[11] simple, "open-box" algorithm is a proposal to achieve just that (Figure 3.1).

Tracheal Intubation and Surgical Airways versus Oxygenation and Ventilation

Tracheal intubation indications and techniques are described in Section 2. There is no consensus of which technique or device is best suited for all situations. However, tracheal intubation requires significant skill and expertise, which is only achieved through regular practice and training to avoid significant morbidity and mortality. This precludes a universal adaptation across specialties in the form of a difficult pediatric airway algorithm. It makes it impossible to dictate an algorithm that will be accepted by various clinicians, pediatric specialists, and pediatric anesthesia care providers. Therefore, an "open-box" algorithm is mandatory (Figure 3.1).

In contrast to tracheal intubation, as suggested above, oxygenation and ventilation saves lives and prevents avoidable harm. The technique of simple mask ventilation and even the use of SGA devices in children can be learned by all specialists.

The emergency front of neck airway (FONA) is a frequently propagated last-resort technique to salvage an impossible oxygenation/ventilation scenario.[17] It is a rare occurrence in pediatric anesthesia and must be considered during complicated and failed intubation attempts before swelling and bleeding make mask ventilation impossible. It is the authors' opinion that (unplanned) emergency FONA should only ever be considered as an option in a desperate scenario rather than a recognized effective treatment of failed airway management in children. However, elective FONA contingency planning in children with a known difficult airway may be considered before the start of a procedure. If time permits (preinduction), it is possible to identify and mark critical airway structures using ultrasound.

Unexpected, Suspected, and Expected Pediatric Difficult Airway

Any universal difficult pediatric airway approach also requires accommodation of three different principal clinical situations:[18]

- *unexpected:* the previously healthy child who develops an unexpected severe airway problem or acutely deteriorates
- *suspected:* the child with a previously normal airway, which is now compromised, such as stridor, foreign body, or acute epiglottitis
- *expected:* the elective, known problematic patient having an expected difficult airway, such as Treacher Collins syndrome, Pierre Robin sequence, or other craniofacial abnormality affecting the airway

The urgency of the clinical situation then dictates the necessary steps: (1) immediate intervention, (2) mobilizing the best existing local expertise (which includes ENT specialists or general surgeons if doubts about the ability to face-mask-ventilate exist), or (3) careful planning and referral to a specialist pediatric center if necessary.

Children who present with an acutely impaired normal airway or known difficult airway must be treated by an experienced (pediatric) anesthesiologist in an appropriately staffed and well-equipped pediatric setting. It is essential to establish a minimum standard of pediatric airway equipment and medication in all places where children are treated.[13] There is no place for pride and not seeking help or advice. Figure 3.2 suggests a simple flow chart to this approach, addressing the pediatric airway, the

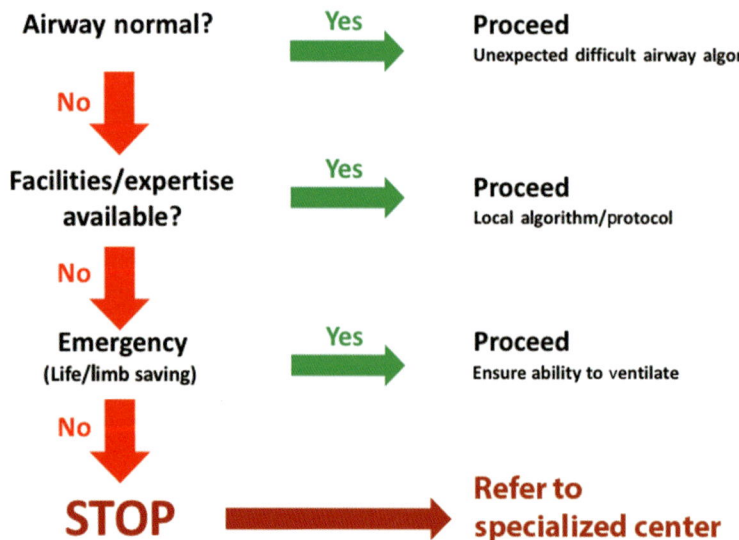

Figure 3.2 Flow chart for approaching pediatric airway management. (Adapted from Marin and Engelhardt. *Algoritmo para el manejo de la vía aérea difícil en pediatría.* 2014, with permission.)

clinical condition, the facilities, and the expertise of the department.

Summary

The overarching goal of a universal, "open-box" difficult airway algorithm is the prevention of perioperative hypoxia and to facilitate adequate ventilation in children. Prevention of a difficult airway through regular practice, teaching, and training with dedicated pediatric staff and equipment is a priority. The first crucial step after encountering difficulties is to prevent, recognize, and treat *anatomical/mechanical* and *functional airway obstructions* with clinical skill and drugs, respectively. A locally accepted algorithm based on simple and common principles with suitable equipment should be established. Such an approach to the difficult pediatric airway may find acceptance across specialist pediatric specialties and pediatric anesthesia societies and groups.

References

1. Sands SA, Edwards BA, Kelly VJ, Davidson MR, Wilkinson MH, Berger PJ. A Model Analysis of Arterial Oxygen Desaturation during Apnea in Preterm Infants. *PLoS Computational Biology* 2009; **5**: e1000588.

2. Hardman JG, Wills JS. The Development of Hypoxaemia during Apnoea in Children: a Computational Modelling Investigation. *British Journal of Anaesthesia* 2006; **97**: 564–70.

3. de Graaff JC, Bijker JB, Kappen TH, van Wolfswinkel L, Zuithoff NP, Kalkman CJ. Incidence of Intraoperative Hypoxemia in Children in Relation to Age. *Anesthesia & Analgesia* 2013; **117**: 169–75.

4. Gencorelli FJ, Fields RG, Litman RS. Complications during Rapid Sequence Induction of General Anesthesia in Children: a Benchmark Study. *Paediatric Anaesthesia* 2010; **20**: 421–4.

5. Bhananker SM, Ramamoorthy C, Geiduschek JM, Posner KL, Domino KB, Haberkern CM, et al Anesthesia-Related Cardiac Arrest in Children: Update from the Pediatric Perioperative Cardiac Arrest Registry. *Anesthesia & Analgesia* 2007; **105**: 344–50.

6. Long E, Sabato S, Babi F. Endotracheal Intubation in the Pediatric Emergency Department. *Pediatric Anesthesia* 2014; **24**: 1204.

7. Poets CF, Roberts RS, Schmidt B, Whyte RK, Asztalos EV, Bader D, et al. Canadian Oxygen Trial Investigators. Association between Intermittent Hypoxemia or Bradycardia and Late Death or Disability in Extremely Preterm Infants. *JAMA* 2015; **314**: 595–603.

8. Engelhardt T. Rapid Sequence Induction has No Use in Pediatric Anesthesia. *Paediatric Anaesthesia* 2015; **25**: 5–8.

9. Eich C, Timmermann A, Russo SG, Cremer S, Nickut A, Strack M, et al. A Controlled Rapid-Sequence Induction Technique for Infants May Reduce Unsafe Actions and Stress. *Acta Anaesthesiologica Scandinavica* 2009; **53**: 1167–72.

10. Fiadjoe JE, Jagannathan N, Hunyady AI, Greenberg RS, Reynolds PI, Matuszczak ME, et al. Airway Management Complications in Children with Difficult Tracheal Intubation from the Pediatric Difficult Intubation (PeDI) Registry: a Prospective Cohort Analysis *The Lancet Respiratory Medicine* 2016; **4**: 37–48.

11. Weiss M, Engelhardt T. Proposal for the Management of the Unexpected Difficult Pediatric Airway. *Paediatric Anaesthesia* 2010; **20**: 454–64.

12. Schmidt AR, Weiss M, Engelhardt T. The Paediatric Airway: Basic Principles and Current Developments. *European Journal of Anaesthesiology* 2014; **31**: 293–9.

13. Engelhardt T, Machotta A, Weiss M. Management Strategies for the Difficult Paediatric Airway. *Trends in Anaesthesia and Critical Care* 2013; **3**: 183–7.

14. Weiss M, Engelhardt T. Cannot Ventilate – Paralyze! *Pediatric Anesthesia* 2012; **22**: 1147–9.

15. Bennett JA, Abrams JT, Van Riper DF, Horrow JC. Difficult or Impossible Ventilation after Sufentanil-Induced Anesthesia is Caused Primarily by Vocal Cord Closure. *Anesthesiology* 1997; **87**: 1070–4.

16. Woodall NM, Cook TM. National Census of Airway Management Techniques Used for Anaesthesia in the UK: First Phase of the Fourth National Audit Project at the Royal College of Anaesthetists. *British Journal of Anaesthesia* 2011; **106**: 266–71.

17. Sabato SC, Long E. An Institutional Approach to the Management of the "Can't Intubate, Can't Oxygenate"

Emergency in Children. *Pediatric Anesthesia* 2016; **26**: 784–93.

18 Engelhardt T, Weiss M. A Child with a Difficult Airway: What do I do Next? *Current Opinion in Anaesthesiology* 2012; **25**: 326–32.

19 Marin, PCE, Engelhardt T. Algoritmo Para el Manejo de la vía Aérea Difícil en Pediatría. *Revista Colombiana de Anestesiología* 2014; **42**: 325–35.

Section 2

Devices and Techniques to Manage the Abnormal Airway

Chapter 4

Direct Laryngoscopy Equipment and Techniques

Maria Matuszczak and Cheryl K. Gooden

The technique of laryngoscopy is essential in the daily delivery of many anesthetics. Direct and indirect methods of laryngoscopy are quite commonly utilized.[1] This chapter will address considerations as they relate to direct laryngoscopy.

History of Direct Laryngoscopy

Laryngoscopy has been used by otolaryngologists since the early 1800s and many different devices allowed the examination of the larynx under indirect vision using mirrors and light reflection. In 1895, the first direct laryngoscopy was performed on an adult patient by the German, Alfred Kirstein, with a device known as an "autoscope," a modified esophagoscope.[2] About 20 years later, in 1913, Chevalier Jackson, from Pennsylvania, USA, and Henry Janeway, an anesthesiologist in New York, USA, developed a laryngoscope with a light source at the distal tip, which could be used by anesthesiologists to intubate patients for surgery. Over time, many modifications were made to the blade designed by Jackson and Janeway. In 1941, Robert Miller designed the Miller blade as we know it today. Two years later, Robert Macintosh designed a curved blade, the Macintosh blade; and subsequently Magill developed a battery-powered laryngoscope.[3] In 1946 and 1947, the adult Miller and Macintosh blades, respectively, were adapted for children.[4,5] Since their introduction more than 50 years ago into airway management, the Macintosh and Miller laryngoscope blades continue to demonstrate their utility in direct laryngoscopy, and are most commonly used for intubation. Many other curved and straight blades have been developed since then; for example, the Wis-Hipple, the Wisconsin, the Robertshaw, the Seward, and the McCoy laryngoscope blades; to name a few.[6,7]

Equipment: Different Blades

The components of a direct laryngoscope are a handle, a blade, and a light source. The variations in the different laryngoscopes will affect the shape, the tip of the blade, and the placement of the illumination. The blade itself is composed of the spatula and flange. The spatula is in direct contact with the tongue, and the left lateral border of the blade is called the flange. The tip of the blade can be placed in the vallecula and therefore lift the epiglottis indirectly or pick up the dorsal aspect of the epiglottis and directly lift the epiglottis. The Miller blade is a straight blade with a slight curve at the tip, which is meant to facilitate lifting of the epiglottis. A direct or indirect insertion of the straight blade to the glottis is an accepted technique in its use. The blade is uniquely configured with a semicircular opening, which can provide a view to the larynx, while the flange size is minimized to decrease injury. Due to the distinct airway features observed in the infant and small child, many laryngoscopists prefer to use a straight blade in this patient population. This is partly due to the fact of how well the straight blade lifts the base of the tongue to visualize the larynx.[8] However, with appropriate training, curved blades can be successfully used in infants and small children as the tip of a curved blade can also pick up the epiglottis if needed.

The Macintosh laryngoscope is the most widely used direct laryngoscope.[9] The curvature of the blade was originally designed to minimize injuries to the upper teeth. The tip of the blade is meant to be placed in the vallecula to indirectly lift the epiglottis. There are different versions of the Macintosh blade, mainly due to variations of the more or less accentuated curvature and the distance between the light source and the tip of the blade.

The Wis-Hipple blade is a straight blade consisting of a spatula with a circular flange, and a wide tip to facilitate lifting of the epiglottis. The Wisconsin blade, developed at the Wisconsin General Hospital, is a straight blade and is very similar to the Wis-Hipple blade, with the flange extending to the distal end, which should allow for a greater visual field.[10] The Wisconsin blade has a large semicircular cross section with a wider tip and is also designed to lift the epiglottis.

On the other hand, the Robertshaw blade is fairly straight, but the distal part has a gentle curve. The blade is designed to be used similar to the Macintosh blade. The tip is to be placed into the vallecula, a fold between the tongue and the dorsal aspect of the epiglottis, and lift the epiglottis indirectly to allow a direct view of the vocal cords. The Seward blade is very similar to the Robertshaw blade in that the distal part of the blade is gently curved and is also designed to be used to indirectly to lift the epiglottis, similar to the Macintosh and Robertshaw blades.

The McCoy blade has the same curve as the Macintosh blade, but contrary to all the blades described above, has an adjustable hinged tip. The handle allows control of the flexible tip, which, during laryngoscopy, serves to gradually elevate the epiglottis. This is particularly useful in a very anteriorly positioned airway and improves direct vision of the vocal cords.[11] However, the McCoy blade is not designed for use in infants and small children.

To be succinct, the laryngoscope blades can be categorized into three groups: (1) straight blades include the Miller, Wis-Hipple, and Wisconsin; (2) curved blades include the Macintosh and McCoy; and (3) semi-curved blades include the Robertshaw and Seward. The Miller blades are available in sizes 00, 0, 1, 2, 3, and 4, and the Macintosh blades in sizes 0, 1, 2, 3, 4, and 5. The Wis-Hipple blade is manufactured in sizes 00, 0, 1, and 1.5; the Robertshaw blade in sizes 0 and 1; the Seward blade in sizes 1 and 2; the Wisconsin and McCoy blades in sizes 2, 3, and 4. There are many factors to consider when deciding to use any one of these laryngoscope blades. These factors may include individual preference, training, clinical experience, availability, the patient's age, and airway anatomy. Currently, there is no study that demonstrates one type of laryngoscope blade is better than another for the management of the normal pediatric airway.

Major changes have occurred in the last 20 years concerning the materials used and illumination for laryngoscopes. The performance of the light system of the laryngoscope is critical as it impacts ease of intubation. The quality of the illumination of the larynx depends on three features, which consist of the distance from the light source to the tip of the blade, the type of light bulb or integrated fiberoptic device, and the battery type and charge status. The light-emitting diode (LED) and fiberoptic-illuminated systems produce a brighter and whiter light as compared to the traditional light bulbs. Since the bovine spongiform encephalopathy outbreak in Great Britain, the production and use of disposable blades has increased significantly.[12,13] This is due to the fact that the infectious agent, a prion, remains viable after the standard laryngoscope sterilization process.[14,15]

Accessory devices such as continuous oxygen ports (Oxyscope), continuous suction devices, and additional light sources have all been incorporated into laryngoscopes in the past, but are no longer commercially available. Nowadays, the benefits of passive oxygenation during laryngoscopy and intubation, as described by Ledbetter and colleagues in 1988, are once again gaining much attention.[16] Some of the literature suggests that the use of oxygen insufflation during laryngoscopy and intubation makes instrumentation of the airway safer.[16]

Equipment: Other Facilitator Devices

Other devices are designed to facilitate the direct laryngoscopy and intubation. These are simple, malleable stylets; articulating stylets; ETT introducers; and tube exchangers. Other devices, namely the lighted stylets and the optical stylets, are designed to be used alone or can facilitate intubation in combination with direct laryngoscopy.

Malleable Stylets

The most commonly used stylet tends to be single-use, malleable metal wire with a protective plastic coating. The stylet is placed into the ETT and allows shaping the tip of the ETT with the purpose to "blindly" place the ETT into the trachea. This will increase the success rate of intubation if only the arytenoids or the epiglottis are visualized, and the vocal cords cannot be seen. The stylet needs to be adapted to the size of the ETT and should slide easily in and out. When loading the ETT, the stylet should not protrude from the tip of the tube and should be securely fixed in a safe position to avoid injury of the trachea during intubation. As soon as the tip of the ETT passes the vocal cords, the stylet should be withdrawn. Several case reports of traumatic tracheal laceration due to inappropriate use of stylets have been reported.[17,18] Any forceful use of a styleted

ETT should be avoided. The withdrawal of the stylet should be smooth, and the stylet should be examined as the plastic coating can be sheared off and can obstruct the lumen of the ETT. The Portex intubation stylet is one example of a malleable stylet and is available for ETTs of all sizes.

Articulating Stylets

The articulating stylets available for clinical use include the Parker Flex-it articulating stylet and the Truflex stylet.[19] The single-use Parker Flex-it stylet (Parker Medical) can be used for oral and nasal intubation and does not need shaping before direct laryngoscopy. The curvature of the ETT can be gradually modified as needed during the intubation process by pressing the proximal end of the stylet with the thumb. The ETT needs to be held with the entire fist to be able to modify the curvature of the stylet during the intubation. The Parker Flex-it stylet is available in four sizes: the smallest size fits a 5.0 ETT. The Truflex stylet (Teleflex) is a reusable device, and its handle, which is located at the distal end, allows control of the flexible tip. While the Parker stylet bends the entire ETT, the Truflex stylet only bends the tip of the ETT. The smallest tube that fits the Truflex stylet is a 6.0 ETT. No matter the choice of stylet, it should always be easy to remove from the ETT. Lubrication of the stylet is ideal, and should always be checked as part of the preparation process for direct laryngoscopy.

Introducers and Exchange Catheters

Tracheal tube introducers differ from stylets as they are not preloaded onto an ETT. Typically, an introducer is placed into the trachea with the aid of direct laryngoscopy and advanced close to the carina. The ETT will then be placed over the introducer and guided into the trachea. The introducer is particularly useful in the clinical scenario where visualization of the glottis is limited. When the epiglottis cannot be identified (Cormack–Lehane grade IV), the use of an introducer is not recommended. At present, there are several introducers that are commercially available.[20] The classic Eschmann introducer, the Frova intubating introducer, and the Cook airway exchange catheter are most commonly used.

The Eschmann introducer is a reusable, plain, malleable "bougie" with a 40-degree bend at the distal tip. It is available in two sizes: for pediatrics, in curved 10 fr × 70 cm long; and for adults, in curved or straight 15 fr × 70 cm long. The Eschmann introducer is also known as a "gum elastic bougie" although to the contrary, it does not have the dilatation function of a bougie.[21] Once the Eschmann introducer is passed through the glottis, a tactile sensation of bouncing off the tracheal rings should be appreciated and indicates correct placement. The ETT can then be loaded on the introducer and advanced into the trachea.

The Frova intubating introducer (Cook Medical) is a single-use, hollow catheter with a rigid metallic stylet and a Rapi-Fit adapter. It has two side ports and a 35-degree bend distal tip. The Rapi-Fit adapter (15 mm) allows for connection to an anesthesia circuit or ventilation bag and the Rapi-Fit Luer lock adapter can connect to a jet ventilation device. There are two sizes of the Frova intubating introducer available: for pediatrics 8 fr × 35 cm long, and for adults 14 fr × 70 cm long. The pediatric size can fit into a 3.0 or larger ETT, while the adult introducer can be placed into a 6.0 or larger ETT.

The Cook airway exchange catheter can be used as an introducer or a tube exchanger. It is similar to the Frova intubating introducer as it is also a single-use, hollow device. However, the longer length of the Cook airway exchange catheter allows for the "exchange" of an ETT. During the exchange of an ETT over the Cook airway exchange catheter, it is advisable to use a laryngoscope to have visual control of the tube exchange. The reason for visualizing this procedure is because the catheter can fold back on itself and exit the trachea. Of note, this can occur when difficulty with the exchange is encountered and force is applied to advance the new ETT. The potential for complications associated with blind airway exchange are not negligible.[22] The exchange catheter comes in four different sizes. The infant size 8 fr × 45 cm long can be used in a 3.0 ETT. The pediatric sizes 11 fr × 83 cm long can fit in a 4.0 ETT, while the 14 fr × 83 cm long fits in a 5.0 ETT. The adult size 19 fr × 83 cm long is appropriate for a 7.0 or larger ETT.

Lighted Stylets

Lighted stylets were introduced as early as 1957 by Sir Robert Macintosh and can be used to facilitate intubation by direct laryngoscopy.[23] The Trachlight stylet (Laerdal Medical) was one example of a lighted stylet that, after 20 years on the market, was phased out in 2009. However, there are still several models of lighted stylets that remain available to the airway provider. The Surch-Lite (Bovie Medical Industries) and the AincA lighted stylet (Anesthesia Associates) can be used in pediatric patients. These stylets can be used for blind intubation and rely on the transillumination effect that occurs when the ETT loaded with the lighted stylet enters the glottis and becomes distinctly visible as a circumscribed glow in the middle of the neck. In the older child and adolescent, the absence of the well-defined glow indicates an esophageal ETT placement. While in infants, because of their small neck size, the transillumination from the esophagus can be mistaken for ETT placement. Therefore, in the infant population, the combined use of the lighted stylet with direct laryngoscopy will help to avoid any misjudgment. In very obese patients, the transillumination effect may not be visible. In order to facilitate endotracheal intubation, the tip of the tube loaded with a lighted stylet needs to be shaped similar to a hockey stick to produce the brightest glow at the level of the glottis. Then the stylet is withdrawn to advance the ETT further into the trachea. Both the lighted stylet and tracheal tube introducer have been used in nasotracheal intubation.[24]

Optical Stylets

There are three reusable optical stylets that are available in pediatric sizes, which fit anywhere from a 2.5 to 5.0 ETT. In the difficult airway, the combined use of an optical stylet with direct laryngoscopy can be beneficial.[25] First, the pediatric Shikani seeing optical stylet (Clarus Medical) has the following dimensions: 2.4 mm × 26.9 cm long. It is a malleable, stainless steel stylet with an atraumatic tip. The light source for the pediatric Shikani is provided by a "turbo LED" or a "GreenLight laryngoscope handle." Next, the Bonfils and Brambrink intubation endoscopes (Karl Storz) are other forms of optical stylets for consideration. The Brambrink has a slightly smaller diameter and length compared to the Shikani: it is 2 mm × 22 cm long, with a 40-degree distal deflection. On the other hand, the Bonfils has somewhat larger dimensions than either the Shikani or Brambrink, at 3.5 mm × 35 cm long. The Brambrink and Bonfils are semirigid, stainless steel stylets with high-resolution fiberoptic bundles, which are equipped with an eyepiece and the option to connect to a camera source. Any attempt made to bend them will result in their breakage. Both these devices are compatible with all cold light sources in the Karl Storz product line or, for more portability, a LED battery light source can be attached to the proximal portion of the stylet. An adjustable ETT stopper with a side port for oxygen will provide passive oxygenation during intubation. The indications for use of any of these optical stylets in combination with direct laryngoscopy are the need for a retromolar or lateral approach to the airway, the presence of a cyst or tumor in the airway, and Cormack–Lehane grade III or IV view. Most commonly, the optical stylet is used as the sole intubation tool.[26,27]

Preparation

Prior to describing the technique of direct laryngoscopy, it is important to emphasize that the careful preparation of all required equipment is essential to the safe management of the pediatric airway. For oral endotracheal intubation with direct laryngoscopy, one needs to make sure that the following items are available and function:

1. Standard ASA monitors: electrocardiogram (ECG), pulse oximeter (SpO_2), noninvasive blood pressure (NIBP), capnography (end-tidal carbon dioxide), and temperature sensor/probe.
2. Oxygen source and a ventilation bag or anesthesia circuit.
3. Age-appropriate face mask.
4. Age-appropriate oropharyngeal/nasopharyngeal airways.
5. Age-appropriate ETTs and one size smaller.
6. Malleable stylet, fitting the age-appropriate ETT.
7. Manometer for cuff inflation.
8. Appropriate induction agents, including muscle relaxants, ready to administer.
9. Appropriately sized Yankauer suction tip with tubing and functioning suction.
10. Two appropriately sized laryngoscope blades, with illumination checked for proper function. It is best to have two different types of blades available (e.g., Miller and Macintosh).
11. Shoulder roll and foam "donut," or the equivalent for positioning.
12. Tape.
13. Stethoscope.

Direct Laryngoscopy

Direct laryngoscopy is a technique of performing laryngoscopy that most laryngoscopists share as "common ground" for endotracheal intubation. As the term "direct" implies, it is a form of laryngoscopy that necessitates a direct visual path from the eyes of the laryngoscopists to an eventual endpoint at the glottic opening. Overall, the concept of direct laryngoscopy is quite easy to grasp. Nonetheless, those of us who manage the airway will probably agree that there are times when use of direct laryngoscopy, whether with a curved or straight blade, can be challenging. Ultimately, the decision by the anesthesiologist to use a Macintosh laryngoscope blade or a Miller laryngoscope blade will depend on their clinical judgment and level of comfort with the specific blade. It is important to have strategies in place to deal with the potential challenges of direct laryngoscopy.

Patient Positioning

The sniffing position is usually not necessary in the neonate, infant, and young child. Typically, in these groups of patients the occiput is large in relation to the torso. The result is that very little needs to be done by the laryngoscopist to obtain anterior flexion of the cervical spine in this patient population. However, there is some benefit to placing a small rolled towel underneath the shoulders. Of course, with the older child, the sniffing position becomes more of a consideration. In this case, a small folded blanket or sheet can be placed under the head to provide elevation (5 to 10 cm) and forward movement of the cervical spine.[28]

The sniffing position has long been linked with the use of direct laryngoscopy as the ideal head position. Quite often, the sniffing position is viewed as the "gold standard" of positions for laryngoscopy.[29,30]

The concept of the sniffing position was first described in 1913 by Chevalier Jackson. He proposed the use of a pillow under the patient's head in a natural position with the head extended.[31] That being said, use of the terminology, "sniffing position," has been credited to Sir Ivan Magill in his description, "sniffing the morning air."[32] He also suggested the use of a pillow under the head for extension and flexion at the neck.[32]

The three axes alignment theory (TAAT) was first described in 1944 by Bannister and Macbeth.[33] These three axes consist of the mouth, pharynx, and larynx; and, when in proper alignment, should constitute what is commonly known as the sniffing position. Bannister and Macbeth illustrated that axial alignment could be achieved by flexion of the neck at the upper cervical joint and extension of the head at the atlanto-occipital joint.[33] The rationale for such positioning of the head and neck was that the three axes alignment would provide a line of sight to the laryngeal opening (Figure 4.1).

Horton and colleagues examined the degree of neck flexion and head extension required for the sniffing position. These investigators identified the best angles for neck flexion as 35 degrees and head extension as 15 degrees.[34] In addition, the authors of

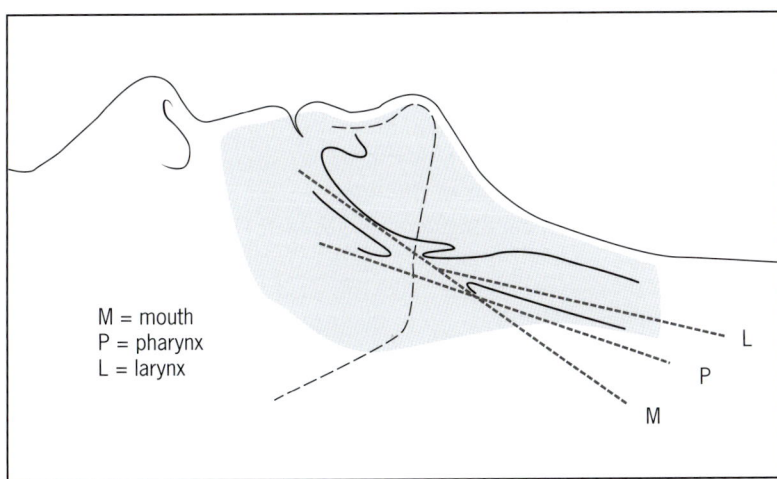

Figure 4.1 Axial alignment for endotracheal intubation.

the study examined the parameter of head elevation, while obtaining the best angles for neck flexion and head extension, as well as airway visualization. In the group studied, head elevation varied from 31 mm to 71 mm.[34] The significance of these results for use in clinical practice are not quite obvious. These are not measurements that are routinely performed by an anesthesiologist in an operating-room setting.

The concept of the sniffing position and its practical considerations, as well as TAAT and head extension, all remain quite robust in the training and practice of anesthesia. This is despite the fact that there is limited evidence to validate the use of any of them.[35-39] The issue of whether or not the sniffing position or TAAT provide the ideal position for intubation has been called into question.[36,38] In a randomized controlled trial, Adnet and colleagues[35] examined the sniffing position compared to simple head extension for laryngoscopic view. The results of their study suggested that there is no benefit for the use of the sniffing position over simple head extension for endotracheal intubation.[35] However, the sniffing position does seem more beneficial in the clinical cases of obesity and limited head extension.

The evidence in the anesthesia literature for the use of the sniffing position or head extension in the pediatric population is far less than in adults. In a prospective study, Vialet and colleagues examined, with the use of MRI, the impact of head extension on the oral, pharyngeal, and laryngeal axes in infants and young children in the presence of an LMA.[39] The investigators concluded that slight head extension enhanced the alignment between the line of sight to the vocal cords and laryngeal axis, but increased the angle of alignment between the pharyngeal and laryngeal axes.

Techniques of Direct Laryngoscopy

Before the laryngoscope blade is inserted into the mouth, the scissors maneuver is performed with the thumb of the right hand pressing downward on the lower lip or teeth while the right index finger applies pressure to the upper lip or teeth to open the mouth as wide as possible. To some extent, the technique of blade insertion into the mouth differs between the Macintosh and Miller laryngoscope blades. There are some clinical airway scenarios that may dictate the need for one blade type over another. The decision-making process involved as to which

Table 4.1 Age-Appropriate Laryngoscope Blade Size

Age	Macintosh	Miller
Very preterm	n/a	00
Preterm	0	0
Neonate/small infant	0	0
Infant to 2 years of age	1	1
2–8 years of age	2	2

n/a: not applicable

type of laryngoscope blade is most ideal will be left to the clinical judgment of the laryngoscopist. The age-appropriate laryngoscope blade size is reviewed in Table 4.1. A technique of direct laryngoscopy that is performed by some laryngoscopists, but not recommended by the authors of this chapter, is to advance the tip of the blade to the esophagus and then withdraw the blade until a view of the laryngeal opening is observed. The potential exists for unnecessary trauma to airway structures.

The Macintosh laryngoscope blade or any other type of curved blade is inserted on the right side of the mouth with the intention of sweeping the tongue leftward, and the blade is positioned in the midline, with a lift forward at a 45-degree angle. The blade is advanced past the base of the tongue, and the tip of the blade is directed into the vallecula while maintaining the 45-degree angle. This action results in an indirect lift of the epiglottis. A view of the glottic opening should be observed.

There are several different techniques for insertion of the Miller laryngoscope blade. The techniques of insertion that will be discussed here may be applied to other types of straight blades. As previously mentioned, the mouth is opened with the scissors maneuver. The Miller blade is inserted into the mouth just right of the midline with a simultaneous sweep of the tongue toward the left side of the mouth. The blade is advanced under visualization past the base of the tongue and directed toward the epiglottis. The distal tip of the blade should directly elevate the epiglottis. The result of lifting the epiglottis should create a view of the glottis. If, for whatever reason, a view of the glottis is not achieved, then another option is to insert the distal tip of the blade into the vallecula. Then the epiglottis is elevated by an indirect approach by elevating the glossoepiglottic ligament. The use of this latter technique may result in the necessary view.

External Laryngeal Manipulation

On occasion, it is not unusual for the laryngoscopist to encounter an airway where a view of the glottic opening is not appreciated with direct laryngoscopy. There can be any number of reasons for a lack of view of the glottis, the details of which will be discussed in a later chapter of this book. That being said, it is important to recognize that some of the reasons for a lack of view of the glottis can be easily corrected. For example, a change of patient position, or the size or type of laryngoscope blade may make a difference in the view.[40] What should not be overlooked is the use of external laryngeal manipulation that may also serve to improve the overall view of the larynx.[8]

Oftentimes, the "back" maneuver is utilized in the form of backward pressure on the thyroid cartilage. This backward pressure will result in dorsal movement of the laryngeal structures. Wilson and colleagues[41] examined the use of the "back" maneuver on the larynx to improve the Cormack–Lehane grade III and IV views. The results of the study by Wilson and colleagues suggested that this maneuver improved the ability of the laryngoscopist to visualize any part of the glottis in the presence of grade III or IV laryngoscopic views.[41]

Another measure that can be taken to improve the view during direct laryngoscopy is referred to as the "BURP" maneuver. BURP is an acronym for backward, upward, and rightward pressure on the thyroid cartilage.[42,43] The description of the BURP maneuver is credited to Knill.[43] The maneuver is performed with the patient in the sniffing position. There should be someone who is familiar with airway management to assist the laryngoscopist by holding the thyroid cartilage between the thumb and index finger or between the thumb and the middle finger.[43] Next, the BURP maneuver is performed by moving the larynx in the three sequential directions of backward, upward, and rightward. More than likely, moving the larynx backward and upward will result in its better exposure, and particularly following the leftward shift of the tongue with direct laryngoscopy. Overall, the benefit of the rightward move of the larynx may be an improved view from the eyes of the laryngoscopist to the glottic opening.

Alternative Techniques of Direct Laryngoscopy

The paraglossal and retromolar techniques are two alternatives that may be utilized for direct laryngoscopy. Typically, these techniques are reserved for use with a straight blade and difficult endotracheal intubation.[44] These techniques may improve the line of vision to the glottis, particularly when there is limited space in the airway.[45]

For the paraglossal laryngoscopy technique, the straight blade enters from the right corner of the mouth. The specific point of entry of the blade is the area between the tongue and tonsil. While inserting the blade into the mouth, the tongue is moved to the left side. The blade is advanced to the epiglottis and elevated. A direct lift of the epiglottis is performed, with exposure of the glottic opening. If the expected view of the glottic opening is not obtained, there may be some benefit to maintaining the position of the blade lateral to the incisors and rotating the head to the left.[45] Overall, the rotation of the head to the left side may improve axial alignment and provide a view of the glottis.

The technique of laryngoscopy is quite similar between the paraglossal approach and retromolar approach. Therefore, the retromolar technique will be described in brief terms. For the retromolar technique,[46-48] the blade is inserted in the mouth just above the molars. The approach most often used with retromolar laryngoscopy is a right-molar approach with a straight blade.[49] However, the left-molar approach has gained interest and has been proven successful.[48] What is more important to note is how these two techniques differ in their approach. In reality, the point of difference is where the blade enters the mouth.

Direct Laryngoscopy for Nasotracheal Intubation

There have been ongoing discussions as to whether or not nasal intubation is the better choice for long-term intubation and ventilation, as well as if there is an increased risk of developing sinusitis and pneumonia.[50] Nasal intubation is most often used when the surgeon requires full access to the mouth or when an oral ETT becomes impossible to secure in place due to the location of the facial injury or surgery.[51] A common indication for nasotracheal intubation is a mandible fracture. On the other hand, the presence of a massive basilar skull fracture or significant maxillofacial trauma is a contraindication for nasal intubation as a false passage into the brain can result.[52] A nasal ETT can be sutured to the nasal septum and is therefore less likely to be dislodged. Many methods have been developed to avoid nasopharyngeal trauma, including lubrication, use of topical vasoconstrictors, thermosoftening the ETT, use of a rubber airway as a guide, occlusion of the tip of the ETT lumen by an inflated esophageal stethoscope, or a combination of all.

The risk of epistaxis remains high with nasotracheal intubation and, based on findings in the literature, at least 40% of patients experience some bleeding.[52] Kwon and colleagues[53] compared fiberoptic nasal inspection before introducing the nasal ETT with a blind nasal introduction of an ETT obstructed with an inflated esophageal stethoscope in 44 randomly assigned adult patients. They found a significant decrease in the incidence of epistaxis in the fiberoptic group.[53]

The preparation for a nasotracheal intubation involves additional steps as compared with an oral intubation. The following items should be available before intubation is initiated: nasal vasoconstrictor, lidocaine gel, nasal trumpets of different sizes, warm water for the nasal ETT, an appropriate-sized Magill forceps, and a laryngoscope. Due to the fact that the nasal passage can be narrow, the ETT that is selected should be a half size smaller than the age-appropriate ETT. The authors of this chapter submit to the reader a technique for nasotracheal intubation, which is associated with minimal to no bleeding. After induction of anesthesia, the mucosa of both nostrils are sprayed with a vasoconstrictor to decrease the risk of bleeding. A nasal trumpet lubricated with lidocaine gel and with an outer diameter smaller than the outer diameter of the chosen ETT is inserted into one nostril, and, if resistance is encountered, the other nostril is used. Meanwhile, the ETT with the cuff completely deflated is placed in warm water to soften it. The first nasal trumpet is exchanged for a lubricated trumpet with an outer diameter larger than the outer diameter of the ETT. If no resistance is felt, the larger trumpet is then switched to the softened ETT. The tip of the ETT should be advanced along the nasal septum, the bevel being directed toward the turbinates to avoid being "hung up" and traumatizing the nasal turbinates.[51] It is important to keep in mind that the ETT should never be forced through the nasopharynx as the result can create a false passage with major bleeding. Whenever resistance is encountered, the ETT should be slightly withdrawn and then advanced with the bevel rotated in a different direction. If there is still resistance, another option is to reinsert the previously successful nasal trumpet and pass a neonatal Cook airway exchange catheter through the trumpet. Once the catheter is visible in the oropharynx, the trumpet can be removed and the ETT advanced over the Cook catheter.[54]

When the ETT enters the oropharynx, the child's head should be positioned for performing direct laryngoscopy. The laryngoscope blade is inserted from the right side of the mouth and the tongue is moved over to the left to appreciate the entire oral cavity as the ETT is sometimes lying behind a mucosal fold. The ETT may need to be pulled back or advanced forward to see the tip that needs to be aligned with the glottic opening. This alignment is rarely possible without additional manipulation as the glottis is in an anterior position in children. Sometimes the only manipulation required is at the area of the neck. Most often, Magill forceps – angled forceps designed for this purpose – are used to pick up the ETT and direct it toward the vocal cords. It is advisable to avoid holding the ETT with the Magill forceps at the level of the cuff as this can result in a cuff rupture. Under the direction of the laryngoscopists, an assistant should facilitate advancing the ETT through the nostril as this will allow for a less forceful grip of the ETT with the Magill forceps. Frequently, when the tip of the ETT passes through the vocal cords, resistance is met as the tip hits the anterior wall of the trachea. Flexing the head may facilitate advancement of the ETT. If laryngoscopy is difficult and the first attempt at intubation is unsuccessful, the tip of the ETT should be left in the supraglottic space, while the ETT is connected to the anesthesia circuit. Then, by closing the mouth and opposite nostril, the patient can be oxygenated and ventilated through the ETT. Using the ETT as a supraglottic device alleviates the need for repeated insertion of the ETT into the nostril.

Summary

Direct laryngoscopy remains quite commonplace in the training and practice of anesthesiology, as well as in other specialties of medicine. Much of the early work associated with the use of direct laryngoscopy is credited to the field of otolaryngology. For the most part, the concept behind direct laryngoscopy is relatively unchanged. However, over time the design of the blades used for direct laryngoscopy have undergone numerous modifications.

The Macintosh laryngoscope blade has the most usage by laryngoscopists.[9] On the contrary, among infants and young children, the Miller laryngoscope blade or other forms of straight blades tend to be commonly utilized. It is somewhat more likely in older children that the choice of laryngoscope blade will depend on the personal preference or experience of the laryngoscopist, as well as airway anatomical considerations. Initially, both the Macintosh and Miller laryngoscope blades were developed for use in adult patients. Later, the evolution of these laryngoscope blades led to their use in the pediatric population. Notably, the technology associated with direct laryngoscopy has advanced significantly over the years.

Most laryngoscopists may agree that the equipment utilized in direct laryngoscopy has undergone change with subsequent generations of both the curved and straight blades. However, the techniques linked to direct laryngoscopy have remained relatively static. This is not to suggest that actual change is required in these techniques. That said, it seems quite evident that direct laryngoscopy as a method of laryngoscopy will continue to maintain its established position in airway management.

References

1. Doherty J, Froom S, Gildersleve C. Pediatric Laryngoscopes and Intubation Aids Old and New. *Pediatric Anesthesia* 2009; **19**: 30–7.
2. Hirsch N, Smith G, Hirsch P, et al. Pioneer of Direct Laryngoscopy. *Anaesthesia* 1986; **41**: 42–5.
3. Sykes K. Entering the 20th Century. In Sykes K. ed. *Anesthesia and the Practice of Medicine*. London: Royal Society of Medicine; 2007: 33–51.
4. Miller R. A New Laryngoscope. *Anesthesiology* 1941; **2**: 317–20.
5. Macintosh R. A New Laryngoscope. *The Lancet* 1943; **1**: 205.
6. Robertshaw F. A New Laryngoscope for Infants and Children. *The Lancet* 1962; **2**: 1034.
7. Levitan RM, Hagberg CA. Upper Airway Retraction: New and Old Laryngoscope Blades. In Hagberg C, ed. *Benumof and Hagberg's Airway Management*. Philadelphia: Saunders, Elsevier; 2013: 508–35.
8. Litman R, Fiadjoe J, Stricker P, et al. The Pediatric Airway. In Coté C, Lerman J, Anderson B, eds. *A Practice of Anesthesia for Infants and Children*. Philadelphia: Saunders, Elsevier; 2013: 237–76.
9. Scott J, Baker P. How did the Macintosh Laryngoscope Become So Popular? *Pediatric Anesthesia* 2009; **19**(Suppl. 1): 24–9.
10. Watanabe S, Suga A, Asakura N, et al. Determination of the Distance between the Laryngoscope Blade and the Upper Incisors during Direct Laryngoscopy: Comparisons of a Curved, an Angulated Straight, and Two Straight Blades. *Anesthesia & Analgesia* 1994; **79**: 638–41.
11. Kulkami AP, Tirmanwar AS. Comparison of Glottis Visualization and Ease of Intubation with Different Laryngoscope Blades. *Indian Journal of Anaesthesia* 2013; **57**: 170–4.
12. Goodwin N, Wilkes A, Hall J. Flexibility and Light Emission of Disposable Paediatric Miller 1 Laryngoscope Blades. *Anaesthesia* 2006; **61**: 792–9.
13. Sudhir G, Wilkes A, Clyburn P, et al. User Satisfaction and Forces Generated during Laryngoscopy Using Disposable Miller Blades: a Manikin Study. *Anaesthesia* 2007; **62**: 1056–60.
14. Bonda DJ, Manjila S, Khan F, et al. Human Prion Diseases: Surgical Lessons Learned from Iatrogenic Prion Transmission. *Neurosurgical Focus* 2016; **41**: E10.
15. Estebe JP. Anesthesia and Non-Conventional Transmissible Agents (or Prion Diseases). *Annales Françaises d'Anesthésie et de Réanimation* 1997; **16**: 955–63.
16. Ledbetter JL, Rasch DK, Pollard TG, et al. Reducing the Risk of Laryngoscopy in Anesthetized Infants. *Anaesthesia* 1988; **43**: 151–3.
17. Tartell P, Hoover L, Friduss M, et al. Pharyngeoesophageal Intubation Injuries: Three Case Reports. *American Journal of Otolaryngology* 1990; **11**: 256–60.
18. Johnson K, Hood D. Esophageal Perforation Associated with Endotracheal Intubation. *Anesthesiology* 1986; **64**: 281–3.
19. Al-Qasmi A, Al-Alawi W, Malik AM, et al. Comparison of Trachel Intubation Using the Storz's C-MAC D-blade™ Videolaryngoscope Aided by Truflex™ Articulating Stylet and the Portex™ Intubating Stylet. *Anesthesiology and Pain Medicine* 2015; **5**: e32299.

Section 2: Devices and Techniques to Manage the Abnormal Airway

20. Frova G. Comparison of Tracheal Introducers. *Anaesthesia* 2005; **60**: 516–17; author reply, 517–18.

21. Viswanathan S, Campbell C, Wood DG, et al. The Eschmann Tracheal Tube Introducer (Gum Elastic Bougie). *Anesthesiology Review* 1992; **19**: 29–34.

22. McLean S, Lnam CR, Benedict W, et al. Airway Exchange Failure and Complications with the Use of the Cook Airway Exchange Catheter: a Single Center Cohort Study of 1177 Patients. *Anesthesia & Analgesia* 2013; **117**: 1325–7.

23. Macintosh R, Richards H. Illuminated Introducer for Endotracheal Tubes. *Anaesthesia* 1957; **12**: 223–5.

24. Davis L, Cook-Sather SD, Schreiner MS. Lighted Stylet Tracheal Intubation: a Review. *Anesthesia & Analgesia* 2000; **90**: 745–56.

25. Young CF, Vadivelu N. Does the Use of a Laryngoscope Facilitate Orotracheal Intubation with a Shikani Optical Stylet? *British Journal of Anaesthesia* 2007; **99**: 302–3.

26. Shurky M, Hanson R, Koveleskie J, et al. Management of the Difficult Pediatric Airway with Shikani Optical Stylet. *Pediatric Anesthesia* 2005; **15**: 342–5.

27. Turkstra TP, Pelz DM, Shaikh AA, et al. Cervical Spine Motion: a Fluoroscopic Comparison of Shikani Optical Stylet vs Macintosh Laryngoscope. *Canadian Journal of Anesthesia/ Journal canadien d'anesthésie* 2007; **54**: 441–7.

28. Westhorpe R. The Position of the Larynx in Children and its Relationship to the Ease of Intubation. *Anaesthesia and Intensive Care* 1987; **15**: 384–8.

29. Isono S. Common Practice and Concepts in Anesthesia: Time for Reassessment: Is the Sniffing Position a "Gold Standard" for Laryngoscopy? *Anesthesiology* 2001; **95**: 825–7.

30. El-Orbany M, Woehlck H, Salem M. Head and Neck Position for Direct Laryngoscopy. *Anesthesia & Analgesia* 2011; **113**: 103–9.

31. Jackson C. The Technique of Insertion of Intratracheal Insufflation Tubes. *Surgery, Gynecology & Obstetrics* 1913; **17**: 507–9.

32. Magill I. Endotracheal Anesthesia. *American Journal of Surgery* 1936; **34**: 450–5.

33. Bannister F, Macbeth R. Direct Laryngoscopy and Tracheal Intubation. *The Lancet* 1944; **2**: 651–4.

34. Horton W, Fahy L, Charters P. Defining a Standard Intubating Position Using "Angle Finder." *British Journal of Anaesthesia* 1989; **62**: 6–12.

35. Adnet F, Baillard C, Borron S, et al. Randomized Study Comparing the "Sniffing Position" with Simple Head Extension for Laryngoscopic View in Elective Surgery Patients. *Anesthesiology* 2001; **95**: 836–41.

36. Adnet F, Borron S, Lapostolle F, et al. The Three Axis Alignment Theory and the "Sniffing Position": Perpetuation of an Anatomic Myth? *Anesthesiology* 1999; **91**: 1964–5.

37. Adnet F, Borron S, Dumas J, et al. Study of the "Sniffing Position" by Magnetic Resonance Imaging. *Anesthesiology* 2001; **94**: 83–6.

38. Adnet F. A Reconsideration of Three Axes Alignment Theory and Sniffing Position. *Anesthesiology* 2002; **97**: 754.

39. Vialet R, Nau A, Chaumoître K, et al. Effects of Head Posture on the Oral, Pharyngeal and Laryngeal Axis Alignment in Infants and Young Children by Magnetic Resonance Imaging. *Pediatric Anesthesia* 2008; **18**: 525–31.

40. Khosla A, Cattano D. Airway Assessment. In Hagberg C, Artime C, Daily W., eds. *The Difficult Airway: a Practical Guide.* New York: Oxford University Press; 2013: 1–8.

41. Wilson M, Spiegelhalter D, Robertson J, et al. Predicting Difficult Intubation. *British Journal of Anaesthesia* 1988; **61**: 211–16.

42. Takahata O, Kubota M, Mamiya K, et al. The Efficacy of the "BURP" Maneuver during a Difficult Laryngoscopy. *Anesthesia & Analgesia* 1997; **84**: 419–21.

43. Knill R. Difficult Laryngoscopy Made Easy with a "BURP." *Canadian Journal of Anesthesia/ Journal canadien d'anesthésie* 1993; **40**: 279–82.

44. Achen B, Terblanche O, Finucane B. View of the Larynx Obtained Using the Miller Blade and Paraglossal Approach, Compared to that with the Macintosh Blade. *Anaesthesia & Intensive Care* 2008; **36**: 717–21.

45. Henderson J. The Use of Paraglossal Straight Blade Laryngoscopy in Difficult Tracheal Intubation. *Anaesthesia* 1997; **52**: 552–60.

46. Saxena K, Nischal H, Bhardwaj M, et al. Right Molar Approach to Tracheal Intubation in a Child with Pierre Robin Syndrome, Cleft Palate, and Tongue Tie. *British Journal of Anaesthesia* 2008; **100**: 141–2.

47. Agrawal S, Asthana V, Meher R, et al. Paraglossal Straight Blade Intubation Technique – an Old Technique Revisited in Difficult Intubations: a Series of 5 Cases. *Indian Journal of Anaesthesia* 2008; **52**: 317–20.

48. Yamamoto K, Tsubokawa T, Ohmura S, et al. Left-Molar Approach Improves the Laryngeal View in Patients with Difficult Laryngoscopy. *Anesthesiology* 2000; **92**: 70.

49 Bonfils P. Difficult Intubation in Pierre-Robin Children, a New Method: the Retromolar Route. *Anaesthetist* 1983; **32**: 363–7.

50 Holzapfel L, Chevret S, Madinier G, et al. Influence of Long-Term Oro- or Nasotracheal Intubation on Nosocomial Maxillary Sinusitis and Pneumonia: Results of a Prospective, Randomized, Clinical Trial. *Critical Care Medicine* 1993; **21**: 1132–8.

51 Cavusoglu T, Yazici I, Demirtas Y, et al. A Rare Complication of Nasotracheal Intubation: Accidental Middle Turbinectomy. *Journal of Craniofacial Surgery* 2009; **20**: 566–8.

52 Marlow T, Goltra D, Schabel S. Intracranial Placement of a Nasotracheal Tube after Facial Fracture: a Rare Complication. *Journal of Emergency Medicine* 1997; **15**: 187–91.

53 Kwon M, Song J, Kim S, et al. Inspection of the Nasopharynx Prior to Fiberoptic-Guided Nasotracheal Intubation Reduces the Risk of Epistaxis. *Journal of Clinical Anesthesia* 2016; **32**: 7–11.

54 Arisaka H, Sakuraba S, Furuya M, et al. Application of Gum Elastic Bougie to Nasal Intubation. *Anesthesia Progress* 2010; **57**: 112–13.

Section 2 Devices and Techniques to Manage the Abnormal Airway

Chapter 5

Supraglottic Airway Equipment and Techniques

Andrea S. Huang, Lisa E. Sohn, Suman Rao, and Narasimhan Jagannathan

Introduction

SGA devices have been used successfully in patients of all ages in various clinical scenarios, including primary airway management under general anesthesia in the operating room, and resuscitation and emergent airway management in the emergency department (ED) and prehospital settings. SGA devices have been used as alternatives to face-mask ventilation and tracheal intubation by healthcare providers with proficient airway management skills, but also by those with less experience, to successfully oxygenate and ventilate the lungs. The clinical efficacy of SGA devices in children has been proven in a large number of clinical studies. Pediatric SGA devices have undergone an evolution in design since their introduction 30 years ago. These newer design features have improved the use of SGA devices to provide positive-pressure ventilation and facilitate fiberoptic-guided tracheal intubation. The evolution, versatility, and utility of the SGA device will be discussed in detail in this chapter.

Basic Principles

The term "extraglottic" may be preferred to "supraglottic" by some medical specialists. To avoid confusion and make a distinction between the two, we will not be discussing all "extraglottic" devices, which include devices that sit *above* the patient's hypopharynx (e.g., Patil oral airway, Mehta's cuffed oropharyngeal airway), and require extracorporeal devices (e.g., a face mask) to facilitate ventilation.[1] Our focus will be on SGA devices that provide a glottic seal, and sit *in* or *below* the hypopharynx and incorporate an apparatus (e.g., airway tube) to allow hands-free ventilation of the patient's lungs. We will also not include SGA devices that do not have pediatric sizes (e.g., streamlined liner of the pharynx airway).

With these considerations, the SGA devices in this chapter will be classified as perilaryngeal or pharyngeal sealers (based on the sealing mechanism and where the distal portion is in relation to the patient's hypopharynx).[2] These two categories are further classified as first- or second-generation devices. Second-generation devices have a built-in gastric tube channel to allow evacuation of gastric contents and gases. This, in theory, may reduce the risk of regurgitation of gastric contents and thus pulmonary aspiration. Applications of SGA devices in pediatric clinical practice include spontaneous ventilation, positive-pressure ventilation, difficult airway management, airway rescue, and resuscitation. See Figure 5.1 and Figure 5.2 for SGA device classification related to this chapter.

Perilaryngeal Sealers

These devices consist of an airway tube attached to a mask. After placement into the patient's pharynx, the mask portion forms a perilaryngeal seal around the patient's larynx. A second seal, the hypopharyngeal seal, is formed by the leading edge of the mask resting against the upper esophageal sphincter. The mask incorporates a cuff, which, for the majority of devices, can be inflated via an inflation line connected to a pilot balloon, valve, and syringe (Figure 5.3). The mask cuff can be inflated for the purpose of improving the perilaryngeal and hypopharyngeal seals, optimizing airway leak pressures, and thus facilitating ventilation of the patient's lungs. The mask is attached to an airway tube with a 15 mm adaptor, which can then be connected to a standard breathing circuit or self-inflating bag. Second-generation perilaryngeal sealers incorporate a gastric tube outlet into the mask cuff, which usually provides a better hypopharyngeal

Diagram 1

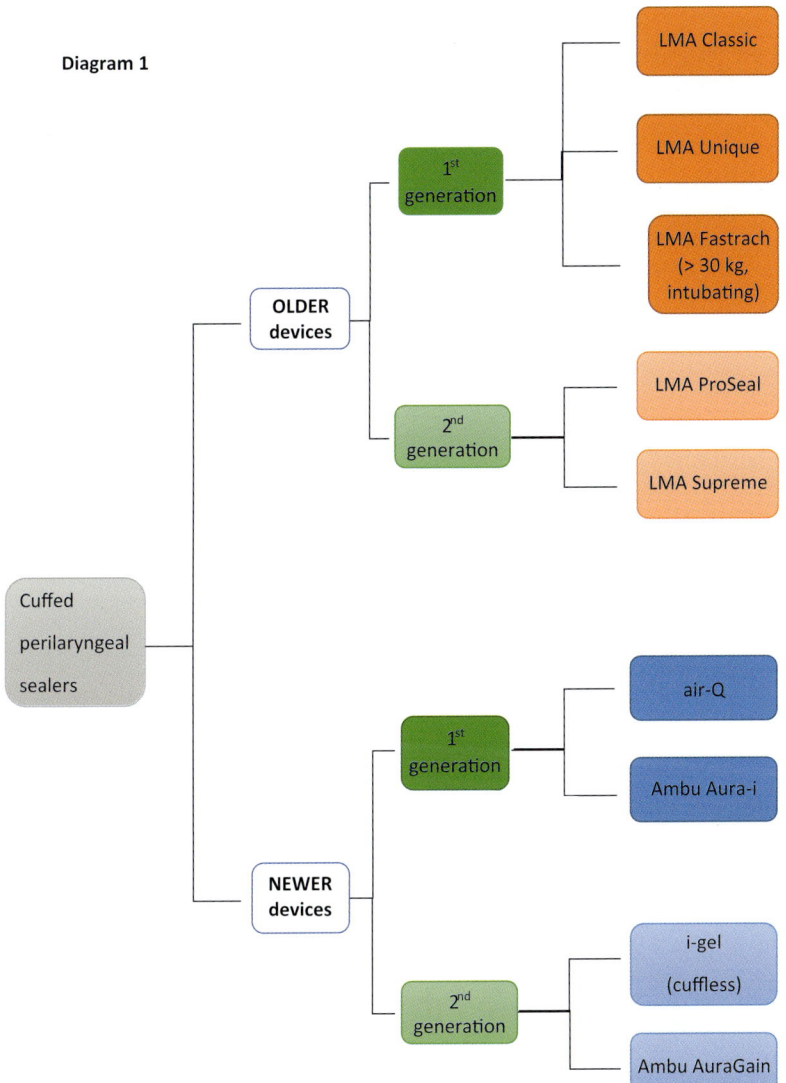

Figure 5.1 SGA device classification for the LMA family.

seal; thus second-generation SGA devices typically have higher airway leak pressures than first-generation SGA devices.

Pharyngeal Sealers

Pharyngeal sealers consist of an airway tube with one or two inflatable cuffs, and a ventilation outlet between the two cuffs to allow for ventilation of the patient's lungs. After placement into the patient's pharynx, the pharyngeal cuff seals the hypopharynx; a second cuff (if present) seals the esophagus. The esophageal cuff is designed to minimize gastric insufflation and regurgitation. Second-generation devices incorporate a gastric channel to allow for drainage of gastric contents. *A significant clinical difference between pharyngeal sealers and perilaryngeal sealers is that they cannot be used to facilitate tracheal intubation in children.*

SGA Device Cuff Volumes and Pressures, and Oropharyngeal Seal Pressures

Almost all SGA devices for children incorporate cuff(s) that can be inflated (the i-gel and air-Q SP

Section 2: Devices and Techniques to Manage the Abnormal Airway

Diagram 2

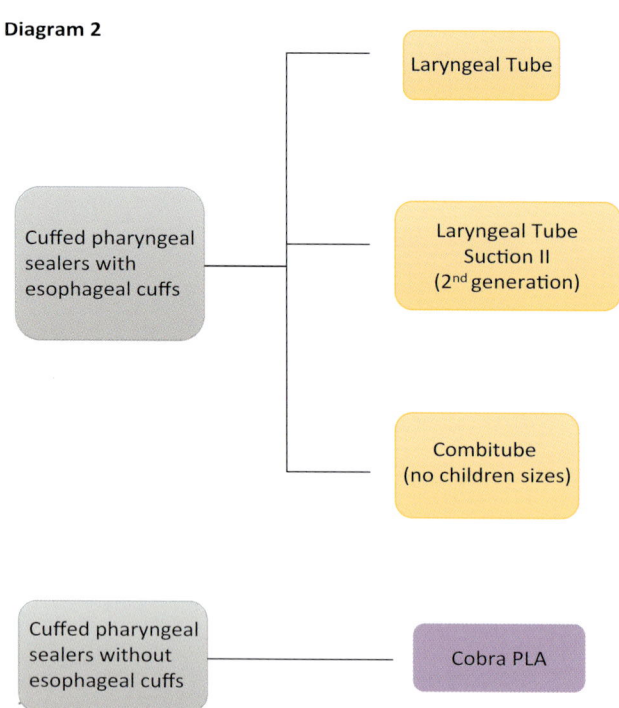

Figure 5.2 SGA device classification of newer SGAs used in children.

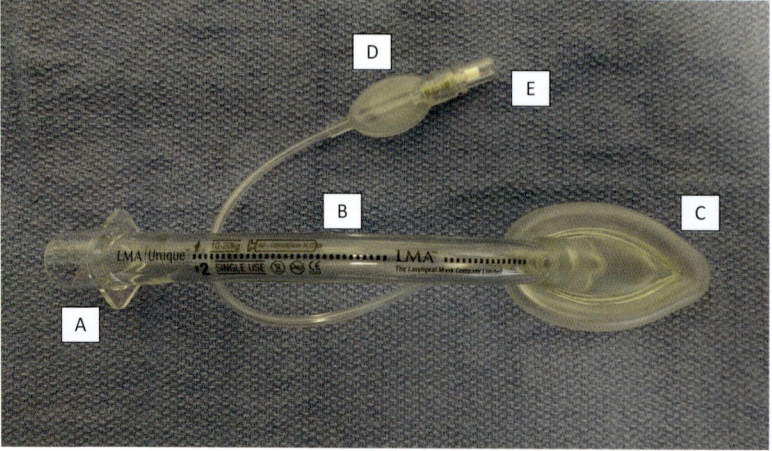

Figure 5.3 Basic perilaryngeal SGA device components:
A. 15 mm adaptor to connect to circuit
B. Airway tube
C. Mask cuff (this one can be inflated)
D. Pilot balloon (connected to mask cuff via inflation line)
E. Valve to connect to syringe

[self-pressurizing] are two exceptions). Therefore, it is important to be aware of the purpose and risk of cuff filling volumes and pressures. SGA device cuffs are inflated with the objective of improving the glottic seal. A good glottic seal facilitates ventilation of the patient's lungs, decreases gastric insufflation, and decreases pollution of the environment with leakage of inhalational agents. When using an SGA device with positive-pressure ventilation, it is important to achieve an oropharyngeal/cuff seal pressure that is greater than the level of positive pressure delivered. However, high cuff filling volumes and resultant high cuff pressures are associated with increased morbidity such as sore throat, hoarseness, nerve palsies, and reduced mucosal perfusion.[3-5] Children's airways may be even more susceptible to

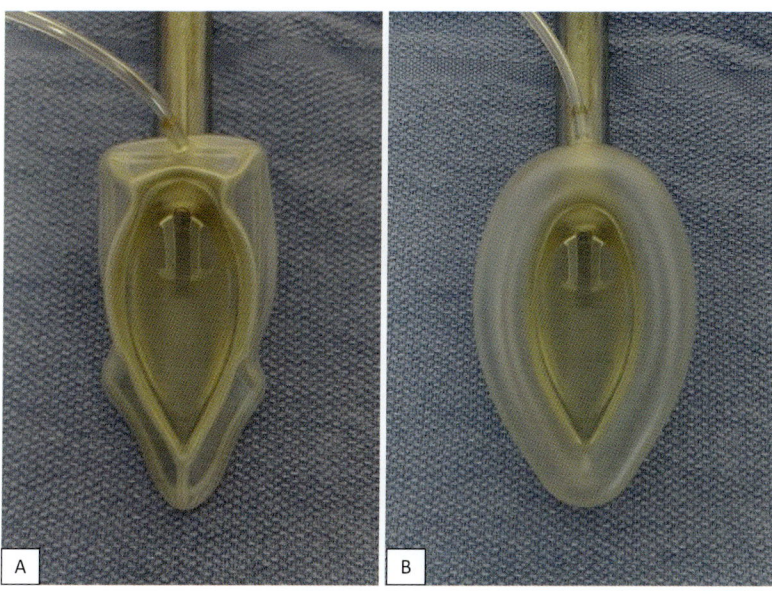

Figure 5.4 SGA device mask cuffs – significant when trying to optimize glottic seal, but overinflation of cuff can cause patient morbidity.
A. Deflated mask cuff
B. Inflated mask cuff

mucosal damage and edema compared to adults (Figure 5.4).

One study in children found that, historically, guided clinical endpoints for "optimal" cuff volumes – such as slowly inflating the cuff until a slight outward shift of the device to a new stationary position was noted – resulted in hyperinflation of the SGA device cuffs. The observed hyperinflation was even more marked in smaller sized devices. It was also noted that the use of nitrous oxide resulted in increased intracuff pressures.[6] Rather than using specific filling volumes, following *maximum* intracuff pressure recommendations may require lower volumes to achieve a sufficient oropharyngeal seal. Reducing the intracuff pressure to 40 cmH$_2$O has been shown to improve oropharyngeal seal, which may result from better molding of the cuff around the airway.[7,8] Titrating cuff pressure to the lowest necessary to achieve an adequate seal may be important for the safe and effective use of these devices in children. Furthermore, the position depth of the mask cuff does not necessarily correlate with ideal sealing pressure or optimal ventilation.[9,10] Therefore, when inflating SGA device cuff(s) in children, the use of a cuff manometer to measure cuff pressures is recommended to prevent morbidity associated with high cuff pressures.[6]

There are a few SGA devices designed to prevent cuff hyperinflation, such as the air-Q SP, which has a self-inflating, low-pressure cuff, and the i-gel, which was designed without an inflatable mask cuff and instead is made of gel-like thermoplastic elastomer designed to conform to the hypopharynx as it warms to body temperature, providing the glottic seal.

Insertion Techniques (see Video 2)

There are two approaches to inserting an SGA device: midline and rotational. In the midline approach, the leading edge of the mask is inserted against the patient's hard palate and into the posterior pharynx (Figure 5.5). However, as the SGA device passes over the patient's tongue with this technique, it may cause a downward displacement of the tongue and epiglottis, causing obstruction and/or suboptimal positioning of the SGA device. Compared to adults, the child's posterior pharyngeal wall is set at a more acute angle to the floor of the mouth, so the rotational technique may allow for easier advancement.[11–13]

In the rotational technique, the SGA device is inserted into the patient's mouth with the mask lumen facing backward, and, as the SGA device is advanced against the hard palate, it is rotated 180 degrees until seated in the pharynx (Figure 5.6). It is important to note that the studies favoring rotational technique were shown using the LMA Classic/Unique, and not with newer devices. Thus, the same conclusions cannot be made for newer devices, especially since they tend to be stiffer.

Section 2: Devices and Techniques to Manage the Abnormal Airway

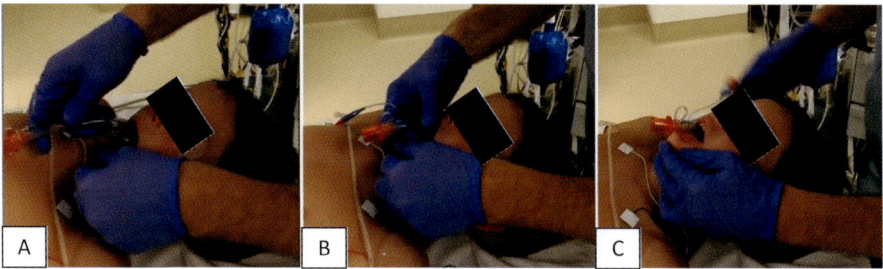

Figure 5.5 SGA device midline insertion technique:
A. The patient's mouth is opened with the SGA device lumen facing forward.
B. The SGA device mask is inserted while pressing against the palate and posterior pharyngeal wall, and advanced downward into the hypopharynx.
C. The SGA device is properly seated before attaching to circuit.

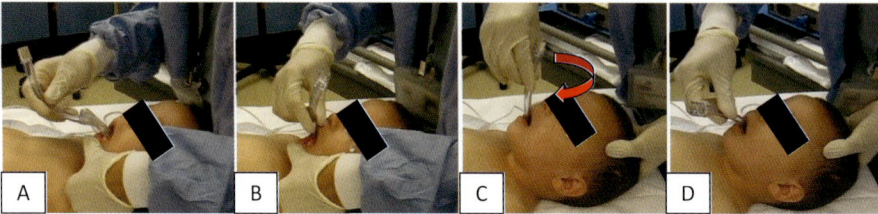

Figure 5.6 SGA device rotational insertion technique:
A. The patient's mouth is opened with the SGA device lumen facing backward.
B. The SGA device mask is inserted while pressing against the palate and posterior pharyngeal wall.
C. and D. The SGA device is rotoated 180 degrees (red arrow) while advancing downward into the hypopharynx.

Basic SGA Device Midline Insertion Technique

1. Position the patient so the neck is flexed and the head extended (maintain a neutral neck position if the cervical spine is unstable).
2. Insert the mask with the tip pressed against the hard palate.
4. Use the index finger to push the mask into the pharynx while maintaining pressure against the palate to avoid the epiglottis.
5. Use the other hand to hold the tube while withdrawing the finger from the mouth.

Types of SGA Devices Used in Children

The advantages and disadvantages of perilaryngeal sealers are shown in Table 5.1.

The LMA family

Dr. Archie Brain invented the very first LMA prototype (a perilaryngeal sealer) in London in the early 1980s. The result was a device that functioned like an "internal face mask," allowing hands-free ventilation and oxygenation of the patient without the invasiveness of tracheal intubation. The LMA first became popular in the UK, and eventually across the world, and has been used successfully in millions of adults and children since its introduction.

LMA Classic

The LMA Classic was released in the UK in 1988, and in the USA in 1992. Its design consists of an airway tube attached to an elliptical-shaped mask, which can be inflated, expanding in all directions. The mask is made of silicone and must be sterilized after each use, and it can be reused up to 40 times. In the bowl of the mask are aperture bars, designed to prevent epiglottic downfolding, which may occur after device placement into the patient's pharynx and cause airway obstruction. The LMA Classic was not designed to facilitate tracheal intubation, but it has been used as a conduit successfully in many patients.[14] Compared to newer devices, the LMA Classic is not ideal as a conduit for tracheal intubation in children. Its airway tube is long and narrow, which cannot accommodate a cuffed tracheal tube, and it is also more difficult to remove the device after successful tracheal intubation.

Chapter 5: Supraglottic Airway Equipment and Techniques

Table 5.1 Perilaryngeal Sealers: Older Devices

Device	Advantages	Disadvantages
LMA Classic	• largest evidence base of safety and efficacy	• in small children (< 10 kg), more complications with poor airway seal, mask displacement, gastric insufflation • no gastric drain provision
LMA Unique	• performs just as well as the LMA Classic • does not require autoclaving	• same as the LMA Classic
LMA ProSeal	• long history of safety and efficacy • gastric drain channel • provides higher airway leak pressure than the LMA Classic • stable in small children	• requires autoclaving • poor conduit for tracheal intubation
LMA Supreme	• single use • gastric drain tube • higher leak pressure than the LMA Classic	• cannot perform fiberoptic-guided intubation due to narrow airway tube
LMA Fastrach	• designed with shorter, wider airway tube to better facilitate fiberoptic-guided tracheal intubation	• only for children bigger than 30 kg

LMA Unique

The LMA Unique was released in 1997. The mask is made of disposable polyvinyl chloride, and it is a single-use version of the LMA Classic.

LMA Classic and Unique: Clinical Evidence

Both the LMA Classic and Unique have been used and studied extensively in children. The LMA Unique was found to perform just as well as the LMA Classic in pediatric patients.[15] There are also many case reports of their successful use in children with difficult airways.[16–18] Significant limitations arise when used in small children, specifically in those less than 10 kg. Its limitations include poor airway seal, mask displacement, and gastric insufflation of air.[19]

LMA ProSeal

The LMA ProSeal was released in 2000, with pediatric sizes made available in 2004. It was the first commercially available second-generation SGA device, meaning its design incorporates a gastric drain channel. This channel runs laterally to the airway tube, through the mask bowl, and ends as a small outlet at the distal end of the mask portion of the device. Other notable differences in its design include wire reinforcement of the airway tube and the presence of a bite block: both to prevent obstruction from the patient biting down on the airway tube. The LMA ProSeal is a reusable device and requires steam autoclaving (Figure 5.7A).

LMA ProSeal: Clinical Evidence

The LMA ProSeal was found to perform similarly to, if not better than, the LMA Classic in children. Second-generation devices usually provide a better hypopharyngeal seal; thus, they provide higher airway leak pressures than first-generation SGA devices. Studies have shown that, in children, the LMA ProSeal had similar or better airway leak pressures and decreased rates of gastric insufflation compared to the LMA Classic.[20,21] There are multiple case reports of its successful use in neonatal resuscitation.[22] Its limitations include the inability to be used as a conduit for tracheal intubation due to its long and narrow airway tube.

LMA Supreme

The LMA Supreme is a second-generation device first released in 2007, and in 2011 for children. Unlike its LMA ProSeal counterpart, it is a single-use device, with an airway tube that is curved and much more rigid to facilitate insertion. Its gastric channel is centrally located, splitting the airway tube into two narrower channels. The mask incorporates fins, rather than aperture bars, to prevent epiglottic downfolding: it has not been shown whether either design

Section 2: Devices and Techniques to Manage the Abnormal Airway

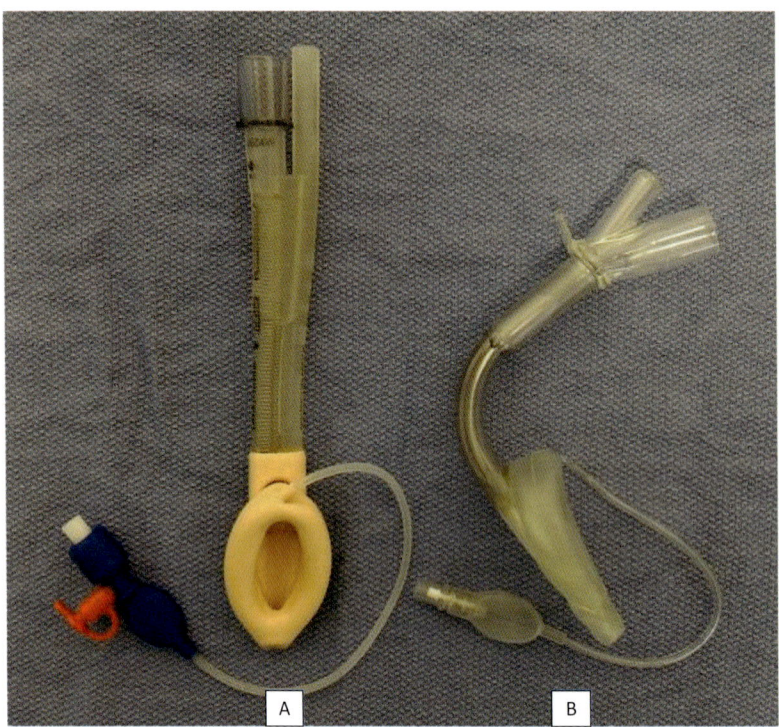

Figure 5.7 Older devices, second-generation SGA devices: LMA ProSeal and LMA Supreme.
A. LMA ProSeal: the airway tube is designed with reinforced wire and is not rigid. The gastric channel runs lateral to the airway tube. Reusable device.
B. LMA Supreme: the airway tube is curved and rigid. The gastric drain runs central to the airway tube. Single-use device.

feature provides any clinical advantage over the other. The narrow airway passages exiting on either side of the gastric channel do not make tracheal intubation through the LMA Supreme feasible in children (Figure 5.7B).

LMA Supreme: Clinical Evidence

As a second-generation device, when compared to the LMA Unique, studies have shown that the LMA Supreme had similar or higher airway leak pressures, and lower rates of gastric insufflation in children.[23,24] However, when compared to a newer SGA device, the i-gel, the LMA Supreme had lower airway leak pressures in children.[25] In a neonatal study, the LMA Supreme was found to be associated with a higher success rate in neonatal resuscitation compared to face-mask ventilation alone (91.5% versus 78% respectively).[26] Most of the difficult airway data with this device are from manikin studies, limiting the applicability of these study results to clinical practice.

Intubating LMA (LMA Fastrach)

The intubating LMA was released in 1995 and is the gold-standard device for blind tracheal intubation in adult patients. Its use is limited in older children weighing 30 kg or more. Unlike the other LMA devices, it was designed with a shorter and wider airway tube to accommodate a cuffed tracheal tube.

Newer SGA devices

The advantages and disadvantages of newer SGA devices and design advancements are shown in Table 5.2.

Air-Q

The air-Q is a newer first-generation SGA device introduced in 2004. Its basic components consist of an oval-shaped mask, which is stiffer than older SGA devices to prevent the tip from folding back on itself during insertion. Its mask design is deeper to improve the perilaryngeal seal and, instead of aperture bars or fins, an elevated keyhole-shaped orifice was designed to prevent epiglottic downfolding. Its airway tube is wider and curved to prevent undesired rotation of the device with resultant mask displacement while in use (Figure 5.8).

After initial clinical studies in small children, the air-Q was redesigned with a deeper mask and a narrower keyhole shape to prevent trapping the epiglottis within the ventilating orifice. After anesthesiologists and

Chapter 5: Supraglottic Airway Equipment and Techniques

Table 5.2 Perilaryngeal Sealers: Newer Devices

Device	Advantages	Disadvantages
Air-Q	• designed to be a conduit for tracheal intubation • can accommodate cuffed tracheal tubes • stable in small children • strong evidence for use in children with difficult airways	• no gastric drain channel
I-gel	• gastric drain channel • favorable fiberoptic position • provides high airway leak pressures • less morbidity from high mask cuff pressures with its non-inflatable mask	• expensive • higher risk of spontaneous dislodgement after placement in small children • long airway tube creates higher risk of unintentional extubation during device removal
Ambu Aura-i	• designed to facilitate tracheal intubation • favorable fiberoptic views	• no gastric drain channel • small sizes 1 and 1.5 cannot accommodate cuffed tracheal tubes
Ambu AuraGain	• gastric drain channel • more stable than the older second-generation device: the LMA Supreme	• few studies comparing it with other newer devices on children

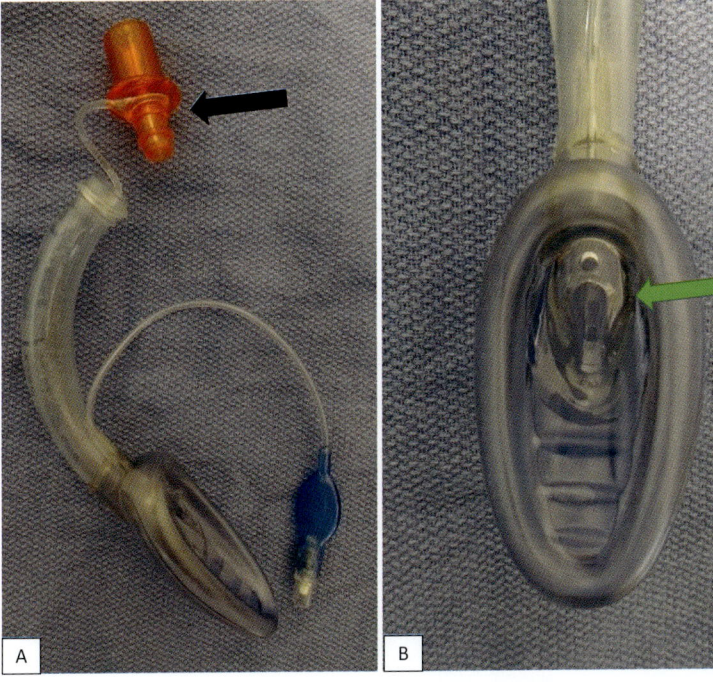

Figure 5.8 Air-Q
A. Detachable 15 mm adaptor (black arrow), which further shortens and widens the airway tube to better accommodate cuffed tracheal tubes (when being used as a conduit for fiberoptic-guided tracheal intubation).
B. Mask bowl design is stiffer and deeper than older SGA devices, with an elevated keyhole-shaped orifice (green arrow) to prevent epiglottic downfolding.

neonatologists suggested the size 1 device was too large for the average neonate, a 0.5 size was designed for the neonate. Furthermore, the air-Q was designed to be a more effective and practical conduit for tracheal intubation: a significant advantage when approaching a difficult airway. The following design features make the air-Q more effective for facilitating tracheal intubation than earlier SGA device versions:

Section 2: Devices and Techniques to Manage the Abnormal Airway

- shorter, wider airway tube: to accommodate a cuffed tracheal tube and facilitate its removal
- detachable 15 mm adaptor: further shortening and widening the airway tube to accommodate a cuffed tracheal tube
- absence of aperture bars in the mask bowl: to improve passage of the tracheal tube through the device
- specially designed removal stylet: to facilitate removal of the air-Q after successful tracheal intubation

Please see the section, "Difficult Airway: Clinical Application of SGA Device Use in Children," below, and refer to Figure 5.11 and Video 3 and Video 4 for a step-by-step technique in tracheal intubation via the SGA device.

Air-Q: Clinical Evidence

The air-Q has been shown to be just as effective as, if not more favorable than, previous SGA devices, especially as a conduit for tracheal intubation in children with normal and difficult airways.[27–29] Case reports have also reported its successful use in neonates with difficult airways.[29] When compared to the LMA Unique in healthy children (10–15 kg), the air-Q had higher airway leak pressures and provided better fiberoptic views of the glottis. Studies in children support the use of fiberoptic-guided tracheal intubation as blind intubation in children is not recommended due to frequent epiglottic downfolding.[30,31] Within the air-Q family, the air-Q SP device was found to be just as effective as the LMA Unique in children, but without the risk of mask cuff overinflation and the morbidities associated with high cuff pressures.[32]

I-gel

The i-gel is a newer second-generation device introduced in 2007, with pediatric sizes released in 2010. Unlike all other SGA devices, the i-gel does not rely on an inflatable mask cuff to modify the oropharyngeal seal. Instead, the mask is made of gel-like thermoplastic elastomer designed to conform to the hypopharynx as it warms to body temperature, improving the airway seal as it envelopes the laryngeal inlet. As a second-generation device, a gastric channel is incorporated on the lateral side of its broader airway tube. Be aware that the smallest size, 1, does not have a gastric channel (Figure 5.9).

I-gel: Clinical Evidence

The i-gel has been shown to be safe and effective in children with normal and difficult airways. It has been

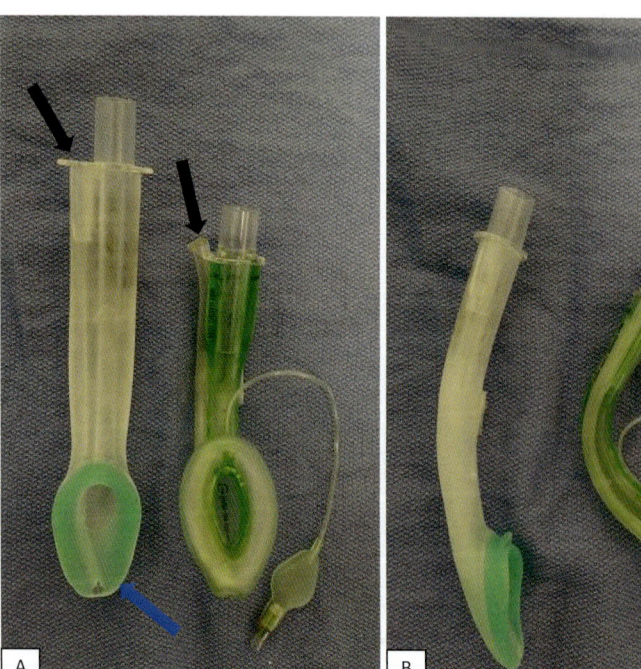

Figure 5.9 Newer, second-generation SGA devices: i-gel and Ambu AuraGain. A. The gastric drains are lateral to each respective airway tube (black arrow). The i-gel mask is non-inflatable (blue arrow): instead it is made of gel-like thermoplastic elastomer. The airway tube of the i-gel is notably wider and longer, which can pose problems when attempting to remove the device after successful tracheal intubation. B. The airway tube of the Ambu AuraGain is more curved and shorter than the LMA Supreme's, with an inflatable mask cuff.

found to have similar, if not better, leak pressures than previous SGA devices, along with providing better fiberoptic views.[25,33–35] Meta-analyses of this device suggest that the i-gel is suitable for positive-pressure ventilation. Although it has been used successfully as a conduit for fiberoptic intubation in many children, reports suggest more problems with its use compared to the air-Q, which include difficulty removing the i-gel after tracheal intubation due to its longer length, and the inability to pass cuffed tracheal tubes in its sizes 1 and 1.5.[36–38] There are also reports of spontaneous mask dislodgement after insertion into the patient's pharynx requiring additional positional adjustments, especially in smaller children.[39,40]

Ambu Aura-i

The Ambu Aura-i, like the air-Q, was designed to facilitate tracheal intubation with its short and wide airway tube to accommodate a cuffed tracheal tube. However, its 15 mm adaptor is molded into the structure of the airway tube, and thus cannot be disconnected. When used as a conduit for tracheal intubation, this fixed proximal portion of the airway tube in sizes 1 and 1.5 can be too narrow to accommodate the inflation pilot balloon of cuffed tracheal tubes during the SGA device removal process[41] (Figure 5.10).

Ambu Aura-i: Clinical Evidence

The Ambu Aura-i is just as effective a conduit for fiberoptic intubation as the air-Q in children, but, as noted, there are limitations with its smaller sizes when using a cuffed tracheal tube.[41] One study in children younger than 12 months of age showed similar fiberoptic views with the air-Q, but lower airway leak pressures, likely due to the Ambu Aura-i's smaller mask cuff.[42] In summary, it performs just as well as its counterpart SGA devices without any additional advantages.

Ambu AuraGain

The Ambu AuraGain is a second-generation device in the Ambu Aura family, with a larger cuff and gastric drain. A recent study in infants and children showed that, compared to the LMA Supreme (another second-generation device), the Ambu AuraGain had similar airway leak pressures, but required fewer airway maneuvers to maintain a patent airway.[43]

The advantages and disadvantages of pharyngeal sealers with esophageal cuffs are shown in Table 5.3.

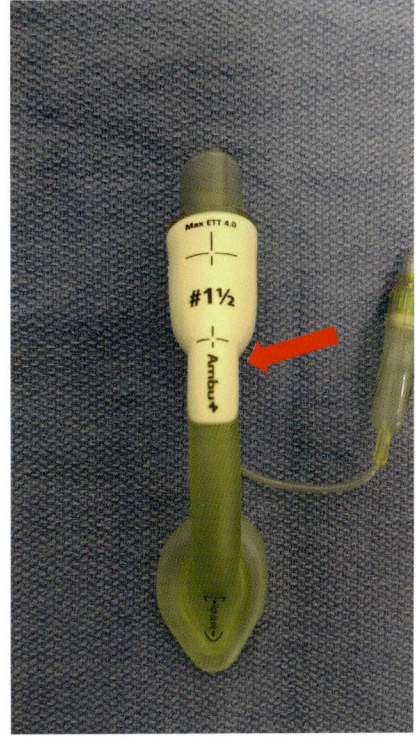

Figure 5.10 Ambu Aura-i
The 15 mm adaptor is molded into the structure of the airway tube, and thus cannot be disconnected (unlike the air-Q). When used as a conduit for tracheal intubation, this fixed proximal portion (red arrow) of the airway tube in sizes 1 and 1.5 can be too narrow to accommodate the inflation pilot balloon of cuffed tracheal tubes during the SGA device removal process.

The Laryngeal Tube and its Advanced Version, LTS II

The Laryngeal Tube (VBM Medizintechnik) was introduced in 1988, around the same time as the LMA Classic. Its sizes range from 0 to 2.5. It differs from the SGA devices mentioned thus far in its sealing mechanism and where its distal portion rests in relation to the patient's hypopharynx. It is made up of a single-lumen silicone tube with two cuffs and a ventilation outlet between the two cuffs. After blind placement into the patient's pharynx, the smaller distal cuff seals the esophagus, and the larger proximal cuff seals the hypopharynx. One study in small children (less than 10 kg) showed an 80% failure rate; for those over 10 kg, the failure rate decreased to 6%.[44]

The LTS II is a second-generation double-lumen device with sizes 1 to 2.5. It was found to have higher success rates in small children compared to

Table 5.3 Pharyngeal Sealers with Esophageal Cuffs

Device	Advantages	Disadvantages
Laryngeal Tube	• can be inserted blindly • effective in out-of-hospital scenarios	• high failure rate in small children (< 10 kg) • cannot be used as a conduit for tracheal intubation
Laryngeal Tube Suction II (LTS II)	• much more effective in small children than first-generation Laryngeal Tube • has been used in children with difficult airways	• cannot be used as a conduit for tracheal intubation
Combitube	• can be inserted blindly • effective rescue device • effective in out-of-hospital scenarios	• pediatric sizes not available

Table 5.4 Pharyngeal Sealer without Esophageal Cuff

Device	Advantage	Disadvantage
Cobra Perilaryngeal Airway (PLA)	• comparable to LMA Unique in a few studies	• not as effective when compared to many other SGA devices available for children

the first-generation device.[45] One study comparing the LTS II and the LMA ProSeal in children showed it was equally effective and had higher seal pressures.[46] The LTS II has been used successfully in both the expected and unexpected difficult airway.[45] The main disadvantage of pharyngeal sealers compared to perilaryngeal sealers is that they cannot be used as a conduit for tracheal intubation, which is advantageous when managing the difficult airway.

The advantage and disadvantage of the perilaryngeal and pharyngeal sealer are shown in Table 5.4.

Cobra PLA

The Cobra PLA (Engineered Medical Systems; 2003) consists of a tube with a tapered striated "cobra head" with ventilating orifices at its distal end, and a large pharyngeal cuff just proximal to it.

Cobra PLA: Clinical Evidence

Two studies in children showed that the Cobra PLA performed just as well as the LMA Unique, with one study showing higher cuff seal pressures.[47,48] However, other studies have also shown increased problems with the Cobra PLA in children, such as epiglottic downfolding in 77%, gastric insufflation in 21%, and device instability, requiring frequent readjustments during eye surgery.[49–51] Given the number of effective SGA devices currently available for children, the Cobra PLA is not recommended for routine use.

Difficult Airway: Clinical Application of SGA Device Use in Children

SGA devices are versatile and have become a critical tool in the management of the difficult airway. They can be inserted quickly to establish rapid ventilation and oxygenation of the lungs. SGA devices are incorporated in the difficult airway algorithms of countries all over the world when difficult mask ventilation and/or laryngoscopy is encountered. In those patients who are difficult to mask-ventilate and/or difficult to intubate, SGA devices may be able to bypass the reasons for the difficulties and allow for successful ventilation. Factors such as a large tongue, airway secretions/blood, airway obstruction, and limited neck mobility may have less of an impact on the successful use of an SGA device than with mask ventilation and tracheal intubation.[52]

Furthermore, design features of newer SGA devices allow them to be more effective conduits for tracheal intubation, and studies have shown them to be a reliable tool for children with both normal and difficult airways.[27–29,36,38] Almost all the SGA devices described in this chapter (except for the Cobra PLA and the Ambu AuraGain) have reports of successful use in children with difficult airways. The use of a visualization method, such as a fiberoptic bronchoscope or optical stylet, is recommended, since blind

Chapter 5: Supraglottic Airway Equipment and Techniques

intubations through SGA devices in children have low success rates.[30]

The SGA Device as a Conduit for Fiberoptic Tracheal Intubation Technique

Refer to Figure 5.11 and Video 3 and Video 4.

1. Prepare the following equipment in the appropriate sizes:
   - SGA device designed for fiberoptic tracheal intubation (e.g., air-Q, Ambu Aura-i).
   - Tracheal tube.
   - Fiberoptic bronchoscope.
   - Stylet for SGA device removal: can be from manufacturer, or, if unavailable, can use uncuffed tracheal tube.
   - Lubricate all necessary parts and test the removability of adaptors/connectors and so on before proceeding.

2. Insert the SGA device into the patient's pharynx (Figure 5.11A).

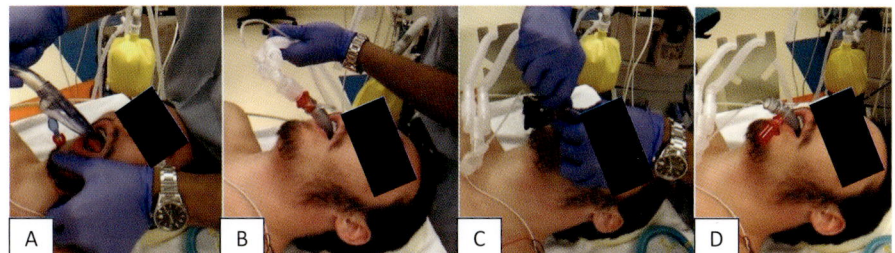

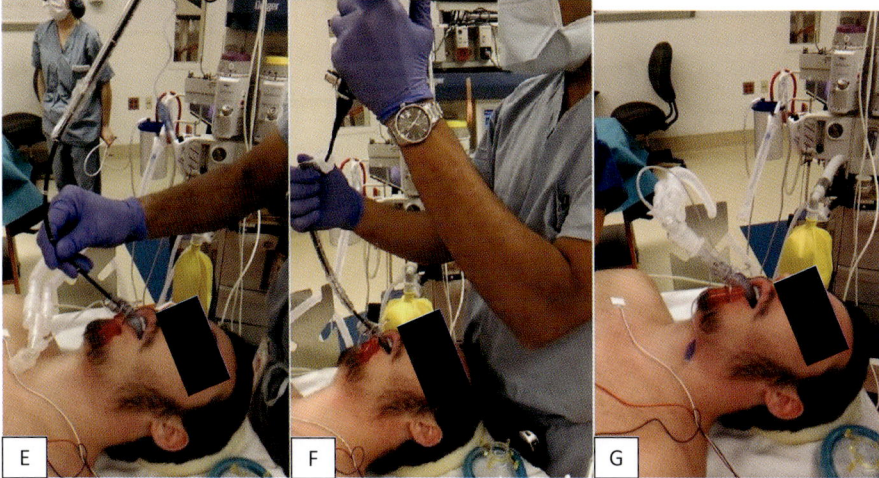

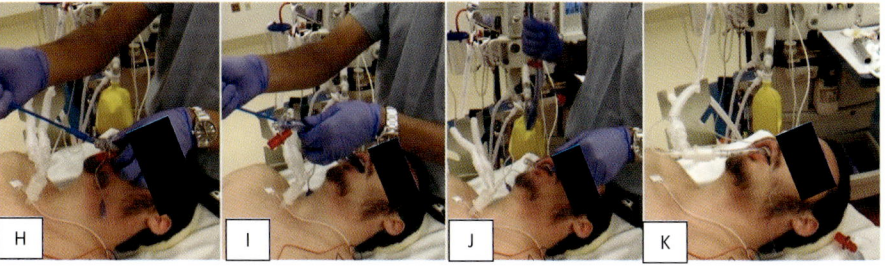

Figure 5.11A–K Directions in how to use the air-Q as a conduit for fiberoptic-guided tracheal intubation.

Section 2: Devices and Techniques to Manage the Abnormal Airway

3. Attach the SGA device to the circuit/oxygen source and confirm effective oxygenation and ventilation of patient's lungs (Figure 5.11B).
4. Remove the detachable 15 mm adaptor if using an air-Q (other SGA devices do not have detachable adaptors) (Figure 5.11C, D).
5. Advance the fiberoptic bronchoscope (loaded with an appropriately sized tracheal tube) through the SGA device tube and ultimately into the patient's trachea (visualize tracheal rings and carina) (Figure 5.11E).
6. Unload the tracheal tube from the fiberoptic bronchoscope and advance until the tracheal tube is in the trachea. Correct tracheal tube placement in the trachea is confirmed as the fiberoptic bronchoscope is withdrawn from the patient's trachea (Figure 5.11F).

   Tip: if you encounter difficulty passing the tracheal tube through the patient's glottis and into the trachea, consider rotating the tracheal tube, or administering jaw thrust.

7. With both the SGA device and tracheal tube in place, connect the circuit to the tracheal tube and again confirm adequate ventilation/oxygenation of patient's lungs (Figure 5.11G).

   Next steps: how to remove the SGA device that is still in patient's pharynx.

8. Detach the adaptor from the tracheal tube and insert a removal stylet (if unavailable, use uncuffed tracheal tube) to maintain traction (Figure 5.11H).
9. As one hand removes the SGA device from the patient's pharynx, the other hand maintains traction and acts as an opposing force on the tracheal tube to prevent unintentional extubation during this process (Figure 5.11I).

   Tip: as the SGA device is being removed from the pharynx, as soon as you see the distal tip of the cuffed tracheal tube, immediately grab hold of the tracheal tube with one hand. Then you must remove the stylet *before* the inflation pilot balloon passes into the SGA device tube, and *before* pulling out the SGA device completely.

10. After successful SGA device removal, confirm the tracheal tube is in the trachea by reattaching the tracheal tube adaptor and circuit, and confirming adequate oxygenation/ventilation of the patient's lungs (Figure 5.11J, K).

Technique: SGA Device Use in the Awake Infant with an Anticipated Difficult Airway

Refer to Video 1 (the Pierre Robin neonate case).

1. Topicalize the infant's pharynx to minimize gagging and facilitate easier placement of the SGA device.

   Tip: there are many ways to do this. One technique involves using a standard infant pacifier. Lidocaine 2% jelly is mixed with either a glucose solution or a surgical lubricant and is injected into the nipple portion of the infant pacier (be aware of recommended lidocaine toxicity and dosing guidelines). Small perforations are then made in the nipple using a 20 G needle. As the infant sucks on the pacifier, there is pharyngeal spread of the lidocaine jelly.

2. Insert the SGA device into the awake infant's pharynx.
3. Connect the SGA device to a circuit and confirm adequate oxygenation/ventilation. If the infant had obstruction at rest due to difficult airway anatomy, the SGA device should result in some relief of the airway obstruction.

   *At this point, consider awake versus asleep intubation.

4. Awake: insert fiberoptic bronchoscope (with appropriately sized tracheal tube) through the SGA device tube. On visualization of the glottic opening, consider giving anesthetic agents (inhalation or intravenous), or continue to advance the fiberoptic bronchoscope and tracheal tube into the trachea of the awake infant.
5. If the decision is to proceed under anesthesia, connect the SGA device (which was placed in the awake infant) to the anesthesia machine circuit and deliver inhalation anesthetic agents, or administer intravenous agents while maintaining spontaneous ventilation.
6. If there is adequate oxygenation/ventilation with general anesthesia, disconnect the circuit from the SGA device, insert the fiberoptic bronchoscope and advance the tracheal tube into the infant's trachea.

Other Clinical Applications and Evidence of SGA Device Use in Children

Spontaneous Ventilation

The first perilaryngeal SGA device by Dr. Brain was developed for the purpose of allowing hands-free, noninvasive ventilation of the spontaneously breathing anesthetized patient. Since then, millions of children have also successfully benefited from the use of perilaryngeal SGA devices. From the first LMA Classic to the newest SGA devices, these have proven to be safe and effective for the anesthetized spontaneously breathing child. In the awake spontaneously breathing child with a difficult airway, SGA devices, such as the air-Q, have successfully relieved airway obstruction during airway management.[27,28]

Positive-Pressure Ventilation

The ability to provide positive-pressure ventilation has improved as SGA device designs have evolved to provide better oropharyngeal seals. Changes to the mask shape, size, material, bowl design, and incorporated gastric channels have been made to improve the airway seal. Studies have shown that second-generation SGA devices and newer SGA devices allow for more effective positive-pressure ventilation and decreased gastric insufflation. SGA devices have been used routinely and safely in children requiring positive-pressure ventilation; for example, in laparoscopic surgeries.[53,54] In surgeries where intubation is considered the gold standard, such as adenotonsillectomies, studies have found SGA devices to be just as safe as endotracheal intubation.[55–58]

Rescue Airway

SGA devices have been used successfully as rescue airway devices by healthcare providers with a wide range of airway management skills. They are more effective than face-mask ventilation alone, and much easier to learn and less traumatic to place by novices when compared with tracheal intubation by direct laryngoscopy.[59,60] Therefore, it is not surprising that the SGA device is used in many out-of-hospital settings by first responders. The effectiveness of SGA devices is well known and therefore many difficult airway algorithms include the SGA device when there is a "can't ventilate, can't intubate" scenario.

Pediatric/Neonatal Resuscitation

It is not uncommon for a newborn to require immediate respiratory support after birth. Many neonatal resuscitation studies have shown that SGA device use in newborns is safe and highly effective. Studies have shown that, when compared with mask ventilation and tracheal intubation, SGA device use was associated with higher appearance, pulse, grimace, activity, and respiration (APGAR) scores and lower newborn intensive care unit (NICU) admission rates. In summary, studies showed higher successful resuscitation rates, shorter required ventilation times, and lower need for tracheal intubation when SGA devices were used.[61] The LMA Classic is the most extensively described SGA device for use in this specific scenario, but there is no current evidence to show one brand of SGA device to be more effective in children.

Conclusion

The small child's airway is uniquely different from that of the adult, and, although SGA devices were initially designed for adult patients, much progress has been made in the design of SGA devices with the child's airway anatomy in mind. Furthermore, the versatility of the SGA device has been proven in multiple studies of children in various clinical scenarios, including the difficult airway.

References

1. Brimacombe J. A Proposed Classification System for Extraglottic Airway Devices. *Anesthesiology* 2004; **101**(2): 559.

2. Miller DM. A Proposed Classification and Scoring System for Supraglottic Sealing Airways: a Brief Review. *Anesthesia & Analgesia* 2004; **99**(5): 1553–9; table of contents.

3. Nagai K, Sakuramoto C, Goto F. Unilateral Hypoglossal Nerve Paralysis following the Use of the Laryngeal Mask Airway. *Anaesthesia* 1994; **49**(7): 603–4.

4. Marjot R. Trauma to the Posterior Pharyngeal Wall Caused by a Laryngeal Mask Airway. *Anaesthesia* 1991; **46**(7): 589–90.

5. Burgard G, Mollhoff T, Prien T. The Effect of Laryngeal Mask Cuff Pressure on Postoperative Sore Throat Incidence. *Journal of Clinical Anesthesia* 1996; **8**(3): 198–201.

6. Ong M, Chambers NA, Hullet B, Erb TO, von Ungern-Sternberg

Section 2: Devices and Techniques to Manage the Abnormal Airway

BS. Laryngeal Mask Airway and Tracheal Tube Cuff Pressures in Children: are Clinical Endpoints Valuable for Guiding Inflation? *Anaesthesia* 2008; **63**(7): 738–44.

7 Licina A, Chambers NA, Hullett B, Erb TO, von Ungern-Sternberg BS. Lower Cuff Pressures Improve the Seal of Pediatric Laryngeal Mask Airways. *Paediatric Anaesthesia* 2008; **18**(10): 952–6.

8 Hockings L, Heaney M, Chambers NA, Erb TO, von Ungern-Sternberg BS. Reduced Air Leakage by Adjusting the Cuff Pressure in Pediatric Laryngeal Mask Airways during Spontaneous Ventilation. *Paediatric Anaesthesia* 2010; **20**(4): 313–17.

9 Inagawa G, Okuda K, Miwa T, Hiroki K. Higher Airway Seal does Not Imply Adequate Positioning of Laryngeal Mask Airways in Paediatric Patients. *Paediatric Anaesthesia* 2002; **12**(4): 322–6.

10 Goudsouzian NG, Denman W, Cleveland R, Shorten G. Radiologic Localization of the Laryngeal Mask Airway in Children. *Anesthesiology* 1992; **77**(6): 1085–9.

11 Nakayama S, Osaka Y, Yamashita M. The Rotational Technique with a Partially Inflated Laryngeal Mask Airway Improves the Ease of Insertion in Children. *Paediatric Anaesthesia* 2002; **12**(5): 416–19.

12 McNicol LR. Insertion of Laryngeal Mask Airway in Children. *Anaesthesia* 1991; **46**(4): 330.

13 Ghai B, Ram J, Makkar JK, Wig J. Fiber-Optic Assessment of LMA Position in Children: a Randomized Crossover Comparison of Two Techniques. *Paediatric Anaesthesia* 2011; **21**(11): 1142–7.

14 Wong DT, Yang JJ, Mak HY, Jagannathan N. Use of Intubation Introducers through a Supraglottic Airway to Facilitate Tracheal Intubation: a Brief Review. *Canadian Journal of Anaesthesia/Journal canadien d'anesthesie* 2012; **59**(7): 704–15.

15 Mathis MR, Haydar B, Taylor EL, et al. Failure of the Laryngeal Mask Airway Unique and Classic in the Pediatric Surgical Patient: a Study of Clinical Predictors and Outcomes. *Anesthesiology* 2013; **119**(6): 1284–95.

16 Walker RW, Allen DL, Rothera MR. A Fibreoptic Intubation Technique for Children with Mucopolysaccharidoses Using the Laryngeal Mask Airway. *Paediatric Anaesthesia* 1997; **7**(5): 421–6.

17 Inada T, Fujise K, Tachibana K, Shingu K. Orotracheal Intubation through the Laryngeal Mask Airway in Paediatric Patients with Treacher-Collins Syndrome. *Paediatric Anaesthesia* 1995; **5**(2): 129–32.

18 Asai T, Nagata A, Shingu K. Awake Tracheal Intubation through the Laryngeal Mask in Neonates with Upper Airway Obstruction. *Paediatric Anaesthesia* 2008; **18**(1): 77–80.

19 Lopez-Gil M, Brimacombe J, Alvarez M. Safety and Efficacy of the Laryngeal Mask Airway. A Prospective Survey of 1400 Children. *Anaesthesia* 1996; **51**(10): 969–72.

20 Shimbori H, Ono K, Miwa T, Morimura N, Noguchi M, Hiroki K. Comparison of the LMA-ProSeal and LMA-Classic in Children. *British Journal of Anaesthesia* 2004; **93**(4): 528–31.

21 Goldmann K, Jakob C. A Randomized Crossover Comparison of the Size 2 1/2 Laryngeal Mask Airway ProSeal versus Laryngeal Mask Airway-Classic in Pediatric Patients. *Anesthesia and Analgesia* 2005; **100**(6): 1605–10.

22 Micaglio M, Ori C, Parotto M, Zanardo V, Trevisanuto D. The ProSeal Laryngeal Mask Airway for Neonatal Resuscitation: First Reports. *Paediatric Anaesthesia* 2007; **17**(5): 499; author reply, 499–500.

23 Jagannathan N, Sohn L, Sommers K, et al. A Randomized Comparison of the Laryngeal Mask Airway Supreme and Laryngeal Mask Airway Unique in Infants and Children: Does Cuff Pressure Influence Leak Pressure? *Paediatric Anaesthesia* 2013; **23**(10): 927–33.

24 Jagannathan N, Sohn LE, Sawardekar A, Chang E, Langen KE, Anderson K. A Randomised Trial Comparing the Laryngeal Mask Airway Supreme with the Laryngeal Mask Airway Unique in Children. *Anaesthesia* 2012; **67**(2): 139–44.

25 Jagannathan N, Sommers K, Sohn LE, et al. A Randomized Equivalence Trial Comparing the i-gel and Laryngeal Mask Airway Supreme in Children. *Paediatric Anaesthesia* 2013; **23**(2): 127–33.

26 Trevisanuto D, Cavallin F, Nguyen LN, et al. Supreme Laryngeal Mask Airway versus Face Mask during Neonatal Resuscitation: a Randomized Controlled Trial. *The Journal of Pediatrics* 2015; **167**(2): 286–91 e281.

27 Jagannathan N, Sohn LE, Eidem JM. Use of the air-Q Intubating Laryngeal Airway for Rapid-Sequence Intubation in Infants with Severe Airway Obstruction: a Case Series. *Anaesthesia* 2013; **68**(6): 636–8.

28 Jagannathan N, Roth AG, Sohn LE, Pak TY, Amin S, Suresh S. The New air-Q Intubating Laryngeal Airway for Tracheal Intubation in Children with Anticipated Difficult Airway: a Case Series. *Paediatric Anaesthesia* 2009; **19**(6): 618–22.

29 Fiadjoe JE, Stricker PA. The air-Q Intubating Laryngeal Airway in Neonates with Difficult Airways. *Paediatric Anaesthesia* 2011; **21**(6): 702–3.

30. Kleine-Brueggeney M, Nicolet A, Nabecker S, et al. Blind Intubation of Anaesthetised Children with Supraglottic Airway Devices Ambu Aura-i and Air-Q Cannot be Recommended: a Randomised Controlled Trial. *European Journal of Anaesthesiology* 2015; **32**(9): 631–9.

31. Jagannathan N, Sohn LE, Mankoo R, Langen KE, Mandler T. A Randomized Crossover Comparison between the Laryngeal Mask Airway-Unique and the air-Q Intubating Laryngeal Airway in Children. *Paediatric Anaesthesia* 2012; **22**(2): 161–7.

32. Jagannathan N, Sohn LE, Sawardekar A, et al. A Randomised Comparison of the Self-Pressurised air-Q Intubating Laryngeal Airway with the LMA Unique in Children. *Anaesthesia* 2012; **67**(9): 973–9.

33. Fukuhara A, Okutani R, Oda Y. A Randomized Comparison of the i-gel and the ProSeal Laryngeal Mask Airway in Pediatric Patients: Performance and Fiberoptic Findings. *Journal of Anesthesia* 2013; **27**(1): 1–6.

34. Goyal R, Shukla RN, Kumar G. Comparison of Size 2 i-gel Supraglottic Airway with LMA-ProSeal and LMA-Classic in Spontaneously Breathing Children Undergoing Elective Surgery. *Paediatric Anaesthesia* 2012; **22**(4): 355–9.

35. Lee JR, Kim MS, Kim JT, et al. A Randomised Trial Comparing the i-gel with the LMA Classic in Children. *Anaesthesia* 2012; **67**(6): 606–11.

36. Dhanger S, Adinarayanan S, Vinayagam S, Kumar MP. I-gel Assisted Fiberoptic Intubation in a Child with Morquio's Syndrome. *Saudi Journal of Anaesthesia* 2015; **9**(2): 217–19.

37. Jagannathan N, Sohn L, Ramsey M, et al. A Randomized Comparison between the i-gel and the air-Q Supraglottic Airways when Used by Anesthesiology Trainees as Conduits for Tracheal Intubation in Children. *Canadian Journal of Anaesthesia/Journal canadien d'Anesthesie* 2015; **62**(6): 587–94.

38. Kim YL, Seo DM, Shim KS, et al. Successful Tracheal Intubation Using Fiberoptic Bronchoscope via an i-gel Supraglottic Airway in a Pediatric Patient with Goldenhar Syndrome – a Case Report. *Korean Journal of Anesthesiology* 2013; **65**(1): 61–5.

39. Hughes C, Place K, Berg S, Mason D. A Clinical Evaluation of the i-gel Supraglottic Airway Device in Children. *Paediatric Anaesthesia* 2012; **22**(8): 765–71.

40. Theiler LG, Kleine-Brueggeney M, Luepold B, et al. Performance of the Pediatric-Sized i-gel Compared with the Ambu AuraOnce Laryngeal Mask in Anesthetized and Ventilated Children. *Anesthesiology* 2011; **115**(1): 102–10.

41. Jagannathan N, Sohn LE, Sawardekar A, et al. A Randomized Trial Comparing the Ambu Aura-i with the air-Q Intubating Laryngeal Airway as Conduits for Tracheal Intubation in Children. *Paediatric Anaesthesia* 2012; **22**(12): 1197–204.

42. Darlong V, Biyani G, Baidya DK, et al. Comparison of air-Q and Ambu Aura-i for Controlled Ventilation in Infants: a Randomized Controlled Trial. *Paediatric Anaesthesia* 2015; **25**(8): 795–800.

43. Jagannathan N, Hajduk J, Sohn L, et al. A Randomised Comparison of the Ambu AuraGain and the LMA Supreme in Infants and Children. *Anaesthesia* 2016; **71**(2): 205–12.

44. Richebe P, Semjen F, Cros AM, Maurette P. Clinical Assessment of the Laryngeal Tube in Pediatric Anesthesia. *Paediatric Anaesthesia* 2005; **15**(5): 391–6.

45. Scheller B, Schalk R, Byhahn C, et al. Laryngeal Tube Suction II for Difficult Airway Management in Neonates and Small Infants. *Resuscitation* 2009; **80**(7): 805–10.

46. Gaitini L, Yanovski B, Toame R, Carmi N, Somri M. Laryngeal Tube Suction II versus the ProSeal Laryngeal Mask in Anesthetized Children with Spontaneous Ventilation: 19AP6-3. *European Journal of Anaesthesiology* 2007; **24**: 203.

47. Szmuk P, Ghelber O, Matuszczak M, Rabb MF, Ezri T, Sessler DI. A Prospective, Randomized Comparison of Cobra Perilaryngeal Airway and Laryngeal Mask Airway Unique in Pediatric Patients. *Anesthesia & Analgesia* 2008; **107**(5): 1523–30.

48. Gaitini L, Carmi N, Yanovski B, et al. Comparison of the CobraPLA (Cobra Perilaryngeal Airway) and the Laryngeal Mask Airway Unique in Children under Pressure Controlled Ventilation. *Paediatric Anaesthesia* 2008; **18**(4): 313–19.

49. Passariello M, Almenrader N, Coccetti B, Haiberger R, Pietropaoli P. Insertion Characteristics, Sealing Pressure and Fiberoptic Positioning of CobraPLA in Children. *Paediatric Anaesthesia* 2007; **17**(10): 977–82.

50. Polaner DM, Ahuja D, Zuk J, Pan Z. Video Assessment of Supraglottic Airway Orientation through the Perilaryngeal Airway in Pediatric Patients. *Anesthesia & Analgesia* 2006; **102**(6): 1685–8.

51. Sunder RA, Sinha R, Agarwal A, Perumal BC, Paneerselvam SR. Comparison of Cobra Perilaryngeal Airway (CobraPLA) with Flexible Laryngeal Mask Airway in Terms of Device Stability and Ventilation Characteristics in Pediatric Ophthalmic Surgery. *Journal of Anaesthesiology, Clinical Pharmacology* 2012; **28**(3): 322–5.

52. Timmermann A. Supraglottic Airways in Difficult Airway Management: Successes, Failures, Use and Misuse. *Anaesthesia* 2011; **66**(Suppl.2): 45–56.

53. Mironov PI, Estekhin AM, Mirasov AA. Anaesthetic Maintenance with Laryngeal Mask for a Laparoscopic Surgery in Pediatric Patients. *Anesteziologija i Reanimatologiia* 2013; 1: 10–14.

54. Sinha A, Sharma B, Sood J. ProSeal as an Alternative to Endotracheal Intubation in Pediatric Laparoscopy. *Paediatric Anaesthesia* 2007; **17**(4): 327–32.

55. Clarke MB, Forster P, Cook TM. Airway Management for Tonsillectomy: a National Survey of UK Practice. *British Journal of Anaesthesia* 2007; 99(3): 425–8.

56. John RE, Hill S, Hughes TJ. Airway Protection by the Laryngeal Mask. A Barrier to Dye Placed in the Pharynx. *Anaesthesia* 1991; **46**(5): 366–7.

57. Peng A, Dodson KM, Thacker LR, Kierce J, Shapiro J, Baldassari CM. Use of Laryngeal Mask Airway in Pediatric Adenotonsillectomy. *Archives of Otolaryngology – Head & Neck Surgery* 2011; **137**(1): 42–6.

58. Sierpina DI, Chaudhary H, Walner DL, et al. Laryngeal Mask Airway versus Endotracheal Tube in Pediatric Adenotonsillectomy. *The Laryngoscope* 2012; **122**(2): 429–35.

59. Alexander R, Chinery JP, Swales H, Sutton D. "Mouth to Mouth Ventilation": a Comparison of the Laryngeal Mask Airway with the Laerdal Pocket Facemask. *Resuscitation* 2009; **80**(11): 1240–3.

60. Timmermann A, Russo SG, Crozier TA, et al. Novices Ventilate and Intubate Quicker and Safer via Intubating Laryngeal Mask than by Conventional Bag-Mask Ventilation and Laryngoscopy. *Anesthesiology* 2007; **107**(4): 570–6.

61. Schmolzer GM, Agarwal M, Kamlin CO, Davis PG. Supraglottic Airway Devices during Neonatal Resuscitation: an Historical Perspective, Systematic Review and Meta-Analysis of Available Clinical Trials. *Resuscitation* 2013; **84**(6): 722–30.

Section 2 Devices and Techniques to Manage the Abnormal Airway

Chapter 6

Oxygenation Techniques for Children with Difficult Airways

Paul A. Baker

Introduction

It is important for the pediatric airway clinician to maintain oxygenation and avoid trauma when managing a child with a difficult airway. While these two objectives are compatible, it is also known that oxygen therapy can lead to significant harm. This chapter will include a discussion of various forms of oxygenation techniques during pediatric airway management, with an emphasis on avoiding hypoxia during all phases of the perioperative process. Included in this discussion will be mention of the deleterious effects of hypoxemia and hyperoxia, and the potential dangers of some oxygenation techniques.

Hypoxemia

Respiratory events are the most common cause of adverse events during pediatric anesthesia.[1] These complications are age dependent, with neonates and infants being at highest risk. Perioperative hypoxia is relatively common during pediatric anesthesia. The reported incidence is dependent on the definition of hypoxemia and the reliability of objective recording using pulse oximetry. In a prospective analysis of 575 non-cardiac surgery patients, aged between 0 and 16 years of age, true hypoxemia (defined as $SpO_2 \leq 90\%$ for at least 1 minute without recording artifact) occurred in 6% of cases. Of these 67 cases, 28% occurred at induction, 46% occurred during maintenance, and 25% occurred during emergence. The incidence of hypoxemia increases significantly in younger patients. The highest incidence was in neonates, where up to 50% of patients suffered some degree of hypoxia.

Patients at risk of hypoxemia included those with:

- respiratory complications (40% of hypoxemic cases), including sputum, atelectasis, and hypoventilation
- complications secondary to procedural problems (24% of cases), including tracheobronchoscopy, laparoscopy, and high ventilation pressures
- intubation-related factors relating to endobronchial intubation, tracheal tube, and SGA device use
- dislodgement of the airway device (19% of cases)
- laryngeal or bronchial spasm (13% of cases)
- hypoxia related to congenital heart disease (1% of cases)
- equipment failure (1% of cases)[2]

The Consequences of Hypoxemia

The clinical consequences of brief periods of hypoxemia during pediatric anesthesia are unknown. Hypoxemia is common and usually well tolerated, provided normal oxygen saturation is rapidly restored. Extreme prolonged hypoxemia, however, has severe consequences. A study of central venous oxygen saturation ($S_{CV}O_2$) measurements in pediatric cardiac patients found that measurements of $S_{CV}O_2 < 60\%$ were associated with poor clinical outcomes and $S_{CV}O_2 < 40\%$ for > 18 minutes was the most predictive indicator of major adverse events.[3]

Infants and neonates are most at risk for adverse respiratory events and consequential cardiac arrest during anesthesia.[4] In a multicenter study of perioperative cardiac arrest, infants accounted for 55% of anesthesia-related cardiac events.[5] Practitioners need to be aware of the warning signs of cardiac arrest in children. Hypoxia is frequently associated with bradycardia, which is the most common warning sign of cardiac arrest in children (54%). This is followed by hypotension (49%), low oxygen saturation (46%), unmeasurable blood pressure (25%), abnormal end-tidal carbon dioxide (21%), cyanosis (21%), and cardiac arrhythmias (16%).[5]

The Perils of Oxygen

Oxygen is the most commonly used gas in medicine and a component of all general anesthetics. Yet, despite the ubiquitous presence of therapeutic oxygen, it is not without adverse effects, particularly when administered in high concentrations to premature neonates.[6,7]

Neonatal Resuscitation and Oxygen Toxicity

Neonates are susceptible to life-threatening hypoxic episodes at birth, which can occur in up to 6–10% of deliveries. Such events can then lead to death or severe morbidity, including hypoxic encephalopathy, developmental delay, epilepsy, and cerebral palsy. Resuscitation of the newborn is now recommended with air due to growing recognition of poor outcomes from neonates resuscitated with 100% oxygen. A Cochrane review found a reduction in mortality in infants resuscitated with room air, but there is insufficient evidence to recommend the ideal oxygen concentration for neonatal resuscitation or to recommend a policy of using air over 100% oxygen or vice versa.[8]

High concentrations of oxygen administered during neonatal resuscitation are associated with oxidative stress, possibly due to oxygen free radicals. Immature neonates are unable to avoid the damage caused by oxygen free radicals because they lack the antioxidant system that is necessary to limit hydroxyl radical formation. A prospective study of severely asphyxiated term neonates, resuscitated with room air or 100% oxygen, found less oxidative stress, less cardiac and less renal damage when neonates were resuscitated with air rather than 100% oxygen.[9] There is also evidence of long-term morbidity following brief exposure to 100% oxygen at birth, including childhood leukemia, indicating potential DNA mutation.[10] These problems seem to be age specific and exposure of 100% oxygen to older children is not associated with the same effects. The groups at most risk of the effects of oxidative stress are preterm neonates (gestational age < 37 weeks). *The International Liaison Committee on Resuscitation (ILCOR) has reiterated concerns about 100% oxygen used during resuscitation of the newborn by stating that air is as effective as 100% oxygen for neonatal resuscitation.*[11]

Retinopathy of Prematurity

The etiology of retinopathy of prematurity (ROP) seems to be multifactorial. A number of factors have been linked to this condition, including extremes of arterial oxygenation (hypoxemia and hyperoxia), antenatal and neonatal exposure to inflammation, and genetic polymorphisms. There are no anesthesia-related cases of ROP, but a reasonable target is to use a minimum inspired oxygen concentration to achieve oxygen saturations between 90% and 94%. *There is no evidence that anesthesia is a causative factor in ROP.*[6]

Bronchopulmonary Dysplasia (BPD)

BPD is a condition of extremely premature infants (< 1000 g, gestation 23–28 weeks). These neonates invariably require mechanical ventilation, which can then lead to interstitial dysplasia of the lung, which is associated with 20–40% mortality. The etiology of BPD is thought to be a combination of external factors (prematurity, postnatal infection, ventilator-induced lung injury, oxygen toxicity) and genetic factors in a susceptible host. The "susceptible host" refers to the presence of a gene that allows an individual to tolerate oxidative stress. An anesthetic plan would aim to minimize airway stimulation, avoid hypoxia and hyperoxia, optimize lung function preoperatively, avoid high airway pressures, and optimize postoperative oxygenation and analgesia.[6]

Atelectasis

High FiO_2 is associated with absorption atelectasis in the lung, which can occur rapidly within 5 minutes after the induction of anesthesia. This, combined with high oxygen consumption, typically seen in neonates and infants, can lead to ventilation perfusion mismatch. Lung inhomogeneity then occurs when closed, recruitable, and overdistended alveolar regions co-exist. This then sets up ventilator-induced lung injury. Protective ventilation strategies can be applied to minimize lung injury by judicious and controlled use of oxygen, low tidal volume ventilation, PEEP and recruitment maneuvers. Alveolar volume recruitment has been applied to children < 2 years of age with beneficial effects using $30\,cmH_2O$ for 10 seconds.[12]

Atelectasis tends to occur in dependent parts of the lungs and is one factor associated with postoperative pulmonary complications. The deleterious effects of atelectasis can be mitigated by limiting FiO_2.

Other Limitations of Oxygen Therapy

The duration and concentration of oxygen therapy should be limited in certain groups of patients. Children receiving chemotherapy agents are at risk of adverse effects from hyperoxia. Bleomycin with high

FiO₂ can cause acute interstitial pneumonia and chronic pulmonary fibrosis. Children at risk of high pulmonary vascular resistance and systemic vascular resistance require careful titration of FiO₂ to maintain oxygenation, but avoid hyperoxia, which is associated with increased vascular resistance.

Oxygen should be treated like any other drug. Concentrations should be measured and titrated to provide the ideal dose to match the condition of the patient. Practitioners should be mindful of the adverse effects and interactions with other drugs before prescribing and administering oxygen. It is equally important to be careful of the extremes of oxygen therapy and understand the chronic effects of hyperoxia, but also the life-threatening impact of hypoxia.

Airway Management Techniques for Children

The following techniques have been developed to maintain oxygenation for the patient, so that the practitioner can more easily provide careful airway management, without trauma.

Preoxygenation

In the presence of a difficult airway, preoxygenation buys valuable time for laryngoscopy and tracheal intubation before the onset of hypoxia, and is recommended by current adult airway management guidelines.[13–15] Preoxygenation techniques increase oxygen reserve in the lungs and therefore increase the duration of apnea without desaturation (DAWD) reaching ≤ 90%.[16] Given the poor predictive value of bedside screening tests in children and adults, it is wise to be prepared for the unexpected difficult airway. It is therefore sensible to preoxygenate all patients. For some uncooperative children, this is not a practical option, but many of these children receive an inhalation induction with 100% oxygen and a volatile agent, which can effectively achieve denitrogenation of the lungs.

Without oxygen, following the induction of anesthesia and the onset of apnea, oxygen desaturation occurs rapidly after the oxygen saturation falls to 94%, particularly if the airway is obstructed during apnea. A study by Hardman and colleagues demonstrated that the onset of oxygen desaturation was age dependent. Modeling healthy virtual children who were 1 month, 1 year, 8 years, and 18 years of age, following apnea, it was found that oxygen desaturation occurred in the order of age, with the 1-month-old neonate exhibiting oxygen desaturation first, followed by the 1-year-old, 8-year-old, and then the 18-year-old. This modeling was conducted with open and obstructed airways, and repeated with preoxygenation periods of 0, 1, and 3 minutes. The rate of oxygen desaturation of hemoglobin from 90% to 40% was approximately the same for all ages (~33%/min for an obstructed airway, and ~26%/min for an open airway). Preoxygenation delayed the onset of oxygen desaturation in all age groups, but the benefit of preoxygenation was least in the 1-month neonate. In the absence of preoxygenation and an open airway, a 1-month-old neonate desaturated in only 6.6 seconds compared to 33.6 seconds for the 8-year-old child. This difference can be explained by the physiology of the neonate, which has a larger minute ventilation to FRC ratio, a high metabolic rate, and low maximal SaO₂ compared to older children.[17]

The DAWD to ≤ 90% depends on the preoxygenation technique, oxygen reserve at the start of apnea, oxygen consumption, and the amount of oxygen required to maintain SpO₂ at 90%. In a theoretical healthy adolescent or adult, that time is 6.9 minutes with 100% oxygen therapy and 1 minute if the patient is breathing air.

Preoxygenation involves tidal volume breathing (TVB), with 100% oxygen through a sealed face mask for 3 minutes. A fast technique of equivalent efficacy to TVB involves eight deep breaths of 100% oxygen for 60 seconds. The endpoint for these techniques is an end-tidal oxygen concentration of 90% (F_EO_2 = 0.9). Another fast technique using four deep breaths of 100% oxygen over 30 seconds is not recommended and is inferior to the TVB 3 minute and eight deep breaths techniques.[16,18] Failure to reach F_EO_2 = 0.9 can be attributed to a decreased fresh gas flow, low FiO₂, inadequate preoxygenation time, and leaks around the mask. The DAWD depends on the quality of the preoxygenation technique, the lung FRC, and oxygen consumption. Preoxygenation can be optimized by sitting the patient up to increase their FRC. Application of PEEP has been studied in this context, and several studies show improved denitrogenation conditions and prolonged DAWD with PEEP.[19] As discussed, infants have a relatively small FRC and high metabolic rate compared to an adult, which aggravates the rapidity of hypoxia onset during apnea, particularly in association with airway obstruction. This physiology reduces the DAWD and explains the benefit of prolonging oxygenation after induction of anesthesia.

Apneic Oxygenation

The concept of delivering oxygen to apneic patients was first described by Holmdahl in 1956.[20] It was recognized that, during apnea, oxygen is taken up by the blood from the FRC at a rate that exceeds the outflow of carbon dioxide. This occurs because of the relatively high solubility of carbon dioxide in the blood. Flow rate differential then occurs between oxygen removal from the alveoli and carbon dioxide excretion. This generates a negative pressure gradient of −20 cmH$_2$O, creating bulk flow of oxygen from the upper airway to the alveoli. Oxygen can be delivered from the nose, face mask, pharynx, or trachea at varying flow rates and FiO$_2$. The effectiveness of apneic oxygenation varies depending on the delivery technique and the age and physical status of the patient.

Using this technique with preoxygenation and apneic oxygenation through a tracheal tube, normal oxygen saturations can be maintained for at least 10 minutes in children, but infants may desaturate after only 3 minutes of apnea. In this study of 28 children and infants, PaO$_2$ decreased at 4.1 kPa/min or 30 mmHg, which is three times faster than an adult.[21] A similar study demonstrated that, after preoxygenation and apneic oxygenation with 0.1 L/(kg min) through a tracheal tube, oxygen desaturation was prevented for 3 minutes. In a control group breathing air, oxygen desaturation occurred after 116 seconds in patients who were 3–10 kg; 147 seconds if weight was 10–20 kg, and 217 seconds if the child weighed > 20 kg.[22]

A limitation of this technique is the steady increase in PaCO$_2$ of 0.4–0.8 kPa/min due to absent ventilation and clearance of carbon dioxide. Over time, this can cause respiratory acidosis and an associated spectrum of complications, including cardiac arrhythmias and vasodilation.

Nasal Cannula for Low Flow Oxygenation

In 1977, Wung described the insufflation of nasal oxygen at 10 L/min via corrugated tubing for newborns with respiratory distress syndrome. A nasal tracheal tube was then intubated via the other nostril. This technique had the desired effect of reducing the incidence of hypoxia and bradycardia.[23] The use of a nasal cannula to extend oxygenation into the postinduction phase of anesthesia is now recommended during laryngoscopy and tracheal intubation by recent adult airway management guidelines.[14] Dry nasal oxygen at 15 L/min for an adult can achieve near 100% FiO$_2$, but has limitations for preoxygenation because of patient intolerance due to nasal desiccation. Despite this limitation, this technique is effective at prolonging apnea time after the administration of sedatives and muscle relaxants.[19] This technique has been given the acronym NO DESAT for nasal oxygen during efforts securing a tube.[24] In adults and adolescents, preoxygenation can comfortably start with 2 L/min nasal oxygen, and the flow can increase to 15 L/min after induction.

Oxygen through nasal prongs has also been used to oxygenate infants during tracheal intubation.[25] The nasal prongs are applied with no flow under the face mask during preoxygenation, without any problems caused by leaks around the mask. After induction of anesthesia with a muscle relaxant and apnea, nasal oxygen flow is turned to 6–8 L/min. With this technique, the author reports infrequent bradycardic and desaturation episodes during airway management. The importance of proper patient positioning is emphasized with neck extension using a shoulder roll to avoid airway obstruction.

Heated Humidified High-Flow Nasal Cannula (HHHFNC)

The upper limit of gas flow through a nasal cannula is primarily limited by patient tolerance. Cool dry gas becomes very uncomfortable at high flows. By heating nasal gas to body temperature and providing humidification to > 99% relative humidity, nasal gas can be administered to patients comfortably, using flow rates equal to or exceeding the patient's inspiratory flow rate.[26] This technique was originally described for pediatric intensive care patients as a form of respiratory support for premature neonates.[27] HHHFNC has also been used successfully to treat infants with bronchiolitis, reducing the need for tracheal intubation and the need for intensive care admission. There is also a role for HHHFNC in transporting critically unwell children where intubation rates have fallen as a result of this treatment. Other benefits in children have been described, including the management of obstructive sleep apnea, post-extubation stridor, and viral-induced wheeze.[26]

Physiological advantages of HHHFNC include decreased work of breathing, partial ventilation with limited carbon dioxide clearance, and CPAP at approximately 0.45 cmH$_2$O pressure per 1 L/min flow rate. As a result of high gas flow and CPAP, improved washout of nasopharyngeal dead space occurs and alveolar ventilation is possible, which allows lung recruitment from positive distending pressure.[26]

Partial carbon dioxide clearance is seen with HHHFNC in adult apneic patients. In an adult study, this clearance resulted in a modest PaCO$_2$ increase during apnea of 0.15 kPa/min compared to PaCO$_2$ of 0.4–0.8 kPa/min without HHHFNC.[28] There is currently no evidence to suggest that this carbon dioxide clearance with HHHFNC occurs in children.

Rare complications have occurred with HHHFNC therapy. Abdominal distension has been reported in two small case reports in children with intra-abdominal pathology requiring restricted use of this therapy in this context. Infection reported in 2005 from *Ralstonia* spp. infection was linked to a Vapotherm 2000i HHHFNC system. This system was temporarily withdrawn and modified to prevent recurrence of this problem. No further infections have been reported since the product was reintroduced. Barotrauma has been reported in a small number of children associated with HHHFNC therapy. Pneumothoraces occurred in two children, pneumomediastinum in one child, and subcutaneous scalp emphysema, pneumo-orbitis, and pneumocephalus without pneumothorax or pneumomediastinum was reported in a premature infant receiving HHHFNC therapy.[26]

To mitigate the risk of barotrauma, it is important that an adequate leak is provided around the nares by ensuring that the nasal prongs do not exceed 50% of the nasal diameter. This provides protection against excessive lung distending pressure. Application of HHHFNC in conjunction with face-mask ventilation is also contraindicated because of the risk of excessive flow and airway pressure due to outflow obstruction. Another practical point is the importance of maintaining an open upper airway during HHHFNC therapy. This may require simple upper airway maneuvers such as a jaw thrust.

The Optiflow (Fisher and Paykel Healthcare) is a heated humidified high-flow delivery system. The nasal cannulas are specifically designed for this purpose to withstand high flows of gas. The cannulas are made of soft silicon and are designed with skin applicators for the face to improve patient comfort during prolonged use.

Adult flow rates of 70 L/min have been described for transnasal humidified rapid-insufflation ventilator exchange (THRIVE).[28] Recommended pediatric flow rates appear in Table 6.1.

An early report of 20 infants less than 3 months old undergoing tracheal intubation with HHHFNC found that the benefit seemed to depend on whether the child was sick or healthy. Oxygen saturation remained normal throughout the intubation for 12 healthy children with normal lungs, but five of the eight sick children desaturated. It is unknown whether the sick children would have been worse without HHHFNC.[29]

The use of HHHFNC therapy during pediatric anesthesia is still novel compared to the extensive experience in pediatric intensive care. Potential applications during pediatric anesthesia might include HHHFNC for preoxygenation, tracheal intubation, laryngeal, and other upper airway surgery, endoscopy, and anesthesia recovery.

In adult patients, HHHFNC has also been used effectively in the ICU during difficult tracheal intubation and as a primary oxygenation mechanism for prolonged periods of apnea during surgery.[28,30] Figure 6.1 shows the nasal cannula apparatus in a 2-year-old child receiving 2 L/(kg min) oxygen flow through the THRIVE Optiflow device for upper gastrointestinal endoscopy.

Table 6.1 Suggested Flow Rates for Children Receiving HHHFNC Oxygen/Air

(Personal communication from Associate Professor Andreas Schibler, Mater Research Institute, University of Queensland, Brisbane, Australia)

Weight	Flow rate
0–15 kg	2 L/(kg min)
15–30 kg	35 L/min
30–50 kg	40 L/min
> 50 kg	50 L/min

Bag-Mask Ventilation

Bag-mask ventilation is a core skill in airway management and is the default technique when all others fail. Airway narrowing is the main cause of difficult

Section 2: Devices and Techniques to Manage the Abnormal Airway

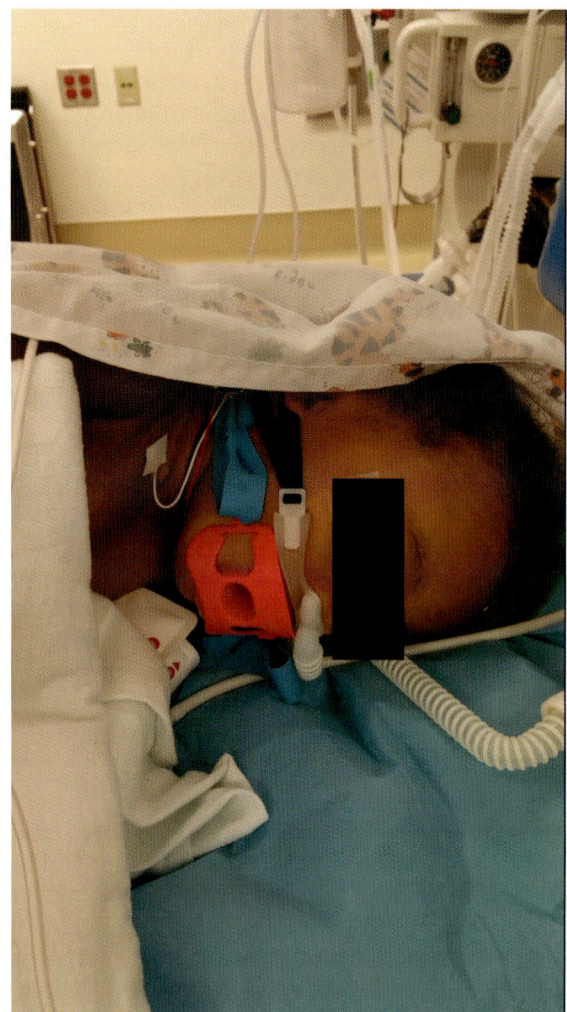

Figure 6.1 Nasal cannula apparatus in a 2-year-old child receiving 2 L/(kg min) oxygen flow through the THRIVE Optiflow device (HHHFNC) for upper gastrointestinal endoscopy.

ventilation, and children with a collapsible upper airway, such as that seen in laryngomalacia, will benefit from CPAP, which stents the airway and increases FRC.

Creating an adequate mask seal can be challenging during bag-mask ventilation for children with dysmorphic features and distorted anatomy. A novel approach to mask seal in a term infant with a frontonasal encephalocele was achieved by using an inverted adult size five face mask over the infant's face.[31]

Maintaining a patent airway during an inhalation induction of anesthesia can be particularly challenging in infants with micrognathia. Optimum bag-mask ventilation techniques may be required in these patients. This technique includes two people: one ventilates the bag using 100% oxygen and a respiratory rate consistent with the resting respiratory rate of the child. A double C-E grip with fingers on the jaw and mask helps to create a jaw thrust and minimizes leaks around the mask. Airway maneuvers include jaw thrust, head tilt, and chin lift. Of these, jaw thrust is the most effective to open the obstructed airway in an anesthetized child.[32] Airway adjuncts can be used to improve airway opening, including Guedel and nasopharyngeal airways.

Tracheal Intubation

An analysis of airway management complications in children with difficult tracheal intubation found that temporary hypoxemia was the most frequent cause of non-severe complications.[36] In this prospective cohort analysis from the PeDI Registry, 1018 children were studied over an interval from 2012 to 2015. Hypoxemia was defined as a 10% decrease from the preintubation oxygenation saturation for more than 45 seconds. The overall finding of hypoxemia during tracheal intubation was 9% (94/1018). Of that number of hypoxemic patients, 65 (8%) were anticipated difficult intubations and 29 (15%) were unanticipated.

Although the incidence of difficult laryngoscopy is lower in children than in adults (1.37% versus 9%), the incidence of difficult laryngoscopy in infants is significantly higher than in older children (4.7% versus 0.7%).[33] The incidence of difficult laryngoscopy is doubled in children undergoing cardiac anesthesia due to the relatively high incidence of concomitant congenital syndromes such as CHARGE and DiGeorge.[34] Difficulty to intubate can change as the child matures. *Children with Treacher Collins syndrome, for example, become more difficult to intubate with age, whereas Pierre Robin sequence improves with age.*[35]

Direct laryngoscopy attempts may be prolonged for infants with difficult airways, increasing the likelihood of patient hypoxia, trauma, and awareness. Administering oxygen and maintaining normal oxygen saturations during an intubation attempt has obvious advantages for the patient by avoiding the adverse effects of hypoxia, which have already been discussed. There are also human-factor benefits because a well-oxygenated child allows the practitioner to remain calm, take time, and perform a less rushed and potentially less traumatic attempt at intubation. The absence of oxygen desaturation during intubation also reduces the need to withdraw the laryngoscope for bag-mask ventilation reoxygenation. This could mean fewer intubation attempts.

Multiple intubation attempts are a leading cause of severe complications in pediatric airway management due to laryngeal trauma and potential airway obstruction.[36] This is particularly relevant to neonates and infants who have lax supraglottic and subglottic mucosae, making them predisposed to swelling. This age group has a relatively narrow airway. From birth to adolescence, the trachea more than doubles in length, triples in diameter, and increases by six-fold in cross-sectional area.[37] The relationship between gas flow and lumen diameter is explained by Poiseuille's law: ($Q = \frac{\pi P r^4}{8 \eta l}$)

(Poiseuille's law: Q: flow; P: pressure; r: radius; η: viscosity; l: length)

For a neonate with a preexisting small tracheal radius, a small amount of mucosal swelling can have a large detrimental impact on gas flow because of the r^4 factor.

A careful, controlled intubation attempt without the stress of hypoxia may lead to improved first-pass success, avoiding multiple airway maneuvers and associated awareness. A study of awareness in children found that the only predictive factor identified for awareness was multiple airway maneuvers.[38]

Another benefit of oxygen treatment during intubation is education.[25] A trainee can safely perform tracheal intubation in a child or infant under supervision without the stress generated by pulse oximeter alarms signaling hypoxia. Awareness is avoided by total intravenous anesthesia, and the educational experience is enhanced by video laryngoscopy where the whole intubation attempt is overseen by the supervisor and potentially recorded and played back for review.

Pharyngeal Oxygenation

There are various ways of administering oxygen during tracheal intubation. Low-flow and high-flow nasal cannula oxygenation have already been discussed, but there are alternative techniques.

Laryngoscopes

Early attempts to add oxygen to a laryngoscope were described by Wung in 1977. A number 8 French suction catheter was taped to a size 0 Miller laryngoscope blade and oxygen was given at 2 L/min^{-1}.[23] Next came the Oxyscope by Todres and Crone in 1978, which had a more robust design involving a built-in modification to size 0 and 1 Miller blades. These laryngoscopes were used to intubate newborn babies with 2 L/min of oxygen, and the same modification was soon added to Macintosh blades. The modification consisted of a metal tube running down the length of the blade to supply oxygen to the tip. A clinical study published in 1981 described a decreased incidence of hypoxia and bradycardia when neonates with hyaline membrane disease were intubated with oxygen rather than air.[39]

The concept of laryngoscope delivery of oxygen applies to other devices including the Bullard laryngoscope with an integrated 3.7 mm working channel suitable for insufflation of oxygen. The Bullard laryngoscope (Circon ACMI) is rigid and anatomically shaped with a viewing lens and a fiberoptic light. It is available in adult and pediatric sizes. It can be used for laryngoscopy without head manipulation, and, because of its very narrow profile, it allows intubation with only 6 mm of mouth opening. This laryngoscope has become less popular and has been superseded by other devices.

Optical Stylets

Several optical stylets are equipped with side ports to attach oxygen for use during tracheal intubation. The oxygen flows inside the tracheal tube to the tip of the stylet. This mechanism is used in the Brambrink and Bonfils optical stylets and the Shikani and Levitan stylets. Optical stylets are used clinically as adjuncts to laryngoscopes during direct laryngoscopy, or as stand-alone intubation devices for patients with difficult airways. The tip of the optical stylet is navigated to the vocal cords and the tracheal tube is then advanced down the trachea. If supplementary oxygen is used with the optical stylet, it is normally delivered via the tip of the laryngoscope blade to the larynx. Apart from treating hypoxia, the oxygen flow can help to clear the lens of the optical stylet from debris or fogging.

Video Laryngoscopes

The Truview PCD optical video laryngoscope (Truphatek International Ltd) has a pediatric-size laryngoscope, which features a channel suitable for oxygen

Section 2: Devices and Techniques to Manage the Abnormal Airway

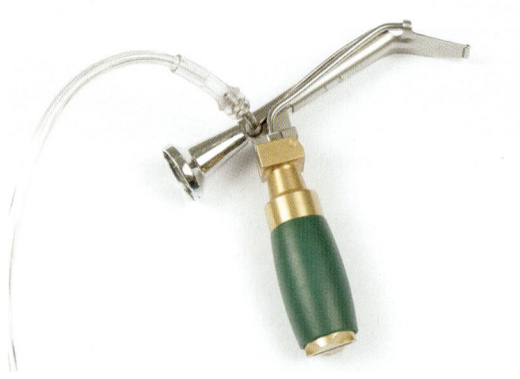

Figure 6.2 The Truphatek Truview video laryngoscope with oxygen tubing attached, allowing for insufflation of oxygen during tracheal intubation.

insufflation to the tip of the blade (Figure 6.2). A study by Steiner and colleagues used laryngoscope apneic oxygenation and measured time for a 1% drop in SpO_2 from baseline. They also measured the slope of overall desaturation versus time in pediatric patients undergoing tracheal intubation. The patients were intubated with either a standard Macintosh laryngoscope without supplementary oxygen in group 1, or a Truview PCD video laryngoscope (VLO_2) with an oxygen attachment in group 2, or a modified Macintosh laryngoscope with an oxygen catheter taped to the side of the blade in group 3. Groups 2 and 3 received oxygen at 2–3 L/min, depending on the size of the blade or catheter, in groups 2 and 3. Patients in groups 2 and 3 with insufflated oxygen demonstrated significant increased times to 1% desaturation and significant reduced overall rate of desaturation compared to group 1 that did not receive oxygen. There was no significant difference in results between groups 2 and 3.[40]

Pharyngeal oxygenation has also been studied by Windpassinger and colleagues[41] with an Airtraq laryngoscope (Airtraq, Prodol Meditec S.A., Vizcaya, Spain). A randomized controlled trial used a standard cuffed RAE tube through the Airtraq. Following induction of anesthesia and preoxygenation, children aged 0 to 2 years were randomized to receive no gas or oxygen at 4 L/min through the tracheal tube throughout the intubation phase. The mean laryngoscopy time was 60 seconds. The trachea was then intubated and the cuff was inflated. The oxygen tubing was then removed and the time for oxygen saturation to drop from 100% to 95% was measured. There was a significant prolonged time before desaturation in the oxygen group.

Tracheal Oxygenation

Great care is required when connecting oxygen to any airway device, particularly when the oxygen is delivered below the vocal cords. Oxygen can be delivered through airway exchange catheters using fittings designed for 15 mm and jet ventilator connections. Examples of airway exchange catheter oxygen fittings are the Cook Rapi-Fit connectors. Airway exchange catheters are used for tracheal tube exchange and as placeholders in the event of failed extubation and reintubation with a tracheal tube. They have also been used as primary ventilation devices for elective surgery in infants and neonates with severe laryngotracheal stenosis,[42] and as a rescue airway device for neonates with severe airway obstruction in conjunction with the Ventrain (Dolphys Medical).[43]

Numerous reports of barotrauma confirm the potential dangers of airway exchange catheters. A review of the use of airway exchange catheters to insufflate or jet ventilate oxygen into the airway found that 11% of adult patients receiving jet ventilation through an airway exchange catheter sustained pulmonary barotrauma.[44] Two pediatric case series collectively reviewed 31 patients.[42,45] All patients received manually assisted or volume-controlled ventilation through the airway exchange catheter. There were no reports of barotrauma. One neonate became hypoxic requiring a tracheotomy.[42]

Oxygen can be administered by high-pressure jet ventilation or low-pressure insufflation. Barotrauma is less common when insufflation is used, but the authors of the systematic review recommend avoiding routine use of oxygen through airway exchange catheters.[44]

Rigid Bronchoscope

A rigid bronchoscope is a recommended instrument to manage a difficult pediatric airway. This device has numerous advantages: it can be used as a ventilation device to deliver 100% oxygen, with or without a volatile anesthetic agent; it can splint open an obstruction in the airway; it can push an obstructing foreign body beyond the trachea; it can facilitate suctioning; and it can accommodate surgical instruments to remove foreign bodies. The Difficult Airway Society pediatric airway guideline recommends the rigid bronchoscope as a final option to secure the obstructed airway before FONA.[46]

Following successful intubation and reoxygenation with the bronchoscope, a definitive intubation can be achieved with a tracheal tube by inserting an airway exchange catheter down the middle of the bronchoscope, removing the bronchoscope and railroading an appropriate-sized tracheal tube.

Flexible Bronchoscopy

Flexible bronchoscopy for tracheal intubation is a valuable technique for management of the difficult pediatric airway. Hypoxia is a common cause of morbidity during flexible bronchoscopy. Older children can tolerate an awake flexible bronchoscope intubation with local anesthetic and sedation. Oxygen treatment during this procedure may include nasal cannula with low- or high-flow oxygen. An adult study using HHHFNC up to 70 L/min through the Optiflow during conscious sedation found that this technique was well tolerated and effective at preventing hypoxia during awake intubation.[50] For nasal flexible bronchoscopy, a Hudson mask can be positioned below the mouth to provide low-flow oxygen. Alternatively, a nasopharyngeal airway can be inserted in one nostril for oxygen insufflation, while the flexible bronchoscope and tracheal tube are intubated via the other nostril.[51]

If the child needs a general anesthetic for flexible bronchoscopy, ventilation with oxygen can be continued through a pediatric endoscopy face mask (VBM Medizintechnik). The flexible bronchoscope and a tracheal tube are passed through the middle of the face mask, through the nose or the mouth, and into the trachea.

Children can present with a range of airway anomalies that create difficulties with ventilation and intubation. Complete airway obstruction can occur during induction with both intravenous and gaseous induction techniques. To avoid this problem, an airway can be secured with awake intubation of an SGA device. This technique was first described in 1994 by Johnson and Sims, who successfully intubated a neonate with Goldenhar syndrome after initially placing a size 1 LMA, having nebulized 2% lignocaine at a dose of 6 mg/kg.[52] Once the LMA is placed in the airway, a swivel connector is applied to the circuit and a gas induction can be completed. Using this technique, two appropriate-sized tracheal tubes were pushed together and mounted onto the flexible bronchoscope. This extra tracheal tube length allowed easy removal of the LMA without dislodging the distally placed tracheal tube. Once the LMA is removed, the proximal tracheal tube is disconnected and the 15 mm connector is replaced on the distal tracheal tube in readiness for ventilation (Figure 6.3). There is now a range of SGA devices, which are suitable as tracheal intubation conduits for awake or anesthetized pediatric patients with difficult airways, including the air-Q, Ambu AuraOnce and Ambu AuraGain.[53] Using these airways and tools designed to push a tracheal tube through the SGA device, intubation through an SGA device has become simpler (Figure 6.4). Local anesthetic techniques have also developed with innovative techniques using local anesthetic in a pacifier,[49] mucosal atomization devices (MAD) (Teleflex), and the DeVilbiss nebulizer.

Some flexible bronchoscopes are designed with a working channel, which has been used as a conduit for insufflation of oxygen. This practice *is not recommended* because of the risk of barotrauma. A case report described a term 4-day-old neonate who was intubated with a 3.1 mm external diameter flexible bronchoscope pre-mounted with a 3.5 mm ID tracheal tube. The flexible bronchoscope had a working channel of 1.2 mm, which was used to insufflate oxygen at 2 L/min. After flexible bronchoscope intubation, skin crepitus, decreased air entry, and hypoxia were noticed. A chest X-ray confirmed bilateral pneumothorax, unilateral tension pneumothorax, pneumopericardium, and surgical emphysema. This life-threatening situation required cardiopulmonary resuscitation and bilateral chest drains. The authors of this case report warn against the use of oxygen treatment through the suction channel of a flexible bronchoscope. They also suggest oxygen can be safely delivered via an endoscopy mask or an SGA device/ swivel connector, and finally they recommend treating pneumothorax immediately with chest drains rather than needle thoracostomy.

Emergency Oxygenation for FONA

Options described to manage an emergency FONA procedure include small bore cannula (< 4 mm in

Section 2: Devices and Techniques to Manage the Abnormal Airway

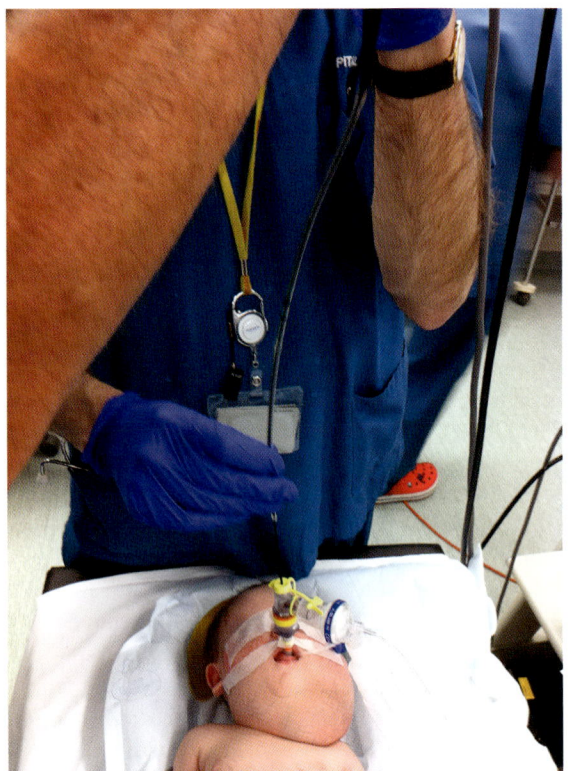

Figure 6.3 A neonate with a large cystic hygroma neck mass. Intubation through an LMA and bronchoscopic swivel connector. Tracheal tubes are mounted on a flexible bronchoscope. Continuous oxygenation and volatile anesthesia are maintained via an anesthetic circuit connected to the bronchoscopic swivel connector.

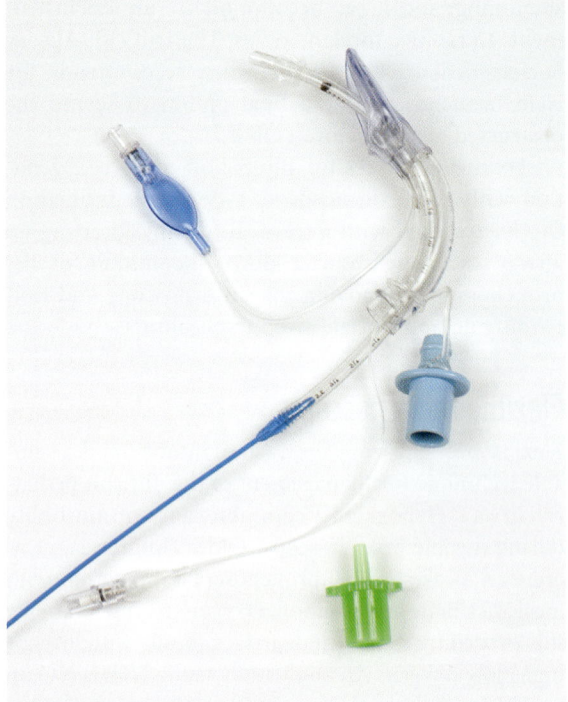

Figure 6.4 air-Q with removal stylet (blue) connected to a tracheal tube.

diameter), large-diameter cannula in kits (> 4 mm diameter), and surgical airway with a scalpel. There is very little evidence to support a decision in favor of one of these options. Most reported successful attempts at FONA have been by surgical tracheotomy, usually performed by a surgeon.

Small Cannula

Ventilation through a small cannula requires a high-pressure gas source to overcome the resistance of the cannula. Various options have been proposed to manage cannula ventilation. Devices can be divided into flow-regulated volume ventilation and pressure-regulated volume ventilation.

Pressure-regulated devices in the presence of small lung volumes and outflow obstruction can deliver potentially dangerous airway pressures, leading to barotrauma and surgical emphysema. Devices such as the Manujet III (VBM Medizintechnik) trans tracheal jet ventilation (TTJV) include pressure ranges on their regulator for different age groups: baby 0–1 bar (0–14.5 psi or 0–100 kPa); infant 1–2.5 bar (14.5–36.3 psi or 100–250 kPa); adult 2.5–4 bar (36.3–58 psi or 250–400 kPa). There is very little published evidence to support the safe use of these devices in children. Two expert panels advised cautious use of the Manujet III starting at the lowest driving pressure and titrating up according to chest movement. Respiratory rate is determined by the time for the chest to recoil and fully expire.[46]

It is essential to down-regulate TTJV prior to use, operating the jet ventilator while holding the cannula and feeling for surgical emphysema. Inspiratory time is kept to a minimum. Start with minimum pressure and increase until chest movement can be seen. Focus should be on the chest, with a goal of restoring oxygenation rather than ventilation. Extreme care must be exercised during use of the jet ventilator, particularly if upper airway obstruction is suspected. Adequate time needs to be allowed for the chest to recoil and expire before giving another breath. Every effort should be used to open the upper airway using jaw thrust or airway adjuncts such as oropharyngeal airways or SGA devices. The patient should have been paralyzed to eliminate laryngospasm. Jet ventilators are associated with a high incidence of complications and are relatively contraindicated for use in neonates, infants, or any other patient with upper airway obstruction.

Flow-regulated volume ventilation includes the Enk oxygen flow modulator (Enk OFM) (Cook Medical) and the Rapid O_2 insufflator (Meditech Systems). These are both Y-connector variants with equivalent outflow diameters. There are no reports of these devices being used for emergency airway management. The Advanced Paediatric Life Support (APLS) guidelines recommend that oxygen flow should be initially set at 1 L/(min year) of age through a Y-connector. An I:E ratio of 1:4 at a rate of 12 breaths per minute is then recommended. The Enk OFM has been experimentally validated with these settings. Care is required with flows through a flowmeter in excess of 15 L/min because of excessive oxygen flow causing the Enk OFM to fail as an on-off device. The Enk OFM is designed with five ventilation holes. All these holes need to be occluded to achieve inflation during inspiration.[54]

Self-made devices for emergency cannula ventilation are potentially very dangerous. A three-way tap in the oxygen line for ventilation is unsafe due to uncontrolled continuous inflation, even during the expiratory phase. This can rapidly lead to barotrauma because of inadequate expiration through the three-way tap side port and therefore *this technique is not recommended*.[55] Bag ventilation through a cannula is inadequate to support oxygenation in adults.[56] There is one report of this technique being used successfully in an 11-month-old, 9 kg child, following an emergency 16 G cannula cricothyroidotomy.[57]

Ventrain

The Ventrain is a flow-regulated oxygen ventilation device, which is capable of limiting high intrathoracic pressure by withdrawing inspired gas during the expiratory phase. This occurs due to the Bernoulli principle. The Ventrain is capable of oxygen insufflation and expiratory ventilation assistance (EVA). EVA occurs when the bypass channel of the Ventrain is occluded, creating a subatmospheric pressure (up to $-217\,cmH_2O$) at the side port. Inspiratory flow is controlled by the oxygen flowmeter. Negative pressure with the Ventrain requires proximal airway obstruction. To assist EVA in this situation, the upper airway may need artificial obstruction.

An animal study using pigs compared the performance of the Ventrain and TTJV during open, partial open, and obstructed airways, and found that minute ventilation and avoidance of high airway pressures were superior with the Ventrain compared to TTJV.[58]

Two cases refer to neonates where the Ventrain was used to ventilate successfully through an 8 French Cook Frova intubating introducer using oxygen flows of 4–6 L/min and respiratory rates of 40–100 breaths per minute. In these cases, conventional tracheal intubation failed due to extreme upper airway obstruction following multiple attempts at direct laryngoscopy. The Frova was used to establish an airway through the vocal cords and the Ventrain ventilated through the Frova intubating introducer applying EVA.[43]

Large-Bore Cannula Emergency Ventilation Devices

Various large-bore cricothyroidotomy kits are available for children, including the pediatric Melker (Cook Medical) and the Quicktrach child device.[59] Animal studies have been conducted on both of these airways.[60,61] There is no clinical evidence to suggest these airways perform better than a scalpel technique.

The Ex Utero Intrapartum Treatment (EXIT) Procedure

The EXIT procedure (see also Chapter 20) is performed by a multidisciplinary team during cesarean section. It is indicated when the neonate's airway is at significant risk of severe obstruction immediately after birth. The technique allows the fetus to be partially delivered and the airway to be controlled while placental perfusion is maintained. It was originally used in 1989 to deliver a fetus with a large anterior neck mass.[62] It then became part of the antenatal treatment of congenital diaphragmatic hernias. In this condition, it was discovered that prenatal obstruction of the trachea using surgical clips could allow expansion and maturation of fetal lungs. The EXIT procedure allowed removal of the tracheal clips prior to delivery while the fetus remained well oxygenated on placental bypass.[63] The EXIT procedure is now indicated for other fetal conditions where airway obstruction immediately after birth is a significant risk. These conditions include giant fetal neck masses, lung or mediastinal tumors, congenital high airway obstruction syndrome (CHAOS), EXIT to extracorporeal membrane oxygenation (ECMO) for certain congenital cardiac conditions and congenital cystic adenomatoid malformation. Recently, EXIT-to-airway for severe micrognathia has been added to this list.[64] An EXIT procedure provides the opportunity to maintain oxygenation for up to 60 minutes prior to placental separation. This window of opportunity can be used to safely intubate the airway prior to delivery.[65]

Conclusion

There are a range of oxygenation techniques that can decrease the incidence of hypoxia during airway management for children with difficult airways. Each of these techniques should be selected to meet the individual requirements of the patient. It is important to be mindful of the potential dangers of some forms of oxygen treatment. The principle goals of managing any child with a difficult airway should be to maintain oxygenation and avoid trauma.

References

1. Bunchungmongkol N, Somboonviboon W, Suraseranivongse S, et al. Pediatric Anesthesia Adverse Events: the Thai Anesthesia Incidents Study (THAI Study) Database of 25 098 cases. *Journal of the Medical Association of Thailand* 2007; **90**: 2072–9.

2. de Graaff JC, Bijker JB, Kappen TH, et al. Incidence of Intraoperative Hypoxemia in Children in Relation to Age. *Anesthesia & Analgesia* 2013; **117**: 169–75.

3. Crowley R, Sanchez E, Ho JK, et al. Prolonged Central Venous Desaturation Measured by Continuous Oximetry is Associated with Adverse Outcomes in Pediatric Cardiac Surgery. *Anesthesiology* 2011; **115**: 1033–43.

4. Gobbo Braz L, Braz JRC, MÓDolo NSP, et al. Perioperative Cardiac Arrest and its Mortality in Children. A 9-Year Survey in a Brazilian Tertiary Teaching Hospital. *Pediatric Anesthesia* 2006; **16**: 860–6.

5. Morray JP, Geiduschek JM, Ramamoorthy C, et al. Anesthesia-Related Cardiac Arrest in Children: Initial Findings of the Pediatric Perioperative Cardiac Arrest (POCA) Registry. *Anesthesiology* 2000; **93**: 6–14.

6. van der Walt J. Oxygen – Elixir of Life or Trojan Horse? Part 2: Oxygen and Neonatal Anesthesia. *Paediatric Anaesthesia* 2006; **16**: 1205–12.

7. van der Walt J. Oxygen – Elixir of Life or Trojan Horse? Part 1: Oxygen and Neonatal Resuscitation. *Paediatric Anaesthesia* 2006; **16**: 1107–11.

8. Tan A, Schulze A, O'Donnell CP, et al. Air versus Oxygen for Resuscitation of Infants at Birth. *The Cochrane Database of Systematic Reviews* 2005: CD002273.

9. Vento M, Moro M, Escrig R, et al. Preterm Resuscitation with low Oxygen Causes Less Oxidative Stress, Inflammation, and Chronic Lung Disease. *Pediatrics* 2009; **124**: e439–49.

10. Naumburg E, Bellocco R, Cnattingius S, et al. Supplementary Oxygen and Risk of Childhood Lymphatic Leukaemia. *Acta Paediatrica* 2002; **91**: 1328–33.

11. ILOR. The International Liason Committee on Resuscitation Consensus on Science with Treatment Recommendations for Pediatric and Neonatal Patients: Neonatal Resuscitation. *Pediatrics* 2006; **117**: 978–88.

12. Marcus RJ, van der Walt JH, Pettifer RJ. Pulmonary Volume Recruitment Restores Pulmonary Compliance and Resistance in Anaesthetized Young Children. *Paediatric Anaesthesia* 2002; **12**: 579–84.

13. Practice Guidelines for Management of the Difficult Airway. An Updated Report by the American Society of Anesthesiologists Task Force on Management of the Difficult Airway. *Anesthesiology* 2013; **118**: 251–70.

14. Frerk C, Mitchell VS, McNarry AF, et al. Difficult Airway Society 2015 Guidelines for Management of Unanticipated Difficult Intubation in Adults. *British Journal of Anaesthesia* 2015; **115**: 827–48.

15. Law AJ, Broemling N, Cooper RM, et al. The Difficult Airway with Recommendations for Management – Part 2: The Anticipated Difficult Airway. *Canadian Journal of Anesthesia/ Journal canadien d'anesthésie* 2013; **60**: 1119–38.

16. Tanoubi I, Drolet P, Donati F. Optimizing Preoxygenation in Adults. *Canadian Journal of Anesthesia/Journal canadien d'anesthésie* 2009; **56**: 449–66.

17. Hardman JG, Wills JS. The Development of Hypoxaemia during Apnoea in Children: a Computational Modelling Investigation. *British Journal of Anaesthesia* 2006; **97**: 564–70.

18. Pandit JJ, Duncan T, Robbins PA. Total Oxygen Uptake with Two Maximal Breathing Techniques

and the Tidal Volume Breathing Technique: a Physiologic Study of Preoxygenation. *Anesthesiology* 2003; **99**: 841–6.

19 Weingart SD, Levitan RM. Preoxygenation and Prevention of Desaturation during Emergency Airway Management. *Annals of Emergency Medicine* 2012; **59**: 165–75.e161.

20 Holmdahl MH. Pulmonary Uptake of Oxygen, Acid-Base Metabolism, and Circulation during Prolonged Apnoea. *Acta Chirurgica Scandinavica Supplementum* 1956; **212**: 1–128.

21 Cook TM, Wolf AR, Henderson AJ. Changes in Blood-Gas Tensions during Apnoeic Oxygenation in Paediatric Patients. *British Journal of Anaesthesia* 1998; **81**: 338–42.

22 Kernisan G, Adler E, Gibbons P, et al. Apneic Oxygenation in Pediatric Patients. *Anesthesiology* 1987; **3**: A521.

23 Wung JT, Stark RI, Indyk L, et al. Oxygen Supplement during Endotracheal Intubation of the Infant. *Pediatrics* 1977; **59**(Suppl.): 1046–48.

24 Levitan RM. (December 9, 2010). NO DESAT! Nasal Oxygen during Efforts Securing a Tube. Emergency Physicians Monthly. Website. http://epmonthly.com/article/no-desat/

25 Bhagwan SD. Levitan's No Desat with Nasal Cannula for Infants with Pyloric Stenosis Requiring Intubation. *Paediatric Anaesthesia* 2013; **23**: 297–8.

26 Hutchings FA, Hilliard TN, Davis PJ. Heated Humidified High-Flow Nasal Cannula Therapy in Children. *Archives of Disease in Childhood* 2015; **100**: 571–5.

27 Sreenan C, Lemke RP, Hudson-Mason A, et al. High-Flow Nasal Cannulae in the Management of Apnea of Prematurity: a Comparison with Conventional Nasal Continuous Positive Airway Pressure. *Pediatrics* 2001; **107**: 1081–3.

28 Patel A, Nouraei SA. Transnasal Humidified Rapid-Insufflation Ventilatory Exchange (THRIVE): a Physiological Method of Increasing Apnoea Time in Patients with Difficult Airways. *Anaesthesia* 2015; **70**: 323–9.

29 Papoff P, Luciani S, Barbara C, et al. High-Flow Nasal Cannula to Prevent Desaturation in Endotracheal Intubation: a Word of Caution. *Critical Care Medicine* 2015; **43**: e327–8.

30 Miguel-Montanes R, Hajage D, Messika J, et al. Use of High-Flow Nasal Cannula Oxygen Therapy to Prevent Desaturation during Tracheal Intubation of Intensive Care Patients with Mild-To-Moderate Hypoxemia. *Critical Care Medicine* 2015; **43**: 574–83.

31 Thomas JJ, Ciarallo C. Facemask Ventilation with a Frontonasal Encephalocele. *Anesthesiology* 2015; **122**(3): 698.

32 von Ungern-Sternberg BS, Erb TO, Reber A, et al. Opening the Upper Airway – Airway Maneuvers in Pediatric Anesthesia. *Paediatric Anaesthesia* 2005; **15**: 181–9.

33 Heinrich S, Birkholz T, Ihmsen H, et al. Incidence and Predictors of Difficult Laryngoscopy in 11 219 Pediatric Anesthesia Procedures. *Paediatric Anaesthesia* 2012; **22**: 729–36.

34 Heinrich S, Birkholz T, Ihmsen H, et al. Incidence and Predictors of Poor Laryngoscopic View in Children Undergoing Pediatric Cardiac Surgery. *Journal of Cardiothoracic and Vascular Anesthesia* 2013; **27**: 516–21.

35 Hosking J, Zoanetti D, Carlyle A, et al. Anesthesia for Treacher Collins Syndrome: a Review of Airway Management in 240 Pediatric Cases. *Paediatric Anaesthesia* 2012; **22**: 752–8.

36 Fiadjoe JE, Nishisaki A, Jagannathan N, et al. Airway Management Complications in Children with Difficult Tracheal Intubation from the Pediatric Difficult Intubation (PeDI) Registry: a Prospective Cohort Analysis. *The Lancet Respiratory Medicine* 2016; **4**: 37–48.

37 Monnier P. Applied Surgical Anatomy of the Larynx and Trachea. In Monnier P, ed. *Pediatric Airway Surgery*. Springer; 2011: 7–29.

38 Lopez U, Habre W, Laurencon M, et al. Intra-Operative Awareness in Children: the Value of an Interview Adapted to Their Cognitive Abilities. *Anaesthesia* 2007; **62**: 778–89.

39 Todres ID, Crone RK. Experience with a Modified Laryngoscope in Sick Infants. *Critical Care Medicine* 1981; **9**: 544–5.

40 Steiner JW, Sessler DI, Makarova N, et al. Use of Deep Laryngeal Oxygen Insufflation during Laryngoscopy in Children: a Randomized Clinical Trial. *British Journal of Anaesthesia* 2016; **117**(3): 305–7.

41 Windpassinger M, Plattner O, Gemeiner J, et al. Pharyngeal Oxygen Insufflation during AirTraq Laryngoscopy Slows Arterial Desaturation in Infants and Small Children. *Anesthesia & Analgesia* 2016; **122**: 1153–7.

42 Fayoux P, Marciniak B, Engelhardt T. Airway Exchange Catheters Use in the Airway Management of Neonates and Infants Undergoing Surgical Treatment of Laryngeal Stenosis. *Pediatric Critical Care Medicine* 2009; **10**: 558–61.

43 Willemsen MG, Noppens R, Mulder AL, et al. Ventilation with the Ventrain through a Small Lumen Catheter in the failed paediatric airway: Two Case Reports. *British Journal of Anaesthesia* 2014; **112**: 946–7.

Section 2: Devices and Techniques to Manage the Abnormal Airway

44 Duggan LV, Law JA, Murphy MF. Brief Review: Supplementing Oxygen through an Airway Exchange Catheter: Efficacy, Complications, and Recommendations. *Canadian Journal of Anesthesia/Journal canadien d'anesthésie* 2011; **58**: 560–8.

45 Wise-Faberowski L, Nargozian C. Utility of Airway Exchange Catheters in Pediatric Patients with a Known Difficult Airway. *Pediatric Critical Care Medicine* 2005; **6**: 454–6.

46 Black AE, Flynn PE, Smith HL, et al. Development of a Guideline for the Management of the Unanticipated Difficult Airway in Pediatric Practice. *Paediatric Anaesthesia* 2015; **25**: 346–62.

47 Jagannathan N, Sequera-Ramos L, Sohn L, et al. Elective Use of Supraglottic Airway Devices for Primary Airway Management in Children with Difficult Airways. *British Journal of Anaesthesia* 2014; **112**: 742–8.

48 Asai T. Is it Safe to Use Supraglottic Airway in Children with Difficult Airways? *British Journal of Anaesthesia* 2014; **112**: 620–2.

49 Jagannathan N, Truong CT. A Simple Method to Deliver Pharyngeal Anesthesia in Syndromic Infants Prior to Awake Insertion of the Intubating Laryngeal Airway. *Canadian Journal of Anesthesia/Journal canadien d'anesthésie* 2010; **57**: 1138–9.

50 Badiger S, John M, Fearnley RA, et al. Optimizing Oxygenation and Intubation Conditions during Awake Fibre-Optic Intubation Using a High-Flow Nasal Oxygen-Delivery System. *British Journal of Anaesthesia* 2015; **115**: 629–32.

51 Holm-Knudsen R, Eriksen K, Rasmussen LS. Using a Nasopharyngeal Airway during Fiberoptic Intubation in Small Children with a Difficult Airway. *Paediatric Anaesthesia* 2005; **15**: 839–45.

52 Johnson CM, Sims C. Awake Fibreoptic Intubation via a Laryngeal Mask in an Infant with Goldenhar's Syndrome. *Anaesthesia & Intensive Care* 1994; **22**: 194–7.

53 Huang AS, Hajduk J, Jagannathan N. Advances in Supraglottic Airway Devices for the Management of Difficult Airways in Children. *Expert Review of Medical Devices* 2016; **13**: 157–69.

54 Baker PA, Brown AJ. Experimental Adaptation of the Enk Oxygen Flow Modulator for Potential Pediatric Use. *Pediatric Anesthesia* 2009; **19**: 458–63.

55 Hamaekers AE, Borg PA, Enk D. A Bench Study of Ventilation via Two Self-Assembled Jet Devices and the Oxygen Flow Modulator in Simulated Upper Airway Obstruction. *Anaesthesia* 2009; **64**: 1353–8.

56 Hooker EA, Danzl DF, O'Brien D, et al. Percutaneous Transtracheal Ventilation: Resuscitation Bags do Not Provide Adequate Ventilation. *Prehospital and Disaster Medicine* 2006; **21**: 431–5.

57 Sandhya VV, Chandra S, Dhanya MR, et al. Cricothyroidotomy in a Pediatric Patient with Upper Airway Foreign Body. *The Airway Gazette* 2013; **17**: 12.

58 Paxian M, Preussler NP, Reinz T, et al. Transtracheal Ventilation with a Novel Ejector-Based Device (Ventrain) in Open, Partly Obstructed, or Totally Closed Upper Airways in Pigs. *British Journal of Anaesthesia* 2015; **115**: 308–16.

59 Sabato SC, Long E. An Institutional Approach to the Management of the "Can't Intubate, Can't Oxygenate" Emergency in Children. *Pediatric Anesthesia* 2016; **26**: 784–93.

60 Prunty SL, Aranda-Palacios A, Heard AM, et al. The "Can't intubate Can't Oxygenate" Scenario in Pediatric Anesthesia: a Comparison of the Melker Cricothyroidotomy Kit with a Scalpel Bougie Technique. *Paediatric Anaesthesia* 2015; **25**: 400–4.

61 Stacey J, Heard AMB, Chapman G, et al. The "Can't Intubate Can't Oxygenate" Scenario in Pediatric Anesthesia: a Comparison of Different Devices for Needle Cricothyroidotomy. *Pediatric Anesthesia* 2012; **22**: 1155–8.

62 Norris MC, Joseph J, Leighton BL. Anesthesia for Perinatal Surgery. *American Journal of Perinatology* 1989; **6**: 39–40.

63 Harrison MR, Adzick NS, Flake AW, et al. Correction of Congenital Diaphragmatic Hernia in Utero VIII: Response of the Hypoplastic Lung to Tracheal Occlusion. *Journal of Pediatric Surgery* 1996; **31**: 1339–48.

64 Morris LM, Lim FY, Elluru RG, et al. Severe Micrognathia: Indications for EXIT-to-Airway. *Fetal Diagnosis and Therapy* 2009; **26**: 162–6.

65 Baker PA, Aftimos S, Anderson BJ. Airway Management during an EXIT Procedure for a Fetus with Dysgnathia Complex. *Paediatric Anaesthesia* 2004; **14**: 781–6.

Section 2 — Devices and Techniques to Manage the Abnormal Airway

Chapter 7

Video Laryngoscopy Equipment and Techniques

Agnes I. Hunyady, James Peyton, Sarah Lee, and Raymond Park

The Evolution of the Concept and Technology of Indirect and Video Laryngoscopy

The term "video laryngoscopy" in its literal sense refers to the airway management technique whereby the larynx is visualized for intubation using a device that has a video camera at the tip of its blade. It is often used interchangeably with the term "indirect laryngoscopy": visualization of the larynx without alignment of pharyngeal, laryngeal, and oral axes, using either "chip-on-tip technology" or a series of reflecting surfaces to look around the corner. The difference between the two terms is best appreciated by briefly looking at the history of laryngoscopy and the evolution of the devices used to facilitate it.

The concept of indirect laryngoscopy is older than direct laryngoscopy. Direct laryngoscopy requires anatomical alignment of the oral, pharyngeal, and laryngeal axes with the laryngoscopist's line of sight.[1] Indirect laryngoscopy involves visualizing the larynx without the need for anatomical alignment. The technique of directing sunlight, then, later, using external light sources for illumination of the larynx was developed in the early 1800s. The use of handheld mirrors made it possible to visualize the larynx in awake patients without discomfort.[2] While these early indirect laryngoscopic techniques led to advances in laryngeal diagnostics, direct laryngoscopy seemed more practical for endotracheal intubation as it created a straight trajectory for ETT delivery. This straight trajectory, however, is not always attainable. The first laryngoscopic devices to attempt to look around the corner for intubation used fiberoptic technology. Fiberoptic bundles built into metal blades provided illumination and transmitted the image through an eyepiece. These devices had acutely curved blades with angles of 50–60 degrees, which hindered the delivery of the ETT. To overcome this problem, the first indirect laryngoscope designed for the intubation of the difficult pediatric airway, the Bullard laryngoscope, was equipped with retractable forceps to help guide the ETT.[3] Other early products, the first channeled indirect laryngoscopes, contained either a tubular (Wu scope) or a C-shaped (Upsher scope) structure to guide the ETT. They, however, did not have pediatric versions.[4,5]

Acute angulation of the blade is not always necessary: simply moving the image sensor to the distal end of the blade results in better visualization, even of a somewhat anterior larynx. A device designed for pediatric intubations consisting of a fiberoptic endoscope inside a metal blade shaped like a conventional straight (modified Miller) direct laryngoscope blade was evaluated by Weiss in the teaching setting. He found that the Cormack–Lehane grade of the view displayed on the monitor was consistently lower than the direct view of the trainee.[6] This concept formed the basis for the Karl Storz V-MAC and C-MAC product lines, where the blades – except for a hyperangulated blade – are shaped like the conventional Macintosh and Miller blades.

The first true video laryngoscope (the GlideScope video laryngoscope [GVL]) was invented by Canadian vascular surgeon, John Pacey. The device integrates a light-emitting diode and a miniature video chip (a complementary metal oxide semiconductor [CMOS] image sensor) on the undersurface of the blade. The image is transmitted via a video cable to an LCD monitor.[7] Because of a lack of fiberoptic elements, the cost of development was lower than for fiberoptic-based devices. This chapter focuses on the video laryngoscopes available for the management of the difficult pediatric airway.

Principles of Video Laryngoscopy

The principles of video laryngoscopy are illustrated in Figure 7.1. "Looking around the corner" is made

69

Section 2: Devices and Techniques to Manage the Abnormal Airway

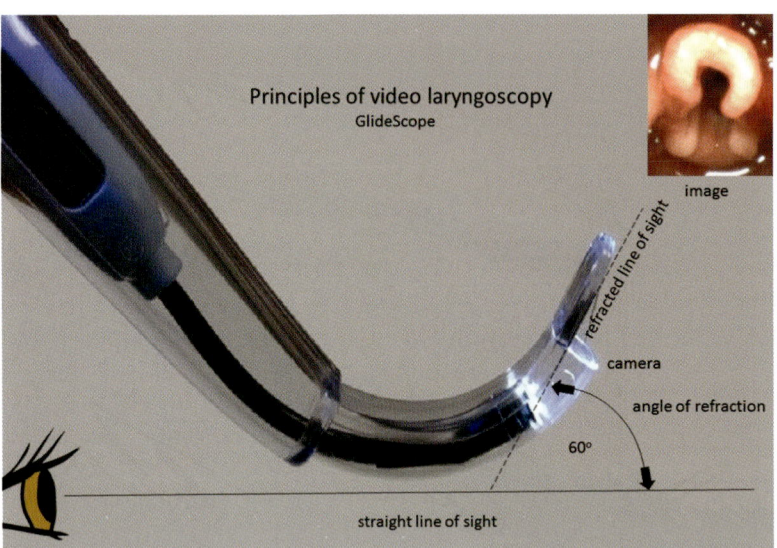

Figure 7.1 The principles of video laryngoscopy.

possible by placing the "eye" (i.e., the camera) at the distal tip (from the laryngoscopist's perspective) of the blade. The greater the curvature of the blade, the greater the refracted angle and the more curved the trajectory of the ETT. In other words, devices with blades with sharp curves might provide better visualization of the "anterior" larynx, but might make the placement of the ETT more difficult compared to devices with lesser blade curvature.

Common Basic Principles

The two main steps in video laryngoscopy-guided intubation are: (1) exposure of the larynx and (2) advancement of the ETT.

Devices vary as to the best approach to insert the blade (or stat) in the patient's mouth and to proximate the larynx. Devices equipped with a blade that closely resembles the Macintosh or Miller blade used for direct laryngoscopy are sometimes also called "enhanced direct laryngoscopes," referring to the fact that the device is equally suitable for direct laryngoscopy and video laryngoscopy. Using these devices, a direct laryngoscopic technique is recommended to achieve a view of the glottis, but if that proves to be difficult, easy conversion to video laryngoscopy is possible. This approach to laryngoscopy is sometimes referred to as video-assisted laryngoscopy and has been extensively utilized in teaching.[6,8,9] Direct laryngoscopy is impossible with devices that have acutely curved blades. The recommended laryngoscopy technique with these devices is quite different from direct laryngoscopy. Instead of a sniffing position or neck extension, a more neutral head position is recommended, and a midline blade/stat insertion is advised. It is important that the laryngoscopist visually follows the insertion of the blade into the mouth before looking at the screen. This will help avoid dental trauma caused by the blade. The degree of airway visualization is most commonly assessed and described by the modified Cormack–Lehane grade widely used in direct laryngoscopy,[10] or – less commonly – by the percent of glottic opening (POGO) visualized.[11]

The lack of a straight trajectory in video laryngoscopy usually makes the advancement of the ETT very difficult or often impossible in non-channeled devices without the help of an adjunct, such as a stylet, fiber-optic bronchoscope, forceps, or a catheter to slide the ETT on. Delivery of the ETT requires dexterity and kinesthetic skill, and is the cause of most failures and complications. It is, therefore, important to strictly follow the general rule that insertion of the styleted ETT into the mouth should be visually followed until it appears on the screen, and never advanced blindly (Figure 7.2).

Challenges of Video Laryngoscopy

View

There are some problems common to video laryngoscopes of various kinds. Insufficient view due to difficult exposure can be approached by repositioning the

Chapter 7: Video Laryngoscopy Equipment and Techniques

Get GlideScope AVL ready by:
Connecting video baton to monitor
Inserting baton into stat
Turning the device on

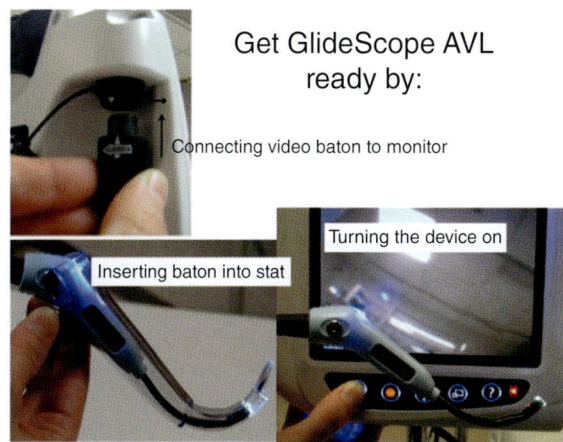

1 MOUTH

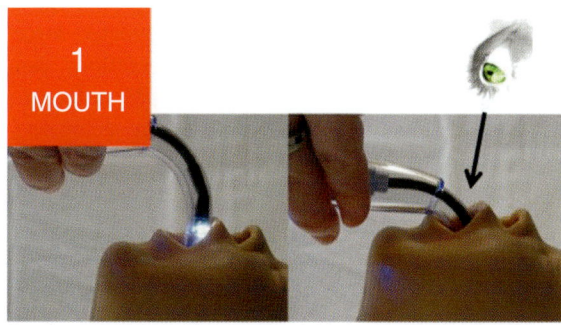

Open the patient's mouth while keeping the neck in the neutral position. Placement of a shoulder roll might be necessary for neonates and small infants. Looking directly into the patient's mouth, with the device in the left hand, introduce the blade of the video laryngoscope into the oropharynx, gliding down along the midline of the tongue, without displacing it.

2 SCREEN

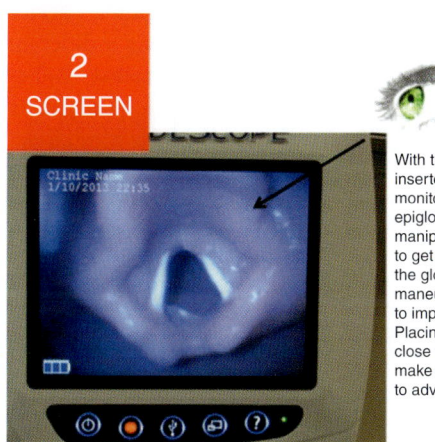

With the laryngoscope inserted, look at the monitor to identify the epiglottis, then manipulate the scope to get the best view of the glottis. BURP maneuver may be used to improve view. Placing the blade too close to the glottis can make it more difficult to advance the ETT.

3 MOUTH

Look directly into the patient's mouth – not at the screen – as you guide the distal tip of the ETT into position next to the tip of the blade, following the curve of the blade as close as possible.

Bend the styleted ETT into a shape that emulates the shape of the stat.

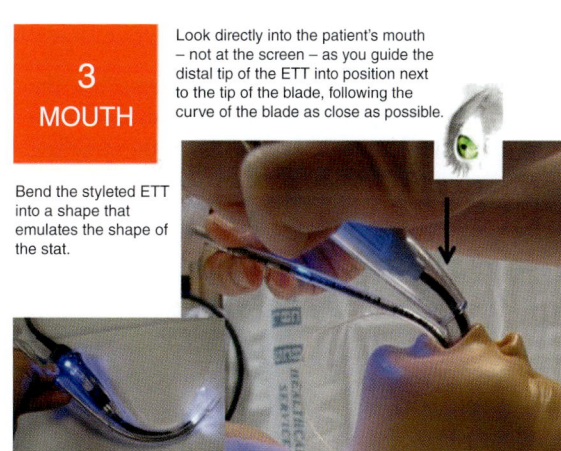

4 SCREEN

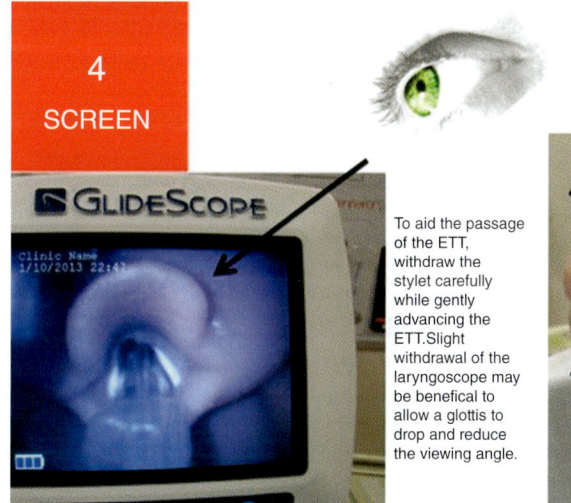

To aid the passage of the ETT, withdraw the stylet carefully while gently advancing the ETT. Slight withdrawal of the laryngoscope may be benefical to allow a glottis to drop and reduce the viewing angle.

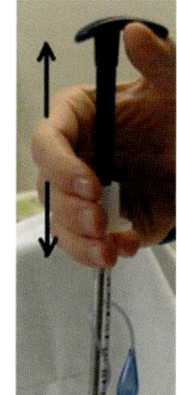

Look at the monitor to complete the intubation.

Figure 7.2A–E Step-by-step use of the GVL.

blade, changing blade size, or switching to a blade with a different curvature. Applying greater force usually does not help. Fogging or secretions can hinder the view, despite good exposure. Manufacturers address this problem with built-in defogging mechanisms facilitated by the device's lamp (GVL: diode-like light source) or using the flow generated by oxygen administration through a side port (Truview). Oxygen insufflation and protecting the camera by the tip of the blade will also prevent soiling of the lens by secretions.

"Red-out" from the lens touching soft tissue and "white-out" caused by refraction has the same etiology and correction as in fiberoptic intubation.

ETT Advancement

View-tube discrepancy is a term that describes the situation where a good view is achieved, but there is difficulty advancing the ETT into the trachea. The greater the curvature of the blade, the higher the likelihood of this happening. Selection of a different blade size or type, or changing the curvature or insertion technique of the stylet can address this issue. When withdrawing an acutely angled stylet, the tip of the ETT may move toward and hit the anterior commissure and be difficult to guide into the larynx. One technique to help address this issue is "reverse loading" the ETT on the stylet (placing the stylet into the ETT then bending it against the inbuilt curve of the ETT, which allows the tip of the ETT to move toward the posterior aspect of the glottis).[12]

Because most of the problems in inserting the ETT into the trachea arise from the tip of the tube abutting laryngeal structures, another suggested solution is to use a different type of ETT with a flexible tip, such as the Parker Flex-Tip ETT, which may allow atraumatic passage of the ETT into the larynx as the tube tip is designed to glide past any obstruction.[13]

In most studies conducted in children with normal airways, video laryngoscopic intubation takes longer than intubation with direct laryngoscopy.[14–20] This increases the risk of hypoxemia and creates a time pressure to secure the airway in the smallest patients.

The efficacy of video laryngoscope devices is usually judged by outcome measures, such as intubation success rate, time to intubation (TTI), time to best view, and best laryngeal view obtained (Modified Cormack–Lehane grade or POGO score). Most comparative evidence regarding the efficacy of video laryngoscopes in pediatric populations comes from manikin studies. While studies on normal pediatric airways are accumulating, there is still a paucity of data on difficult pediatric airways.

The challenges in evaluating the evidence include the following: (a) lack of standardization in assessment of the quality of the glottic view, (b) the inability to correct for varying skill levels of laryngoscopists (emergency physician versus anesthesiologist, trainee versus experienced attending), (c) difficulty accounting for translational changes in the pediatric airway with increasing age and development (some studies focus on infants and neonates; others broaden the inclusionary age), (d) within the same device category, different studies are often using a different generation of the same device. Controlled studies can be very difficult, if not impossible, particularly in pediatric populations, and it is unclear how clinically applicable the results from manikin studies are. Thus, the results of the available studies need to be interpreted with these methodological issues in mind.

A meta-analysis of 14 studies conducted mostly on normal pediatric airways showed that the use of a video laryngoscope generally improved the view of the glottis, but, in the case of all non-channeled devices, TTI was longer, and overall failure rate was higher compared to direct laryngoscopy. First-attempt success rate and complication rate was not different.[16] Small studies suggest that video laryngoscopes improve the view significantly in children with known difficult airways.[21,22]

Devices

Originally, pediatric video laryngoscopes were simply scaled-down versions of adult devices. This was unsatisfactory due to the unique characteristics of the neonatal, infant, and pediatric airways, meaning that poor laryngoscopic views were obtained and high failure rates of intubation were experienced. Pediatric-specific designs have been produced by several manufacturers[23] (Table 7.1).

Bullard Laryngoscope (Circon ACMI)

The Bullard laryngoscope was the first indirect laryngoscope designed not only for adults, but also for children. It is not a true video laryngoscope as it does

Chapter 7: Video Laryngoscopy Equipment and Techniques

Table 7.1 Pediatric Video Laryngoscopes

Device	Comments
Airtraq (Prodol)	Channeled device with an eyepiece that can be connected to a camera. Available in all sizes from neonate to adult.
GlideScope (Verathon Medical)	Hyperangulated 60-degree blade with an inbuilt camera. Available in all sizes from neonate to adult.
McGrath (Aircraft Medical)	Battery-operated device with an inbuilt camera and a small viewing screen attached to the handle. Only available down to the equivalent of a MAC 2 blade size.
Pentax AWS (Pentax)	A channeled, hyperangulated device with an eyepiece that can attach to a camera. Available in all sizes from neonate to adult.
Storz C-MAC (Karl Storz)	The C-MAC is available in Miller and MAC blade configurations down to a Miller 0. A hyperangulated 60-degree "D-blade" is also available down to a size 2 MAC blade equivalent.
Truview PCD (Truphatek International)	A channeled device with an eyepiece that can be connected to a camera, and also has a port to enable oxygen insufflation. Available in all sizes from neonate to adult.
Unremitting Efforts UESCOPE (UE Medical)	A hyperangulated device, similar to the McGrath, using a blade with a 40-degree angle to view the larynx down to a MAC 2 equivalent size, but also available in Miller blade configuration to size 0.

not use CMOS technology, but its historical importance demands a place in this chapter.

This reusable metallic device features an approximately 55-degree-curved blade at the end of a long metal rod that contains the optical elements – fiberoptic cables and a series of mirrors – and two channels. One of the channels has a Luer lock connector for supplemental oxygen administration, suction, or local anesthetic administration; while the other one houses the retractable intubating forceps designed to aid advancement of the ETT into the glottis. The forceps can only be used with ETTs with a Murphy eye as it grabs the ETT tip through the eye. A standard direct laryngoscope handle can be attached to serve as a light source. The eyepiece sits on an arm placed ergonomically in a 45-degree angle from the body of the device. The Bullard comes in three sizes (adult, pediatric, and infant), with the smallest being suitable for intubation of a newborn as small as 1.2 kg.[3] Studies conducted on manikins with simulated difficult airways and in children with normal airways made difficult by in-line neck stabilization documented higher success rates of intubation than with direct laryngoscopy using the Macintosh blade. The TTI, however, was longer than with direct laryngoscopy.[24–26]

The lack of a disposable version, its bulky nature, and the introduction of lightweight and easier-to-use true video laryngoscopes on the market has made this device less popular.

GVLs

The GVL, currently one of the most widely used pediatric video laryngoscopes, has undergone several modifications since it was first sold in 2000. The most widely used variation, the AVL-S, a single-use, digital device, consists of a "baton" (adult and pediatric version) and a series of disposable, low-profile plastic blades called "stats," which come in sizes small enough to use in premature neonates (Figure 7.2). GVL stat size 0 (GVL 0) is intended for intubation of patients weighing less than 1.5 kg, the GVL 1 for patients 1.5–3.6 kg, GVL 2 for 1.8–10 kg, and GVL 2.5 for 10–28 kg.

The tip of the baton houses the color video chip, the performance of which is enhanced by an inbuilt defogging mechanism. Unlike the Storz DCI and the Truview EVO2, the stats have an angulation of 60 degrees, making it unsuitable for direct laryngoscopy. The baton connects to a 6.4″ digital color monitor, which has an integrated real-time video recording capability. The more portable and sturdier version – GlideScope Ranger – has a rechargeable lithium-ion battery and was designed for military and emergency

Section 2: Devices and Techniques to Manage the Abnormal Airway

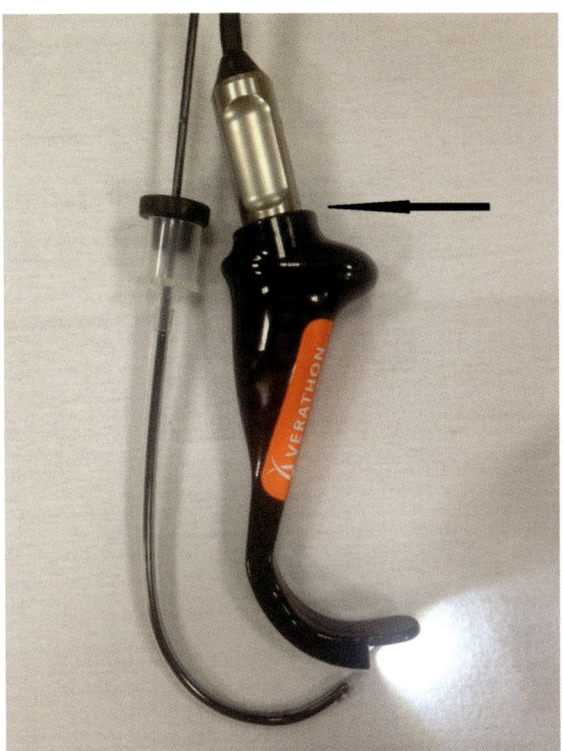

Figure 7.3 The GlideScope Spectrum and the pediatric GlideRight stylet. The black arrow points to the connection of the disposable blade to the smart cable.

medical services use. The same pediatric stats can be attached to the baton.

The newest generation of pediatric GVL, the Spectrum, features several improvements. The optical elements are all encased into the disposable blade, which connects to the smart cable via an HDMI connector (Figure 7.3). The ultrathin blade – colored black to minimize reflection – has a small lip to help guide the ETT.

Figure 7.3 gives a step-by-step approach to using the GlideScope AVL.

Insertion of the blade (stat) into the mouth should be done with the head kept in a neutral position: no neck extension is necessary. A shoulder roll is usually helpful for neonates. The exposure of the larynx should be done from a midline approach. Care should be taken not to push the blade too close to the glottis as it would hinder the maneuverability of the ETT. If the tongue is very large, one might want to insert the stat perpendicular to the lips. In case of a small mouth, positioning the blade slightly to the left (but without sweeping the tongue) gives more room for the ETT.

Due to the 60-degree curvature of the GVL stat, delivering the ETT to the glottis usually requires more dexterity than intubation with direct line of sight, even in normal airways, and is best aided with a stylet.[27] It is generally recommended that the styleted ETT be inserted into the mouth alongside the stat, but an approach from the corner of the mouth or turning the ETT slightly to the right may be necessary to maintain view of the glottis.

While most authors agree on the usefulness of a malleable stylet as an aid with GVL intubation, opinions differ on how the stylet should be bent and whether it should be inserted into the mouth congruently with the stat or from the corner of the mouth. The largest pediatric study, by Kim and colleagues, used C-shaped stylets, which followed the curvature of the stat – like the GlideRight stylet sold for the use of adult intubations by the manufacturer – inserted congruently with the stat. In some cases, the curvature needed to be increased at the tip to about 90 degrees for the styleted ETT to be successfully inserted in the glottis from an approach still congruent with the blade.[14] Fiadjoe and colleagues reported high success rates in infants and neonates with the C-shaped stylet.[28] Milne reports a case where a conventional stylet bent about 90 degrees just above the cuff – hockey-stick-shaped – did not help, while the C-shaped stylet, congruent with blade, successfully aided the ETT into the glottic opening.[29]

Conversely, in their pediatric study, Redel and colleagues attribute the 100% success rate and an intubation time shorter than that in Kim's study to the hockey-stick-shaped stylet, inserted non-congruently.[30] In Ilies' study, the hockey-stick stylet worked in most cases, but in others a Magill forceps or a BURP maneuver was needed. They describe the "weak maneuverability of the stylet armed ET especially in very young children."[31] The company has recently released the pediatric GlideRight stylet, which is similar to the adult version and mimics the shape of the blade, and is more rigid than the malleable 6 Fr stylets. Clinical research to support its superiority is not currently available (Figure 7.3).

Common Challenges and Tips to Overcome Them

Insufficient View

Despite the sharp angulation of the GVL blade, rarely a poor view (Cormack–Lehane grade of more than II) happens.[32] The anatomical features, device characteristics, and the operator practices that cause this have not been systematically studied. In a small study using the first-generation GVL in patients with difficult glottic exposure, Lee and colleagues found that using a GVL stat one size smaller than recommended by the manufacturer improved the view.[22] They attributed the insufficient view to the presence of the previously described blind spot caused by the tip of the blade overhanging the camera.[33] Lee and colleagues speculated that the smaller blade allowed for more rotation around the tongue, allowing the camera to look at the glottis from such an angle that the blind spot was decreased or eliminated. The problem of the blind spot has not been described with the second-generation stat design, suggesting that the manufacturer's recommendations for stat selection are appropriate. In fact, one must be careful in downsizing the blade, as too short a blade might not be able to slide all the way around the tongue, causing an indentation in the tongue base, which in turn could block the view. On the other hand, too long a blade could slide too close to the glottis, wedging the camera into the vallecula, causing the epiglottis to block the view. In cases of an insufficient view, our first step is to withdraw and drop the blade slightly to allow a greater distance from the glottis. External manipulation of the larynx or BURP maneuver may also improve the view with the GVL.[14,22,33]

View-Tube discrepancy

Advancing the ETT into the trachea can be challenging with the GVL, even with a good view of the glottis. This is especially true in young children because of the small airway size and the limited space available to manipulate the styled tube. When the glottic opening is too close to the device, the right arytenoid often obstructs the advancement of the ETT. Withdrawal of the device, even if it results in a grade 2 view, will provide a better trajectory.[23]

Another common scenario, especially in children with severe micrognathia and glossoptosis resulting in very "anterior larynx," is that the tip of the ETT reaches the glottic opening at an acute angle with the plane of the vocal cords, and is directed toward the anterior wall of the trachea, preventing it from sliding into the trachea. To overcome this problem, and to prevent injury to the tracheal wall, the laryngoscopist should stop advancing the stylet beyond a few millimeters away from the glottic opening and should slide the ETT off into the trachea while holding the stylet in place at the glottic opening, allowing the ETT tip to bend in the opposite direction from the curvature of the stylet (Figure 7.2). This is more easily done with an ETT with a curved tip, like the Parker Flex-Tip tube as described earlier. One can also rotate the styleted ETT 90–180 degrees clockwise once the glottic opening is reached to facilitate smooth passage into the trachea.[27] Lillie and colleagues described a technique whereby the stylet was twisted into a spiral shape, which allowed for an easy passage of the ETT into the trachea while rotating clockwise off the stylet.[34] Reverse loading helps overcome view-tube discrepancy by bending the stylet 180 degrees against the natural curvature of the ETT.[23] It is easier done when the difference in diameter between the ETT and the stylet is small, otherwise the ETT tends to spring back.

The new pediatric GlideRight stylet (Figure 7.3) was designed to tackle some of the causes of view-tube discrepancy, but evaluations of this new stylet have not been done.

Efficacy

The GVL has been the most studied video laryngoscope to date. Table 7.2 summarizes the results of randomized trials that compare the efficacy of the pediatric GVL to a direct laryngoscope.

As shown, most studies used manikins for subjects, and it is not completely clear how the results of manikin studies translate to human subjects, especially those with difficult airways. Most studies document an improved view with the GVL compared to direct laryngoscope.[14,21,31] There is strong evidence to support the use of the GVL in children with difficult airways from the PeDI Registry. Data from there showed that the GVL accounted for over 80% of intubation attempts and was more successful than standard direct laryngoscopy in this population. Initial (464/877 1/4 53% versus 33/828 1/4 4%, z-test 1/4 22.2, p < 0.001) and eventual (720/877 1/4 82% versus 174/828 1/4 21%, z-test 1/4 25.2, p < 0.001) success rates for GVL were significantly higher than direct laryngoscopy.

Table 7.2 Efficacy of the GVL Compared to the Direct Laryngoscope

Subjects	Study by first author	Type of study	Number of intubations	Median age of subjects	GVL compared to	Laryngoscopist	Results
Manikins with NA and simulated pediatric DA (SimBaby, Laerdal Medical Ltd)	White 2009[35]	Randomized crossover	32 × 4	n/a Approximately 3–6 months	DL (Miller)	Pediatric anesthesiologists and intensivists	No difference in TTI; DA took longer with both; In DA, GVL had no advantage
Manikins with NA and simulated pediatric DA (Megacode junior manikin, Laerdal)	Rodriguez-Nunez 2010[36]	Randomized crossover	18 × 4	n/a Approximately 5–8 years	DL (Macintosh)	Pediatric residents inexperienced in VL	Success rate not different; TTI longer with GVL; GVL DA longer than GVL NA
Manikin with simulated neonatal DA (ALS baby trainer, Laerdal)	Iacovidou 2011[37]	Randomized crossover	? (45 laryngoscopists)	n/a Infant size	DL (Macintosh)	Inexperienced providers (previous year's undergraduate medical and nursing students)	TTI: longer with GVL; Number of attempts: same
Manikins with NA and simulated DA	Hippard 2016[38]	Randomized crossover	30 × 18	n/a	DL (Miller) Truview	Experienced laryngoscopists	TTI longer with GVL; Success rate lower
Manikin with NA and simulated DA (SimBaby, Laerdal)	Fonte 2011[39]	Randomized	16 × 2 × 4	n/a	DL (Miller 1)	Pediatric residents	TTI longer in GVL
Pediatric patients with NA	Kim 2008[14]	Randomized	203 (100/103)	3 months to 17 years	DL (Macintosh)	Anesthesiologists (3) skilled in VL	View better with GVL; More intubation attempts with GVL; TTI greater with GVL, but not for CL III, IV
Pediatric patients with NA	Redel 2009[30]	Randomized (blinded to airway classification)	60 (30/30)	7 months to 10 years	DL (Macintosh)	Anesthesiologists skilled in VL and DL	TTI not different

Nasotracheal intubation	Kim 2011[40]	Randomized controlled	80	< 10 years	DL (Miller, Macintosh)	Two pediatric anesthesiologists	TTI similar; View similar; Better performance with GVL in second 20 compared to first 20
Pediatric patients with NA	Fiadjoe 2012[28]	Randomized	60	< 12 months	DL (Miller)	Two experienced anesthesiologists	TTI not different
Pediatric patients with NA	Riveros 2013[15]	Randomized	134 (44, 45, 45)	0–10 years	DL (Macintosh)	Anesthesiologists (three) with experience with VL	View with GVL slightly worse; TTI longer
Pediatric patients with NA	Ilies 2012[31]	Non-randomized sequential crossover	24 (48 laryngoscopies)	1–142 months	DL (Macintosh)	A resident and an attending anesthesiologist	View improved or remained unchanged with GVL (except for one)
Pediatric patients with DA	Armstrong 2010[21]	Non-randomized sequential crossover	18 (36 laryngoscopies)	2–16 years	DL (Macintosh)	Anesthesiologists	View better with GVL; Time to optimal view longer
Pediatric patients with DA	Lee 2013[22]	Randomized open crossover	23 x 3	0.5–18 years	DL	Single anesthesiologist experienced with VL	No difference in view between DL and GVL with stat sized by weight, but improved view with one size smaller stat

DA: difficult airway; NA: normal airway; n/a: not-applicable; GVL: GlideScope video laryngoscope; TTI: time to intubation; VL: video laryngoscope; DL: direct laryngoscope; CL: Cormack–Lehane

GVL for Intubation of Infants, Neonates, and Premature Neonates

Infants and neonates, especially the ones with difficult airways, represent a vulnerable population, where the complication rate of tracheal intubation is high.[41] The GVL has been shown to be a suitable device for intubation of infants and neonates, including premature neonates of 23 weeks' gestation.[28,32,42,43] The rate of failed intubation in a small case series is high, and is attributed to hypoxemia, blade size and configuration, and lack of a stylet specifically designed for that population.[32,43] In an equivalence trial of infants and neonates with normal airways, TTI with the GVL was not different from that with the Miller blade. Albeit the placement of the ETT took longer, it was compensated by the shorter time to achieve best view, resulting in a mean TTI of 22.6 seconds.[28] Experience in infants and neonates with difficult airways is very limited.[34,44]

Storz Video Laryngoscopes: C-MAC

Karl Storz Endoskope, manufacturer of several generations of indirect laryngoscopes, is another pioneer in the field of difficult airway management. This company is unique in that it offers a family of difficult airway devices – Storz video laryngoscope (SVL), Bonfils optical stylet, flexible bronchoscopes – which can be operated from the same DCI platform. Earlier versions of the SVL (V-MAC) featured fiberoptic cables built into the blade for illumination and image capture. The newer generation product, the C-MAC Boedeker-Dörges video laryngoscope, is a true video laryngoscope as it applies CMOS technology for image capture. It is more portable than the earlier version, with an 18 cm HD monitor powered by lithium-ion battery. The company's newest release, the C-MAC Pocket Monitor, targets EMS needs with its extreme portability and quick-to-switch-on ("open-to-intubate") 2.4″ display. Despite its simplicity, it has recording capability. Recorded images and videos can be retrieved via an USB port.

All SVLs are suitable for use in the pediatric population. In fact, the SVL was one of two first video laryngoscopy devices with models created for the pediatric population in 2005. It was unique at that time in comparison with other video laryngoscopes in that the size and shape of the blades were based on standard pediatric direct laryngoscopy blades, including pediatric straight blades. The LED light source is more distal on the SVL compared to the direct laryngoscope blade.

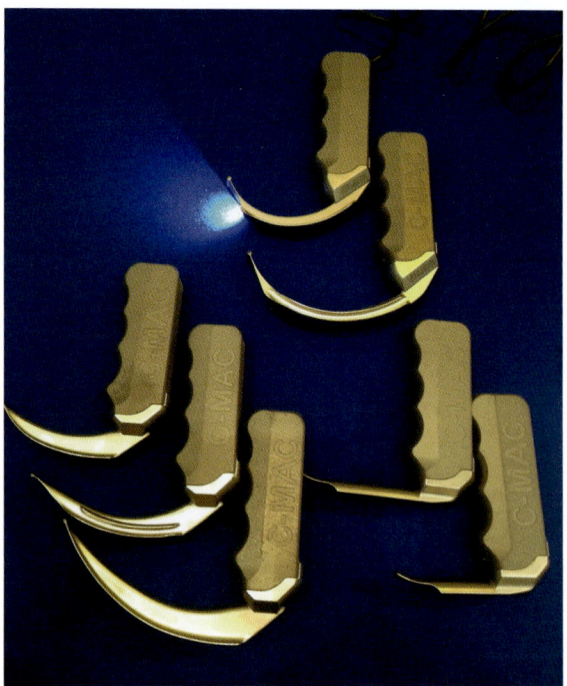

Figure 7.4 SVL blades. The hyperangulated blade (D-Blade) is now available in pediatric size, too.

Currently, the pediatric SVL is available with four different pediatric stainless steel blades (Figure 7.4). The smallest – equivalent in size to a Miller 0 direct laryngoscope blade – is used for neonates approximately 0–4 months in age and is suitable for use in babies as small as 750 g. The Miller 1 blade is suitable for infants approximately 4 months to 1 year of age. Small differences exist between the standard Miller 1 blade and the SVL Miller 1 blade. While both have a slight approximate 10-degree tip angulation and similar widths, the video laryngoscope Miller 1 blade is 0.5 cm longer and does not have the flange. For providers who prefer a curved blade, the Macintosh 2 (Berci-Kaplan) blade is available for use in children approximately 4 to 8 years in age. The pediatric D-blade (Dörges) is available in one pediatric size for patients weighing between 10 and 25 kg, and has a hyperangulated curve, which can be helpful in very anterior airways. The blade's hollow handle is a receptacle for the device's electronic module. Besides image capture and transmission, it can record still images as well as videos, which are stored in an SD memory card in the monitor.

The advantage of a straight blade video laryngoscope – compared to the GVL for use in smaller children and infants – is that it allows for better navigation of the more anteriorly placed glottis behind a typically larger, floppier epiglottis. The blade tip can be inserted into the vallecula or can be used to lift the epiglottis. The blade has a low profile with a height of 5 mm and distal location of the lens. The smaller blade width also allows it to be inserted using a retromolar approach from the side of the mouth, thereby sweeping the often larger tongues that limit intraoral space.[45] Unlike the GVL, the straight angle between the blade at the entrance of the mouth and the blade tip displaying the glottis allows for easier placement of smaller ETTs without use of a curved or any stylet, which decreases the risk of airway trauma.

The design closely resembles the standard DL blade, making it easy for clinicians to learn to use. This is one of the reasons the SVL is particularly popular in critical care and emergency care settings where the number of intubations performed per year per trainee is relatively low. It is also often argued by educators that replicating a view on the screen that is visualized directly enhances the effectiveness of skills training.[46] A study by Weiss and colleagues described the benefits of using the SVL as a teaching tool, highlighting that its versatility for use as both a direct view and a screen view made it useful for teaching normal intubations to trainees. The shared view allowed for quick recognition of problems with the trainee's technique, and facilitated immediate correction by the attending without need for multiple intubation attempts.[6]

It should be pointed out the video laryngoscopic view only replicates the direct view in normal airways with good laryngeal exposure. From the principles of video laryngoscopy (see above), it follows that, when the larynx is "above" the line of sight (difficult; i.e., "anterior" airway or insufficient exposure due to operator error), only the video eye, due to its larger viewing angle, can visualize it.

The SVL is a video-enhanced direct laryngoscope; therefore, initial placement of the blade into the pharynx can be performed similarly to the placement of the direct laryngoscopy blade, in the right of the oropharynx. Some people, however, prefer to use it similarly to the GVL; that is, inserting it midline. In a retrospective study by Green-Hopkins and colleagues involving emergency medicine trainees, right-sided blade insertion resulted in equal success rate as the midline approach, but the right-sided insertion was associated with significantly longer TTI.[47]

Regardless of the mode of insertion, the laryngoscopist should look directly at the patient's mouth and not at the screen when inserting the blade to ensure the blade is positioned properly without causing damage to lips, teeth, or palate. After the blade has been positioned, the laryngoscopist should look up at the screen to identify the appropriate glottic structures. To improve the view of the glottis, the blade can be lifted upwards to elevate the vallecula and epiglottis, and/or external laryngeal pressure or cricoid pressure can be applied in a manner like that used in direct laryngoscopy.

Once a view of the glottic opening has been achieved, the user then focuses on placement of the ETT just right of the blade, once again looking directly at the patient's mouth during insertion to ensure that it is performed without damage to oropharyngeal structures. The ETT is advanced coaxially to the blade until the tip is visualized on the screen and can be placed into the glottic opening. Intubation with an SVL often requires a styleted ETT with a bend at the tip (resembling a hockey stick), mimicking the angle of the blade tip. The stylet provides the rigidity often necessary to navigate past the arytenoids. The stylet can be withdrawn just after the tip of the ETT passes the vocal cords to avoid subglottic injury.

Common Challenges and Tips to Overcome Them

Obtaining the View

While there are many similarities between the SVL and the direct laryngoscopes, the dissimilarities can present or contribute to difficulties in obtaining a view of the glottis. The SVL's bulky handle can abut against the chest in some patients, making it difficult to place the blade into the mouth.[48] Turning the device to the left, so that the handle is parallel to the lips, can facilitate placement in such cases.

Particularly with inexperienced users, the slightly longer blade can lead to placement too deep in the oropharynx such that the esophagus is visualized. To prevent this, the laryngoscopist should advance the blade cautiously and not too quickly while looking at the screen so that the glottic view is not missed.[49] Generally, once the blade tip reaches the uvula, the blade can gently be lifted and visualization can be shifted from the mouth to the screen to avoid placing the blade too deep. If, after the SVL blade is placed, only the esophagus is seen, the laryngoscopist should slowly pull the blade back until the glottis comes into view.

The lack of an antifogging system on early versions was particularly problematic in spontaneously breathing patients.[50] Application of antifogging solution and/or prewarming of the SVL blade have been employed to reduce this problem. A related problem involves challenges with obtaining a view because of mucous or bloody secretions. One solution is thorough preintubation suctioning for patients who appear to have a significant amount of secretions or pretreatment with an antisialagogue agent such as glycopyrrolate. Of note, the newest video laryngoscope system released by Storz features a reportedly improved antifog lens, as well as the option to connect a small suction catheter onto the blade. There has been no reported evidence of the efficacy of these changes.

View-Tube Discrepancy

Although the SVL provides a better, clearer view of the glottis than direct laryngoscopy, similarly to GVL intubation, the ETT tip can get caught on the anterior wall of the trachea. Maneuvers described for GVL – "reverse loading": rotating the ETT 180 degrees, as described above – can be applied.[51]

Because of the very distally placed camera and light source at the end of the SVL blade, the glottis is magnified in such a way that small movements of ETT translate to large movements on screen.[23] The result is that it may take additional time to "find" the ETT tip on the screen and the magnified image may make tube manipulation on screen more challenging. If this is problematic, one described technique involves placing a non-styleted tube in the groove of the straight SVL blade and advancing it using the groove as a track directly into the field of view.[45] Diligent preoxygenation will also help to maintain oxygen saturation if the TTI is slightly increased compared with direct laryngoscopy.

Efficacy of SVL

Studies documenting the efficacy of the SVL compared to direct laryngoscopy are summarized in Table 7.3. Most studies consistently demonstrate that the SVL provides a significantly improved view of the glottis in all groups (manikin, normal pediatric airway, and difficult pediatric airway) compared to direct laryngoscopy.[16–18,51–53] However, the TTI was longer with the SVL.[16–18]

There is only a small case series and a case report documenting the SVL's efficacy in pediatric patients with difficult airways.[51,55] They suggest that, while the SVL may have a limited advantage in patients with normal airways, the SVL has a clear advantage when used in difficult and anatomically abnormal airways, and the likelihood of successful intubation is increased using the SVL in this group.

SVL in Infants and Neonates

The SVL is particularly popular in neonatal ICUs because of its standard blade configuration. The standard blade allows a shared laryngoscopic view between trainee and supervisor, which helps accelerate the steep learning curve in this setting. Vanderhal and colleagues report 48 successful intubations of 42 premature neonates with one of the first prototypes of the SVL. The smallest neonate weighed 530 g. Most of these infants and neonates presumably had normal airways, but five of them previously failed direct laryngoscopy. The intubations in this case series were completed without a stylet. The ETT was advanced in the groove of the blade while visualizing the glottic opening.[56]

In the case series from Hackell and colleagues, five of the seven patients with difficult airways successfully intubated with the SVL were infants, and the successful SVL rescue in Wald's case report was a neonate with a difficult airway.[51,55]

A study on freshly euthanized extremely premature baboons (200–400 g) demonstrated the C-MAC's efficacy in intubation of primates the size of human micro preemies, although the intubation took longer for novices with SVL than with direct laryngoscopy. The difference was not significant when the laryngoscopist was an experienced provider.[57]

McGrath MAC Video Laryngoscope (Aircraft Medical Ltd)

The McGrath video laryngoscope is a portable, battery-powered video laryngoscope, which requires the use of disposable blade sheaths. It has a sheath shape similar to a standard MAC blade, meaning it is also possible to perform direct laryngoscopy using this device. It is advertised as being suitable for ages from infancy to adult, with blade sizes ranging from the equivalent of a MAC 2 up to a MAC 4. Use of the size 2 blade is limited to larger children, restricting its

Table 7.3 Efficacy of SVL Compared to the Direct Laryngoscope

Subjects	Study by first author	Type of study	Number of intubations	Age of subjects	SVL compared to	Intubating person	Results
Manikin (Laerdal)	Fiadjoe 2009[52]	Randomized crossover	32 × 2	n/a Infant manikin	DL	Pediatric anesthesiologist	SVL improved glottic view; No difference in TTI
Pediatric and adult simulator with NA	Donaghue 2013[54]	Randomized crossover	148	n/a Newborn, infant, adult simulator	DL	Pediatric emergency medicine faculty	No difference in first-attempt success rate
Manikin with simulated DA	Kalbhenn 2012[24]	Randomized crossover	30 × 4	n/a Infant	DL (Macintosh), Airtraq, Bullard	Anesthesia residents	TTI longer with SVL; Dental injury same (frequent)
Manikin AirSim Pierre Robin	Saracoglu 2014[53]	Randomized crossover	45 × 4	n/a 3–6 months' manikin	DLs (Miller, Macintosh), McGrath	Anesthesiology residents, nurse anesthetists	SVL improved glottic view; Shorter TTI; Decreased number of attempts and dental trauma compared to all DL blades
Pediatric patients with NA	Vlatten 2009[46]	Randomized	56	≤ 4 years	DL	Attending and resident anesthesiologists	SVL improved view; Increased TTI
Pediatric patients with MIS	Vadi 2016[17]	Randomized	93	2–23 months	DL, GVL	Anesthesiology residents	SVL improved glottic view; Increased TTI with manual in-line stabilization
Pediatric patients with prior DA	Hackell 2009[51]	7 case series	7	3–13 months	DL	Attending anesthesiologists and nurse anesthetists	Improved glottic view; Successful intubation in patients with previously failed DL

SVL: Storz video laryngoscope; DL: direct laryngoscope; NA: normal airway; DA: difficult airway; MIS: manual in-line stabilization; n/a: non-applicable; TTI: time to intubation usefulness in infants. A size 1 blade has been developed and its use described in neonates and small infants,[58] but it is not currently available commercially in the USA. It is designed to be used as a MAC blade with a view to enabling the user to perform an "enhanced direct laryngoscopy", so can be inserted either in the midline into the vallecula or by sweeping the tongue laterally before sitting in the vallecula. If the direct view is suboptimal, the 2.5" color LCD screen attached to the handle allows for easy conversion to video laryngoscopy. This approach to laryngoscopy is sometimes referred to as video-assisted laryngoscopy and has been extensively utilized in teaching.[6] This brings up the question whether the intubation technique should be the one customary for direct laryngoscopy with a curved blade, or the one customary for video laryngoscopy; for example, the GVL. Kim and colleagues compared a patient position most often used in video laryngoscopy, where the head is resting in the neutral position on the table without a pillow (the "head-flat" position) to the traditional sniffing position ("head-elevation" position), where the external auditory meatus is aligned with the sternal notch in 46 pediatric patients with normal airways for intubation with the McGrath video laryngoscope. They found higher POGO scores in the sniffing position, but only a very small reduction in TTI.[59]

Not surprisingly, view-tube discrepancy commonly seen using other video laryngoscopes in children with severe micrognathia has been described with the McGrath, too.[60]

Truview PCD

The Truview PCD consists of an integrated optical lens system built into a straight blade that ends in a 46-degree angulated tip. The proximal end has an eyepiece that allows quick magnetic attachment of a monitor for magnification and a shared view, but also allows indirect laryngoscopy without the monitor. In addition, the blade's standard clip-on connector allows the attachment of the traditional direct laryngoscope handle, further contributing to the portability. The blade also contains a side port for oxygen delivery. This port allows supplemental oxygenation during intubation and additionally serves as a defogging and secretion control mechanism. The oxygen-delivery system has been found to significantly prolong time before desaturation occurs.[20,45] The smaller blade profile, at a height of 8 mm, allows for its use in smaller airways and restricted mouth openings.

In a randomized study of 60 neonates the Truview provided an improved glottic view and similar TTI compared to direct laryngoscopy.[61] In another study on 50 children of 2–8 years of age, it again provided an improved view, but showed a longer TTI (13.8 seconds versus 6.36 seconds) compared to direct laryngoscopy.[19] Other studies have shown that, compared to direct laryngoscopy and other video laryngoscopes, the Truview did not provide an improved glottic view, but required a significantly increased TTI.[15] A study on manikins with simulated difficult airway demonstrated a decreased intubation success rate and longer TTI with the Truview compared to the direct laryngoscope.[38] Only one study, looking at intubation of a manikin by novice paramedics in code scenarios, demonstrated improved glottic views and TTI when the Truview was compared to direct laryngoscopy.[62] There have been no studies evaluating the Truview in live pediatric patients with difficult airways. This device is no longer sold in the USA.

The Unremitting Efforts UESCOPE (UE Medical)

The UESCOPE is a relatively new video laryngoscope, which can be used in a variety of different guises. It is a battery-powered, rechargeable, portable device with a detachable video monitor, similar to the McGrath series 5 video laryngoscope. It has multiple different attachments available, which connect to the monitor. These include reusable size 0 and 1 Miller blades and size 1–4 reusable MAC blades, which can be used for both direct laryngoscopy and indirect video laryngoscopy, as well as disposable blade sheaths. The disposable blade sheaths come in sizes 2–4 and have an acutely angled tip (sitting at 40 degrees compared to the 60-degree angle of the GVL), meaning they cannot be used for direct laryngoscopy, but enabling a view of the larynx to be obtained without the need for anatomical alignment. It has a guidance channel to facilitate ETT placement. It also has a rigid video stylet attachment, so is potentially the most versatile of video laryngoscope systems currently available. There are no studies examining its use in children or adults at the time of writing and, as such, it cannot be recommended over any other video laryngoscope:

more information is currently only available from the manufacturer.[63]

Pentax AWS

The Pentax AWS is a portable, battery-operated video laryngoscope, which is designed for use solely as an indirect laryngoscope. The unit has attached a small 2.4″ video screen and has video output capability to allow viewing on an external monitor.

The AWS is used in conjunction with disposable blades of various sizes: a standard adult and a thinner lower profile adult, as well as pediatric and neonatal sizes. The device is inserted midline and, once the glottis is visualized, an ETT is passed through a channel embedded in the blade. The video monitor displays a cross hair, which illustrates the anticipated ETT trajectory. All blade sizes feature a separate channel for passage of suction catheters. There is limited literature comparing the AWS with other video laryngoscopes, but one study comparing AWS with GVL and Truview in adult size manikins showed higher rates of success with the AWS in the setting of simulated airway pathology (tongue edema with c-spine immobility). The authors posited that the increased efficacy of the AWS compared with other video laryngoscopy devices was the presence of a side channel that facilitated ETT passage.[64] It should be emphasized, however, that there is limited evidence comparing AWS with other video laryngoscopes and that there is insufficient evidence to specifically recommend its use over other devices.

Airtraq

The Airtraq SP video laryngoscope can be used in neonates, infants, children, and adults. The sizes range from neonatal size 0 to adult size 4, and they can be used to insert ETTs from size 2.5 to 8.5. It has a guidance channel to aid intubation and an antifogging system, which warms the camera lens to body temperature. It has an eyepiece at the top of the handle, which can be used directly or can be attached to a camera to allow the image to be viewed on a screen. It is designed to be inserted via the midline of the mouth into the vallecula. It has been shown to improve the view of the larynx when compared to direct laryngoscopy in children with normal airways,[11] but, despite good views, there can be difficulties guiding the ETT into the larynx due to the shape of the blade.[14,15] The time taken to intubate appears to be increased when compared to direct laryngoscopy,[16] but the same or less when compared to other video laryngoscopes.[17] It is portable, but relatively bulky when compared to other video laryngoscopes, and there is currently not enough clinical evidence to recommend its use over any of the other devices available.

Other Video Laryngoscopes

New non-channeled video laryngoscopes suitable for pediatric use are continuously appearing on the market. The Coopdech video laryngoscope portable (VLP) 100 (Daiken Medical Co Ltd) is equipped with a Miller 0, 1, Mac 2, 3, 4, and a J-blade.

TUORen (Changyuan) comes with an assortment of disposable Miller-shaped blades, starting with #00, and a reusable 3″ LCD monitor.

The King Vision video laryngoscope (Ambu) and the Medan video laryngoscope (Supporting Healthcare) also have pediatric blades, but the smallest are equivalent to a Macintosh 2 blade; thus, not suitable for intubation of infants and neonates.

Comparison of Video Laryngoscopes

Studies comparing the efficacy of different video laryngoscopes in children are few, small, and were conducted on manikins or on patients with normal airways (Table 7.4). Even the studies on the most commonly used devices, the GVL and SVL, say very little on success rates and are inconclusive on TTI. A meta-analysis of studies of children with normal airways comparing video laryngoscopes to direct laryngoscope showed a similar intubation success rate of all devices (except for the Bullard), and all non-channeled video laryngoscopes required a longer TTI compared to direct laryngoscopy. The difference in TTI compared to direct laryngoscopy is similar for GVL and SVL.[16] Thus, current evidence does not give guidance for device selection in children with normal airways. Data on children with difficult airways are lacking.

Complications Related to the Use of Video Laryngoscopes

Overall Complications

Eisenberg and colleagues studied a large cohort of pediatric patients who were intubated in the ED with

Table 7.4 Studies Comparing the Efficacy of Different Video Laryngoscopes

Subjects	Study by first author	Type of study	Number of intubations	Age of subjects	Compared devices	Intubating person	Results
Manikin with NA and with simulated DA (SimBaby)	Hurford 2010[65]	Randomized crossover	32 × 4	n/a 3–6 months	GVL, SVL	Anesthesiology consultants and trainees	No difference in TTI; Field of view, ease of use; Willingness to use it in emergency; Overall satisfaction
Manikins with NA and DA, with and without manual in-line stabilization	Hippard 2016[38]	Randomized crossover	30 × 3 × 2 × 3	n/a	GVL, Truview	Experienced laryngoscopists	No difference in success rate and TTI, but preference for Truview
Manikin with simulated DA	Kalbhenn 2012[24]	Randomized crossover	30 × 4	n/a Infant size	Macintosh, Airtraq, Storz, Bullard	Anesthesia residents	Bullard highest success rate: shortest TTI
Manikin with DA	Saracoglu 2014[53]	Randomized crossover	45 × 4	n/a AirSim Pierre Robin manikin	Storz McGrath	Anesthesia residents and nurse anesthetists	Better view with Storz; Success rate higher with Storz; TTI shorter with Storz
Pediatric patients with NA with manual in-line stabilization	Vadi 2016[17]	Randomized	93 (31, 31, 31)	2–23 months	GVL, Storz, DL	Senior anesthesia residents new to VL	TTI longer with Storz than GVL and DL; No difference in success rate; Better view in VL
Pediatric patients with NA	Lees 2013[66]	Randomized crossover	397	0.5–18 years	GVL, Storz, DL	Pediatric anesthesiologists	TTI longer in GVL than in SVL, failure higher in GVL Identical view*
Pediatric patients with NA	Sun 2014[16]	Meta-analysis	14 studies	0–10 years	SVL, GVL, DL	Varied	SVL and GVL improved glottis view; Increased TTI

*Primary purpose of the study was to establish anesthesiologists' ability to learn the use of VL
NA: normal airway; DA: difficult airway; GVL: GlideScope video laryngoscope; SVL: Storz video laryngoscope; VL: video laryngoscope; DL: direct laryngoscope

the C-MAC video laryngoscope, where the device was used either for video-assisted laryngoscopy or for direct laryngoscopy. They found no difference in the overall incidence of complications between the two groups in the 452 patients. Mainstem intubation and recognized esophageal intubation were the most common complications in both groups.[8]

Weiss and colleagues documented several problems during video-assisted laryngoscopy by trainees, which were noted and remedied by the supervisor using the shared view, and claim that video-assisted laryngoscopy possibly prevented several endobronchial and esophageal intubations.[6] In their meta-analysis, Sun and colleagues found similar complication rates for all video laryngoscopies and direct laryngoscopies.[16]

In pediatric studies comparing video laryngoscopy to direct laryngoscopy, the reported complications are heterogeneous.[16] Multiple studies include some measure of hypoxemia, although regardless of the exact definition, rates of hypoxemia did not differ between direct laryngoscopy and video laryngoscopy. However, serious complications are relatively rare events, and it is possible that the available studies were simply not powered to discern differences in complications between the two techniques.

Among adult literature, oropharyngeal injury is the most often cited complication from video laryngoscopy. In a prospective study comparing video laryngoscopy and direct laryngoscopy in patients predicted to be difficult intubations, there was no difference in rates of airway trauma or desaturation.[50] When used as a rescue technique for failed direct laryngoscopy, video laryngoscopy has a reported rate of oropharyngeal trauma of 0.3–1%.[28,51] With the GVL in particular, there are numerous reports of palatopharyngeal arch injury. Injuries of this nature can be minimized by directly visualizing ETT insertion into the mouth and to avoid advancement against resistance. Only when the tip of the ETT appears on the video monitor should the user divert their full attention from the oropharynx to screen.[31]

Oropharyngeal and Laryngotracheal Complications

In a large study analyzing the success rate of the GVL in adults, Aziz and colleagues found a 1% incidence of minor, and a 0.3% incidence of severe oropharyngeal and laryngotracheal injuries associated with the use of the device. The severe complications included vocal cord trauma, tracheal injury, hypopharyngeal and dental trauma, and tonsillar perforation. Another adult study found higher incidence of pharyngeal wall injuries with video laryngoscopy than direct laryngoscopy.[67] Due to the paucity of large studies in children, similar incidence figures are lacking in the pediatric population. In a retrospective analysis of 105 recorded pediatric video laryngoscopic intubations by trainees, the incidence of mucosal injury – defined as "visualization of bleeding from the mucosal surface following passage of the laryngoscope blade" – was 13%. This figure was higher (24%) when a right-sided blade insertion method was used by the trainee, and lower (6%) when a midline approach was used.[47]

Severe tonsillar injury has been described during GVL intubation of a 6-year-old child.[68] Manikin studies aiming to quantify the risk of dental injury by measuring the force trainees exerted on the manikin's upper jaw/front teeth found either no difference in dental injury index, or a lower dental injury index to the advantage of video laryngoscopy compared to direct laryngoscopy.[36,39]

Summary

The last two decades saw a quick proliferation of indirect laryngoscopy. True video laryngoscopes are indirect laryngoscopes equipped with a camera chip on the distal tip of the blade. Most studies show that video laryngoscopy results in better glottic view than direct laryngoscopy in children with normal airways, but TTI is longer with video laryngoscopy.

Video laryngoscopy is superior to direct laryngoscopy when it comes to visualizing the larynx and intubating children, particularly those who are difficult to intubate.

The more hyperangulated the video laryngoscope blade is, the higher the likelihood of visualizing an "anterior glottis," but the insertion of the ETT is more difficult, and the blade becomes unsuitable for direct laryngoscopy..

No video laryngoscopy device proved to be superior to others in comparative studies. While use of video laryngoscopy might prevent certain complications common with DL, especially when the view is shared with a second, more experienced person, soft tissue injury may occur with incorrect technique.

Section 2: Devices and Techniques to Manage the Abnormal Airway

References

1. Karsli C. Managing the Challenging Pediatric Airway: Continuing Professional Development. *Canadian Journal of Anesthesia/Journal canadien d'anesthésie* 2015; **62**(9): 1000–16.

2. Pieters BM, Eindhoven GB, Acott C, van Zundert AA. Pioneers of Laryngoscopy: Indirect, Direct and Video Laryngoscopy. *Anaesthesia and Intensive Care* 2015; (**43**Suppl.): 4–11.

3. Borland LM, Casselbrant M. The Bullard Laryngoscope. A New Indirect Oral Laryngoscope (Pediatric Version). *Anesthesia & Analgesia* 1990; **70**(1): 105–8.

4. Wu TL, Chou HC. A New Laryngoscope: the Combination Intubating Device. *Anesthesiology* 1994; **81**(4): 1085–7.

5. Pearce AC, Shaw S, Macklin S. Evaluation of the Upsherscope. A New Rigid Fibrescope. *Anaesthesia* 1996; **51**(6): 561–4.

6. Weiss M, Schwarz U, Dillier CM, Gerber AC. Teaching and Supervising Tracheal Intubation in Paediatric Patients Using Video Laryngoscopy. *Paediatric Anaesthesia* 2001; **11**(3): 343–8.

7. Cooper RM. Use of a New Video Laryngoscope (GlideScope) in the Management of a Difficult Airway. *Canadian Journal of Anesthesia/Journal canadien d'anesthesie* 2003; **50**(6): 611–13.

8. Eisenberg MA, Green-Hopkins I, Werner H, Nagler J. Comparison between Direct and Video-Assisted Laryngoscopy for Intubations in a Pediatric Emergency Department. *Academic Emergency Medicine* 2016; **23**(8): 870–7.

9. O'Shea JE, Thio M, Kamlin CO, McGrory L, Wong C, John J, et al. Video Laryngoscopy to Teach Neonatal Intubation: A Randomized Trial. *Pediatrics* 2015; **136**(5): 912–19.

10. Yentis SM, Lee DJ. Evaluation of an Improved Scoring System for the Grading of Direct Laryngoscopy. *Anaesthesia* 1998; **53**(11): 1041–4.

11. Levitan RM, Ochroch EA, Kush S, Shofer FS, Hollander JE. Assessment of Airway Visualization: Validation of the Percentage of Glottic Opening (POGO) Scale. *Academic Emergency Medicine* 1998; **5**(9): 919–23.

12. Dow WA, Parsons DG. "Reverse Loading" to Facilitate Glidescope Intubation. *Canadian Journal of Anesthesia/Journal canadien d'anesthésie* 2007; **54**(2): 161–2.

13. Radesic BP, Winkelman C, Einsporn R, Kless J. Ease of Intubation with the Parker Flex-Tip or a Standard Mallinckrodt Endotracheal Tube Using a Video. *AANA Journal* 2012; **80**(5): 363–72.

14. Kim JT, Na HS, Bae JY, Kim DW, Kim HS, Kim CS, et al. GlideScope Video Laryngoscope: a Randomized Clinical Trial in 203 Paediatric Patients. *British Journal of Anaesthesia* 2008; **101**(4): 531–4.

15. Riveros R, Sung W, Sessler DI, Sanchez IP, Mendoza ML, Mascha EJ, et al. Comparison of the Truview PCD and the GlideScope Video Laryngoscopes with Direct Laryngoscopy in Pediatric Patients: a Randomized Trial. *Canadian Journal of Anaesthesia/ Journal canadien d'anesthesie* 2013; **60**(5): 450–7.

16. Sun Y, Lu Y, Huang Y, Jiang H. Pediatric Video Laryngoscope versus Direct Laryngoscope: a Meta-Analysis of Randomized Controlled Trials. *Paediatric Anaesthesia* 2014; **24**(10): 1056–65.

17. Vadi MG, Roddy KJ, Ghazal EA, Um M, Neiheisel AJ, Applegate RL 2nd. Comparison of the GlideScope Cobalt and Storz DCI Video Laryngoscopes in Children Younger than 2 Years of Age during Manual In-Line Stabilization: a Randomized Trainee Evaluation Study. *Pediatric Emergency Care* 2017; **33**(7): 467–73.

18. Vlatten A, Aucoin S, Litz S, Macmanus B, Soder C. A Comparison of the STORZ Video Laryngoscope and Standard Direct Laryngoscopy for Intubation in the Pediatric Airway – a Randomized Clinical Trial. *Paediatric Anaesthesia* 2009; **19**(11): 1102–7.

19. Inal MT, Memis D, Kargi M, Oktay Z, Sut N. Comparison of TruView EVO2 with Miller Laryngoscope in Paediatric Patients. *European Journal of Anaesthesiology* 2010; **27**(11): 950–4.

20. Mutlak H, Rolle U, Rosskopf W, Schalk R, Zacharowski K, Meininger D, et al. Comparison of the TruView Infant EVO2 PCD and C-MAC Video Laryngoscopes with Direct Macintosh Laryngoscopy for Routine Tracheal Intubation in Infants with Normal Airways. *Clinics (Sao Paulo)* 2014; **69**(1): 23–7.

21. Armstrong J, John J, Karsli C. A Comparison between the GlideScope Video Laryngoscope and Direct Laryngoscope in Paediatric Patients with Difficult Airways – a Pilot Study. *Anaesthesia* 2010; **65**(4): 353–7.

22. Lee JH, Park YH, Byon HJ, Han WK, Kim HS, Kim CS, et al. A Comparative Trial of the GlideScope(R) Video Laryngoscope to Direct Laryngoscope in Children with Difficult Direct Laryngoscopy and an Evaluation of the Effect of

Blade Size. *Anesthesia & Analgesia* 2013; **117**(1): 176–81.

23 Fiadjoe JE, Kovatsis P. Video Laryngoscopes in Pediatric Anesthesia: What's New? *Minerva Anestesiologica* 2014; **80**(1): 76–82

24 Kalbhenn J, Boelke AK, Steinmann D. Prospective Model-Based Comparison of Different Laryngoscopes for Difficult Intubation in Infants. *Paediatric Anaesthesia* 2012; **22**(8): 776–80.

25 Komiya K, Inagawa G, Nakamura K, Kikuchi T, Fujimoto J, Sugawara Y, et al. A Simple Fibreoptic Assisted Laryngoscope for Paediatric Difficult Intubation: a Manikin Study. *Anaesthesia* 2009; **64**(4): 425–9.

26 Nileshwar A, Garg V. Comparison of Bullard Laryngoscope and Short-Handled Macintosh Laryngoscope for Orotracheal Intubation in Pediatric Patients with Simulated Restriction of Cervical Spine Movements. *Paediatric Anaesthesia* 2010; **20**(12): 1092–7.

27 Levitan RM, Heitz JW, Sweeney M, Cooper RM. The Complexities of Tracheal Intubation with Direct Laryngoscopy and Alternative Intubation Devices. *Annals of Emergency Medicine* 2011; **57**(3): 240–7.

28 Fiadjoe JE, Gurnaney H, Dalesio N, Sussman E, Zhao H, Zhang X, et al. A Prospective Randomized Equivalence Trial of the GlideScope Cobalt Video Laryngoscope to Traditional Direct Laryngoscopy in Neonates and Infants. *Anesthesiology* 2012; **116**(3): 622–8.

29 Milne AD, Dower AM, Hackmann T. Airway Management Using the Pediatric GlideScope in a Child with Goldenhar Syndrome and Atypical Plasma Cholinesterase. *Paediatric Anaesthesia* 2007; **17**(5): 484–7.

30 Redel A, Karademir F, Schlitterlau A, Frommer M, Scholtz LU, Kranke P, et al. Validation of the GlideScope Video Laryngoscope in Pediatric Patients. *Paediatric Anaesthesia* 2009; **19**(7): 667–71.

31 Ilies C, Fudickar A, Thee C, Dutschke P, Hanss R, Doerges V, et al. Airway Management in Pediatric Patients Using the Glidescope Cobalt: a Feasibility Study. *Minerva Anestesiologica* 2012; **78**(9): 1019–25.

32 Trevisanuto D, Fornaro E, Verghese C. The GlideScope Video Laryngoscope: Initial Experience in Five Neonates. *Canadian Journal of Anaesthesia/Journal canadien d'anesthesie* 2006; **53**(4): 423–4.

33 Hirabayashi Y, Otsuka Y. Apparent Blind Spot with the GlideScope Video Laryngoscope. *British Journal of Anaesthesia* 2009; **103**(3): 461–2.

34 Lillie EM, Harding L, Thomas M. A New Twist in the Pediatric Difficult Airway. *Paediatric Anaesthesia* 2015; **25**(4): 428–30.

35 White M, Weale N, Nolan J, Sale S, Bayley G. Comparison of the Cobalt Glidescope Video Laryngoscope with Conventional Laryngoscopy in Simulated Normal and Difficult Infant Airways. *Paediatric Anaesthesia* 2009; **19**(11): 1108–12.

36 Rodriguez-Nunez A, Oulego-Erroz I, Perez-Gay L, Cortinas-Diaz J. Comparison of the GlideScope Video Laryngoscope to the Standard Macintosh for Intubation by Pediatric Residents In Simulated Child Airway Scenarios. *Pediatric Emergency Care* 2010; **26**(10): 726–9.

37 Iacovidou N, Bassiakou E, Stroumpoulis K, Koudouna E, Aroni F, Papalois A, et al. Conventional Direct Laryngoscopy versus Video Laryngoscopy with the GlideScope (R): a Neonatal Manikin Study with Inexperienced Intubators. *American Journal of Perinatology* 2011; **28**(3): 201–6.

38 Hippard HK, Kalyani G, Olutoye OA, Mann DG, Watcha MF. A Comparison of the Truview PCD and the GlideScope Cobalt AVL Video-Laryngoscopes to the Miller Blade for Successfully Intubating Manikins Simulating Normal and Difficult Pediatric Airways. *Paediatric Anaesthesia* 2016; **26**(6): 613–20.

39 Fonte M, Oulego-Erroz I, Nadkarni L, Sanchez-Santos L, Iglesias-Vasquez A, Rodriguez-Nunez A. A Randomized Comparison of the GlideScope Video Laryngoscope to the Standard Laryngoscopy for Intubation by Pediatric Residents in Simulated Easy and Difficult Infant Airway Scenarios. *Pediatric Emergency Care* 2011; **27**(5): 398–402.

40 Kim HJ, Kim JT, Kim HS, Kim CS, Kim SD. A Comparison of GlideScope Video Laryngoscopy and Direct Laryngoscopy for Nasotracheal Intubation in Children. *Paediatric Anaesthesia* 2011; **21**(4): 417–21.

41 Fiadjoe JE, Nishisaki A, Jagannathan N, Hunyady AI, Greenberg RS, Reynolds PI, et al. Airway Management Complications in Children with Difficult Tracheal Intubation from the Pediatric Difficult Intubation (PeDI) Registry: a Prospective Cohort Analysis. *The Lancet Respiratory Medicine* 2016; **4**(1): 37–48.

42 Hirabayashi Y, Otsuka Y. Early Clinical Experience with GlideScope Video Laryngoscope in 20 Infants. *Paediatric Anaesthesia* 2009; **19**(8): 802–4.

43 Muldowney BL, Stephenson LL, Volz LM, Bilen-Rosas G. Failed Airway Management with the GlideScope: It is Not the Same Tool in Infants. *Journal of Clinical Anesthesia* 2015; **27**(6): 534–5.

44 Byun SH, Lee SY, Hong SY, Ryu T, Kim BJ, Jung JY. Use of the GlideScope Video Laryngoscope for Intubation during Ex Utero Intrapartum Treatment in a Fetus with a Giant Cyst of the 4th Branchial Cleft: a Case Report. *Medicine (Baltimore)* 2016; **95**(39): e4931.

45 Holm-Knudsen R. The Difficult Pediatric Airway – a Review of New Devices for Indirect Laryngoscopy in Children Younger than Two Years of Age. *Paediatric Anaesthesia* 2011; **21**(2): 98–103.

46 Vlatten A, Aucoin S, Gray A, Soder C. Difficult Airway Management with the STORZ Video Laryngoscope in a Child with Robin Sequence. *Paediatric Anaesthesia* 2009; **19**(7): 700–1.

47 Green-Hopkins I, Werner H, Monuteaux MC, Nagler J. Using Video-Recorded Laryngoscopy to Evaluate Laryngoscopic Blade Approach and Adverse Events in Children. *Academic Emergency Medicine* 2015; **22**(11): 1283–9.

48 Oakes ND, Dawar A, Murphy PC. Difficulties Using the C-MAC Paediatric Video Laryngoscope. *Anaesthesia* 2013; **68**(6): 653–4.

49 Xue FS, Tian M, Liao X, Xu YC. Safe and Successful Intubation Using a Storz Video Laryngoscope in Management of Pediatric Difficult Airways. *Paediatric Anaesthesia* 2008; **18**(12): 1251–2.

50 Xue FS, Liao X, Liu JH, Zhang YM. Comparison of the Intubation with the Storz Video Laryngoscope and Standard Direct Laryngoscopy in Pediatric Patients. *Paediatric Anaesthesia* 2009; **19**(12): 1245–6.

51 Hackell RS, Held LD, Stricker PA, Fiadjoe JE. Management of the Difficult Infant Airway with the Storz Video Laryngoscope: a Case Series. *Anesthesia & Analgesia* 2009; **109**(3): 763–6.

52 Fiadjoe JE, Stricker PA, Hackell RS, Salam A, Gurnaney H, Rehman MA, et al. The Efficacy of the Storz Miller 1 Video Laryngoscope in a Simulated Infant Difficult Intubation. *Anesthesia & Analgesia* 2009; **108**(6): 1783–6.

53 Saracoglu KT, Eti Z, Kavas AD, Umuroglu T. Straight Video Blades are Advantageous than Curved Blades in Simulated Pediatric Difficult Intubation. *Paediatric Anaesthesia* 2014; **24**(3): 297–302.

54 Donoghue AJ, Ades AM, Nishisaki A, Deutsch ES. Video Laryngoscopy versus Direct Laryngoscopy in Simulated Pediatric Intubation. *Annals of Emergency Medicine* 2013; **61**(3): 271–7.

55 Wald SH, Keyes M, Brown A. Pediatric Video Laryngoscope Rescue for a Difficult Neonatal Intubation. *Paediatric Anaesthesia* 2008; **18**(8): 790–2.

56 Vanderhal AL, Berci G, Simmons CF, Jr., Hagiike M. A Video Laryngoscopy Technique for the Intubation of the Newborn: Preliminary Report. *Pediatrics* 2009; **124**(2): e339–46.

57 Moreira A, Koele-Schmidt L, Leland M, Seidner S, Blanco C. Neonatal Intubation with Direct Laryngoscopy vs Video Laryngoscopy: an Extremely Premature Baboon Model. *Paediatric Anaesthesia* 2014; **24**(8): 840–4.

58 Ross M, Baxter A. Use of the New McGrath MAC Size-1 Paediatric Video Laryngoscope. *Anaesthesia* 2015; **70**(10): 1217–18.

59 Kim EH, Lee JH, Song IK, Kim JT, Kim BR, Kim HS. Effect of Head Position on Laryngeal Visualisation with the McGrath MAC Video Laryngoscope in Paediatric Patients: a Randomised Controlled Trial. *European Journal of Anaesthesiology* 2016; **33**(7): 528–34.

60 Kim Y, Kim JE, Jeong DH, Lee J. Combined Use of a McGrath MAC Video Laryngoscope and Frova Intubating Introducer in a Patient with Pierre Robin Syndrome: a Case Report. *Korean Journal of Anesthesiology* 2014; **66**(4): 310–13.

61 Singh R, Singh P, Vajifdar H. A Comparison of Truview Infant EVO2 Laryngoscope with the Miller Blade in Neonates and Infants. *Paediatric Anaesthesia* 2009; **19**(4): 338–42.

62 Szarpak L, Truszewski Z, Czyzewski L, Gaszynski T, Rodriguez-Nunez A. A Comparison of the McGrath-MAC and Macintosh Laryngoscopes for Child Tracheal Intubation during Resuscitation by Paramedics. A Randomized, Crossover, Manikin Study. *The American Journal of Emergency Medicine* 2016; **34**(8): 1338–41.

63 UEScope (2015). Website. https://www.uescope.com

64 Malik MA, O'Donoghue C, Carney J, Maharaj CH, Harte BH, Laffey JG. Comparison of the Glidescope, the Pentax AWS, and the Truview EVO2 with the Macintosh Laryngoscope in Experienced Anaesthetists: a Manikin Study. *British Journal of Anaesthesia* 2009; **102**(1): 128–34

65 Hurford DM, White MC. A Comparison of the Glidescope and Karl Storz DCI Video Laryngoscopes in a Paediatric Manikin. *Anaesthesia* 2010; **65**(8): 781–4.

66 Lees M, Seal RF, Spady D, Csanyi-Fritz Y, Robinson JL. Randomized Trial of Success of Pediatric Anesthesiologists Learning to Use Two Video Laryngoscopes. *Paediatric Anaesthesia* 2013; **23**(5): 435–9.

67 Greer D, Marshall KE, Bevans S, Standlee A, McAdams P, Harsha W. Review of Video Laryngoscopy Pharyngeal Wall Injuries. *The Laryngoscope* 2017; **127**(2): 349–53.

68 Rodney JD, Ahmed Z, Gupta D, Zestos MM. Straight to Video: Tonsillar Injury during Elective GlideScope – Assisted Pediatric Intubation. *Middle East Journal of Anaesthesiology* 2015; **23**(1): 101–4.

Section 2 **Devices and Techniques to Manage the Abnormal Airway**

Chapter 8

Flexible Bronchoscopy Techniques: Nasal and Oral Approaches

Paul Stricker and Pete G. Kovatsis

Introduction

Flexible fiberoptic intubation was first described in 1967 and has since become a mainstay in intubations of the difficult airway.[1] The first flexible fiberoptic scope for ETTs greater than 4.5 mm ID was developed in the early 1970s. In the late 1980s, an ultrathin flexible fiberoptic laryngoscope was introduced, allowing intubation with ETTs as small as 2.5 mm ID. Multiple authors have since described the flexible fiberoptic bronchoscope's safe and effective use in both normal and difficult pediatric airways.[2–5] Others have described a variety of intubating methods using the flexible fiberoptic bronchoscope.[6–13] The flexible fiberscope is a device born of innovations in fiberoptic technology.

Since the introduction of the fiberscope, significant improvements in fiberoptic technology have occurred and, more recently, in the advancement of digital technologies, such that these digital scopes have excellent image quality. Yet, despite these advancements, the basic design and features remain the same. Given the changes in design, a more apt name for these scopes is "flexible bronchoscope" and will be used as such in this chapter. Over this same time period, numerous other techniques have been developed to facilitate tracheal intubation, including indirect/video laryngoscopes, optical stylets, ultrasound-guided techniques, and lighted stylets. Despite these developments, the flexible bronchoscope remains the cornerstone tool for airway management as it is the most versatile intubation instrument available. For example, although video/indirect laryngoscopes have simplified airway management for many children with difficult direct laryngoscopy, these tools require access via the oral cavity, which renders them ineffective in children with severe limitations in mouth opening. In these and other scenarios, the flexible bronchoscope may be the only reliable tool for tracheal intubation. As such, the flexible bronchoscope is an indispensable tool for the pediatric anesthesiologist; making acquiring and maintaining the skill set for its use mandatory. In this chapter we present principles and techniques for the successful use of this airway management tool in infants and children.

Equipment

The flexible bronchoscope has three major components: the insertion cord, the handle, and the universal cord. The insertion cord is the flexible portion that is advanced into the patient's airway. The handle is composed of the control lever for flexing the scope, the eyepiece with a dial for focus in older models or a video interface with various function buttons, and access port(s) to the working channel, if present. The universal or umbilical cord either houses the video and light connections or, in older models, inserts into the light source. Some models offer a battery-powered light source, which can replace the universal light cord, resulting in excellent portability. The insertion cord is encased in a waterproof sheet and houses the light and video or optic channels, a cable system for angulation of the tip, and if present, a working channel. The working channel is a hollow conduit for suctioning, injecting medications or saline, and passing instruments (e.g., wires in retrograde intubations). The cable system permits manipulation of the tip of the bronchoscope in a single plane via the angulation lever located on the handle.

Manipulation of the bronchoscope involves three basic movements:

1. Single plane flexion of the distal tip of the insertion cord using the angulation lever
2. Advancement and withdrawal of the insertion cord
3. Clockwise or counterclockwise movement of the insertion cord by rotating the insertion cord and handle using both hands in unison

Pediatric flexible bronchoscopes are available in sizes ranging from 2.2 mm to 4.1 mm diameter. The smallest of these bronchoscopes lacks a working channel, and in general, image quality improves with increasing diameter. A tracheal tube with an internal diameter that exceeds the diameter of the bronchoscope by at least 0.3–0.5 mm is required to effectively pass over and minimize potential damage to the bronchoscope. Flexible bronchoscopes used in adult practice generally have diameters larger than 4.1 mm. These adult-sized bronchoscopes are suitable for use in older children and adolescents in whom corresponding larger tracheal tubes may be used.

Historically, insertion cords encased fiberoptic fibers for their light and optic bundles, and this still remains true for ultrathin 2.2 mm bronchoscopes. These traditional bronchoscopes deliver an image from the bronchoscope tip to an eyepiece via fiberoptic threads in the optic bundle, which run the full length of the scope such that a fiber at the tip of the scope is in precisely the same position or pixel at the eyepiece (i.e., coherent). This is essential to maintain image integrity and accounts for the significant expense associated with repairs. The image produced has a pixelated appearance, where each "pixel" represents a visual image component conducted over a single fiber. Pre-display image processing can reduce the pixelated quality of the displayed image. However, the overall quality and detail of the image is not actually improved, but instead is slightly blurred to remove the borders of the individual fiberoptic threads.

More recently, digital image technology has advanced whereby an image is acquired through a micro lens, converted to an electronic digital signal in a chip located in the tip of the endoscope, and then transmitted through the handle and universal cord of the scope to a monitor for display. This advancement provides a dramatic improvement in image quality over fiberoptic images. Another advantage is that these scopes may be more durable since there are no fiberoptic threads delivering the image within the scope that are prone to breakage during use, improper handling, and storage. Fiberoptic thread breakage is difficult to repair, and poor durability is one of the costly limitations of flexible fiberoptic scopes, particularly for the ultrathin pediatric scopes.

Viewing

Traditional fiberoptic scopes may be used by connecting the scope to an external light source and directly viewing the image using the scope's eyepiece or attaching a video head to the eyepiece for displaying the image on a screen. Some manufacturers incorporate a small display screen mounted on top of the handle combined with a battery-powered LED light source, which creates an extremely portable scope unencumbered by cable connections to an external light source and display. At the time of writing, this universal cable-free system is not yet available for the ultrathin pediatric scopes. Modern digital bronchoscopes no longer afford this cable-free possibility as these scopes are designed to display the image on an external monitor. Future advancements in wireless connectivity will hopefully provide a cable-free system that may be sent to multiple screens within or even out of the procedural suite.

Size Selection

Selection of the appropriate bronchoscope is a key factor for successful airway management in infants and children. In general, the largest size that can be readily accommodated by the desired tracheal tube is selected which provides improved stability for passage of the tracheal tube. Utilizing a larger scope also minimizes the space between the scope and the leading edge of the tracheal tube's bevel, which in turn decreases the chance of tissue entrapment as the tracheal tube is advanced over the scope. As shown in Figure 8.1, a larger space between the tracheal tube and the scope forms a V-shaped hook, which can be jammed onto laryngeal structures during tube advancement, impeding passage and potentially causing injury.

One scenario in which a smaller scope size may be preferred is when delivering ventilation while performing tracheal intubation through an SGA device using bronchoscopic guidance (see Chapter 5 and Videos 3 and 4). In this circumstance, the use of a bronchoscope that occupies most of the lumen of the tracheal tube effectively occludes the tube, thus not allowing effective ventilation to be delivered.

Preparation

Preparation begins with a thorough review of the patient's history and physical exam, followed by the formation of comprehensive management plans and alternative strategies.

To the greatest extent possible, airway equipment should be thoroughly checked and prepared prior to use. This allows for troubleshooting unforeseen issues

Section 2: Devices and Techniques to Manage the Abnormal Airway

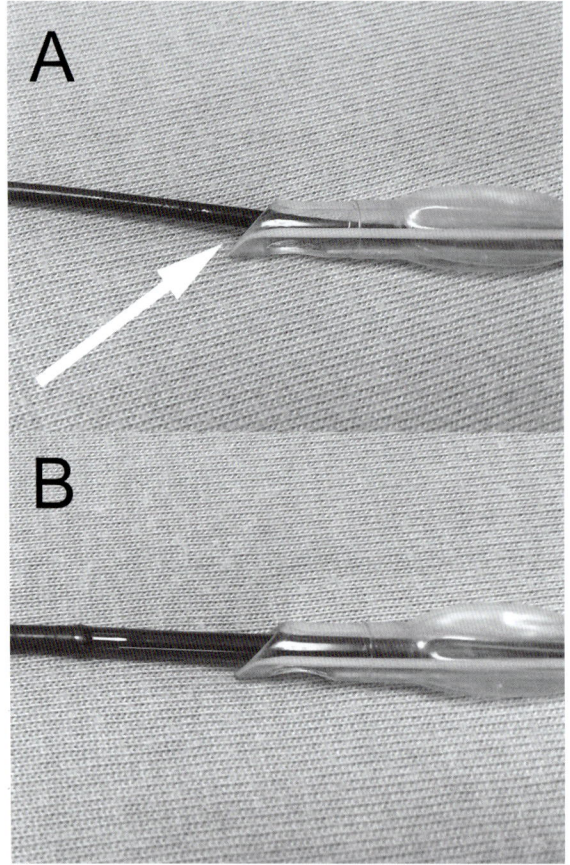

Figure 8.1 The greater size discrepancy between the smaller-diameter bronchoscope and the larger-diameter tracheal tube (A), creating a V-shaped hook (white arrow), which can lead to "hang-up" on airway structures during tracheal tube passage. Selecting a larger-diameter bronchoscope to reduce the size discrepancy between the bronchoscope and the tracheal tube minimizes this hook (B), improving the success in tracheal tube advancement.

with device functionality and verification of the availability of adjunctive tools and backup equipment. Of utmost importance is the application of adequate lubrication to the bronchoscope and interior of the selected tracheal tube, and if required, orientation of the video relative to the scope tip. Preparation should not only include the patient, plan, and bronchoscope preparation, but also preparation of additional backup equipment, and ensuring the availability of additional personnel as necessary according to the clinical scenario. Ideally, there would be three individuals involved in the intubation process: the first performs the intubation. The second helps with head position, jaw, and tongue manipulation, and, in awake or sedated patients, provides gentle restraint.

This second person may be any trained operating-room personnel. The third and most important person only focuses on the patient to control the anesthetic or sedation in a safe and effective method. Too often, all in the room are watching the intubation process such that monitoring the patient and the anesthetic become a reactive rather than a proactive maneuver.

Anesthetic Management

Key management decisions must be made prior to tracheal intubation. These include whether to manage the airway following induction of general anesthesia versus managing in the awake or sedated child.

General Anesthesia versus Sedated/Awake Intubation

An inhalation technique with the patient spontaneously ventilating is the method most often employed for difficult intubations in children. Many pediatric patients who have "difficult airways" are labeled so because tracheal intubation with direct laryngoscopy is difficult, but they are easy to ventilate with a face mask, and tracheal intubation is readily accomplished by other means. Given a patient with an acceptable mask airway, most anesthesiologists will agree that advanced airway management is best performed following the induction of anesthesia, which provides the most optimal conditions and a high degree of safety. This provides the least stressful conditions for the child and the practitioner. Particularly in the spontaneously breathing patient, a general anesthetic still should be supplemented with topical anesthesia. Applying topical anesthesia to the oropharynx and hypopharynx prior to induction will allow early non-stimulating introduction of an oral airway. If intubation proves unsuccessful, the patient may then be allowed to emerge. Reevaluation of the situation is undertaken and recommendations are given to the family and the surgeon. But clearly, the safest course if the patency of the mask airway is in doubt is an awake or sedated intubation.

Two questions play the greatest role in determining that an "awake"/sedated approach to intubation should be pursued:

1. Is ventilation anticipated to be difficult? If ventilation via a natural airway with or without adjuncts, a face mask, or an SGA device is not

expected to be difficult, in most circumstances, an approach to tracheal intubation under general anesthesia can be pursued. In those children in whom ventilation is known or anticipated to be difficult, the safest course is to manage the airway under sedated/awake conditions.

2. Is access to the oral cavity and/or upper airway blocked either by a severely limited mouth opening, tumor, or tissue? Extra consideration should be given to pursuing an awake/sedated approach to intubation in those patients in whom access to the mouth is severely limited, which precludes the use of ventilation rescue devices such as SGA devices.

Sedation for Intubation

In children, there are numerous scenarios in which induction of general anesthesia prior to securing the airway is unsafe. However, most children (with the exception of some adolescents) are unable to cooperate with intubation performed while awake or with minimal sedation. Therefore, deep levels of sedation must be provided to effectively manage the airway, making airway management in these children especially challenging. Sedation requirements may vary tremendously depending on the child's age and medical condition. Neonates are more often done with little-to-no sedation, while a toddler may require a significant amount of sedation just to separate from the family. It is important to titrate sedation to the desired effect. This desired effect is not a motionless child since preventing all movement may mean crossing over to general anesthesia. Thus, gentle restraint may be necessary to prevent head movement and to keep arms at the patient's side. The sedatives used are best determined by a practitioner's experience with those drugs and by the clinical scenario. A description of commonly used regimens follows, with emphasis on remaining very mindful of the synergisms within the various regimens.

- *Dexmedetomidine + benzodiazepine:* Dexmedetomidine has pharmacological properties that make it attractive. It provides sedation while preserving respiratory drive. The sedation it produces is one from which patients can be generally be aroused if needed. It has analgesic properties, and is an antisialagogue, but has the least blunting of airway reflexes. The addition of a benzodiazepine provides amnesia and additional sedation, which is reversible if needed with flumazenil. Dexmedetomidine can be administered in 1 mcg/kg boluses titrated for sedation up to 4 mcg/kg (usually at least 2 mcg/kg is required); boluses are preferred to an infusion for speed of onset. A small dose of opioid can also be added if needed for additional analgesic effects with the preparation for reversal of respiratory depression with an antagonist.

- *Benzodiazepine + opioid:* The combination of a benzodiazepine and an opioid provide the requisite effects to facilitate sedated tracheal intubation: sedation, amnesia, analgesia, and suppression of airway reflexes. The principal disadvantage is a dose-dependent depression of respiratory drive. Careful, patient titration of these agents, allowing enough time for the peak effect to occur before giving additional doses or adjusting infusions, may help avoid excessive sedation and respiratory depression. Both classes of drugs have reversal agents, which must be readily available. Commonly used agents include remifentanil or fentanyl combined with midazolam or diazepam.

- *Ketamine:* Although the use of ketamine is often proposed as a suitable agent for sedated airway management, it has notable disadvantages for this indication. Ketamine is a general anesthetic in doses as low as 1 mg/kg, and, when administered to establish levels adequate for airway management, a state of unintended general anesthesia may be produced, with attendant airway obstruction in those predisposed. As sedation was chosen in a patient predisposed to obstruction and potential loss of airway with general anesthesia, then ketamine is a poor choice for sedation. Ketamine as a supplement for other sedative regimens in divided doses up to a maximum dose of 0.5 mg/kg may be reasonable with the caveats that there is no reversal agent available for ketamine, and it is usually not possible to effectively communicate with patients under its effects even at these low doses.

- *Propofol:* Propofol is also advocated as a suitable agent for sedated airway management, but, like ketamine, propofol has similar disadvantages for this indication. Propofol is more often administered as a general anesthetic to establish levels adequate for airway management, with resultant depressant effects on the upper airway muscles similar to inhalation agents, and attendant airway obstruction in those predisposed. As sedation was chosen in a patient predisposed to obstruction and potential loss of airway with a general anesthesia, then propofol is also a poor choice as a primary sedative for airway management. Propofol infusions with a usual dose of 20–30 mcg/(kg min) and maximum dose of 50 mcg/(kg min) may be utilized as an adjuvant with other sedatives and the appreciation of higher doses increasing airway obstruction. Also, there is no available reversal agent.

With any sedation technique, patience is a necessity, allowing the technique to effectively and safely sedate the patient. Avoiding production pressure is a must in these elective difficult airway scenarios. An effective approach for our colleagues awaiting the intubation is to state a longer time estimate. Then, when the intubation occurs in less time, gratitude is generally the response versus frustration if a short time estimate is given and then exceeded.

Airway Anesthesia and Preparation

The process of airway management often begins in the preoperative area. More effective preparation pays dividends by providing a more effective and efficient intubation sequence. Minimizing crying in children who are anxious and uncooperative with a sedative premedication is an essential start to improving intubation conditions and safety. An intravenous line can be placed and an antisialagogue given (when indicated). A topical mucosal vasoconstricting agent (e.g., oxymetazoline, phenylephrine) can be administered following sedation or in the cooperative patient prior to arrival in the operating room. This can be achieved with an atomizer or even a nebulizer having the child breathe through the nose and/or mouth. These important steps have a number of effects that facilitate successful airway management. Fewer secretions improves visualization with a bronchoscope. Vasoconstriction may prevent or reduce severity of epistaxis. Vasoconstriction and fewer secretions may enhance the effectiveness of topically applied local anesthetics. Dry, vasoconstricted mucosa also allow lower concentrations of local anesthesia to be effective, increasing the volume, but not the dose, that may be given to a smaller patient.

If a nasal approach to flexible bronchoscopic intubation is planned, excellent topical anesthesia of the nasopharynx is needed. This can be achieved by first spraying lidocaine with a mucosal atomizer device into the nostrils. After allowing for this to take effect, lidocaine-soaked pledgets can be inserted to the posterior nasopharynx along the medial septum and left in place for 3–5 minutes to achieve anesthesia of the sphenopalatine ganglion.

Oropharyngeal anesthesia can be achieved by delivering lidocaine via a malleable atomizer device to the hypopharynx and posterior pharynx. Alternatively, topical lidocaine can be delivered via a nebulizer prior to airway management. Care must be taken to avoid exceeding maximum dose limits and toxicity. If a lower lidocaine concentration is desired, diluting the lidocaine with an antisialagogue and/or a vasoconstrictor are options. Atropine is preferred as it will cross membranes more readily than glycopyrrolate. Dosing limits for all administered medications must be kept in mind. Glossopharyngeal and superior laryngeal nerve blocks may also be performed, although many practitioners favor the techniques outlined above, particularly in uncooperative children.

Topical anesthesia of the larynx and trachea is usually achieved by spraying lidocaine through the working channel of the bronchoscope onto the vocal cords and into the trachea. If proceeding with an awake or sedated case in a small infant with a scope that does not have a working channel, using a larger scope with a working channel to assess the airway and spray the larynx is a reasonable two-step process for topicalization. Although a transtracheal injection is feasible, most pediatric anesthesiologists are wary of this technique, especially in our smallest patients because of the potential morbidity from inadvertent needle puncture/injection into the more adjacent structures of a smaller larynx.

The anesthesiologist must exercise caution to avoid excessive local anesthetic doses in children. Often 2% lidocaine or even 0.5–1% in early infancy is best used instead of 4% lidocaine so that sufficient volumes can be delivered. The pharmacokinetics of topical lidocaine in children are not well defined; conservative practice is to limit the total dose to 5 mg/kg. The maximum dose allowed should be calculated and then drawn and divided up for its various applications. Once this dose has been administered, no more should be available as all other local anesthetic should be removed from the clinically active workspaces. This will minimize the potential for "toxicity creep" that may occur due to difficulty remembering how much has been given during an attention-consuming intubation.

General Anesthesia for Airway Management

General anesthesia can be maintained using inhaled agents, intravenous agents, and other adjuvants (e.g., dexmedetomidine), depending on anesthesiologist preference and the clinical circumstance. Whether or not spontaneous ventilation will be maintained influences maintenance drug selection the most.

Muscle Relaxants

There are a variety of circumstances where administration of a muscle relaxant greatly facilitates airway management. For example, when performing bronchoscopic-guided intubation through an SGA device, a muscle relaxant can prevent coughing, laryngospasm, and vocal cord closure around the scope, facilitating tracheal tube passage.

Muscle relaxants also carry disadvantages. Preservation of spontaneous ventilation can be used as a method to maintain oxygenation and deliver anesthetic, and gives the bronchoscope operator more time to navigate the airway. The technique of "following the bubbles" to guide bronchoscope navigation is one that requires air movement across the larynx to be present.

Whether or not muscle relaxant administration is part of the primary airway management plan, administration of muscle relaxants should be considered for every patient. For example, if the primary plan is airway management under general anesthesia with spontaneous ventilation, laryngospasm may occur and completely obstruct the airway. The anesthesiologist should have a plan for how this is managed; administration of succinylcholine may be required and there is value in careful consideration of the dose to be given with the smallest dose to achieve the effect desired preferred (e.g., ~0.2 mg/kg for vocal cord relaxation). In some circumstances, succinylcholine may be the muscle relaxant of choice for pediatric difficult airway management. The potential advantage of succinylcholine is its rapid clearance and offset of action, which may be helpful should attempts fail and a return to spontaneous ventilation is desired. Sugammadex may have a similar role in airway management, where it theoretically allows for rapid reversal of nondepolarizing neuromuscular blockade. Concerns have arisen, however, in recent reports where reversal of profound neuromuscular blockade with sugammadex precipitated laryngospasm in adults.[14]

Flexible Bronchoscopic Intubation: Challenges and Tips

The major contributing factor to failure is inexperience with the flexible bronchoscope.

Challenges

Simple and common mistakes during flexible bronchoscopic intubation that can lead to prolonged attempts or failure:

- advancing too deep before looking
- advancing too quickly and overcompensating by pulling back too far
- advancing without an adequate view
- failing to keep the bronchoscope midline during an oral approach
- failing to keep the bronchoscope taut for proper manipulation (Figure 8.2)
- inadequate topical anesthesia
- lack of assistants for airway manipulations and patient care
- not recognizing the anatomy, particularly in abnormal airways

Most of the mistakes of inexperience can be overcome by practicing on manikins first and then on normal patients under general anesthesia. After performing 20 fiberoptic laryngoscopic intubations in patients, residents were able to intubate in less than one minute on average.[15]

Tube Hang-Up (Table 8.1)

One of the most common intubation challenges encountered after the flexible bronchoscope has been navigated into the trachea is meeting resistance with tracheal tube advancement over the bronchoscope. Generally, bronchoscopic intubation is regarded as a visualization technique, yet the tracheal tube is passed blindly over the scope. When obstruction to tube advancement occurs, the clinician is unable to see what the obstruction is. *The most common cause is thought to be from arytenoid or other perilaryngeal tissue getting caught in the gap between the leading edge of the tracheal tube bevel and the bronchoscope* (also see Figure 8.1). For this reason, select a bronchoscope size that minimizes the size of this gap, as discussed previously. Other possibilities can account for resistance to tube passage, including a tube that is too large for the larynx (i.e., the cricoid cartilage in smaller children and infants, and the vocal cords for

Table 8.1 Methods to Facilitate Tube Entry into the Trachea During Fiberoptic Intubation

Suggestion	Why it works
Bronchoscope diameter should closely approximate the internal diameter of the tracheal tube selected	Less hang-up during tracheal tube passage/advancement
Parker Flex-Tip tube	Bevel of this tracheal tube closely articulates with the insertion cord of the bronchoscope, reducing hang-up
Warmed tracheal tube	Moldable, softened plastic less likely to abut laryngeal structures
External laryngeal manipulation	Downward pressure on the larynx may improve the laryngeal geometry
Bevel orientation	Posteriorly facing bevel or turned 90 degrees counterclockwise will prevent the bevel hitting the right arytenoid cartilage
Video laryngoscope	Use of a video laryngoscope with fiberoptic bronchoscope (hybrid) allows for adequate tongue displacement and the practitioner to visualize tracheal tube entry

A
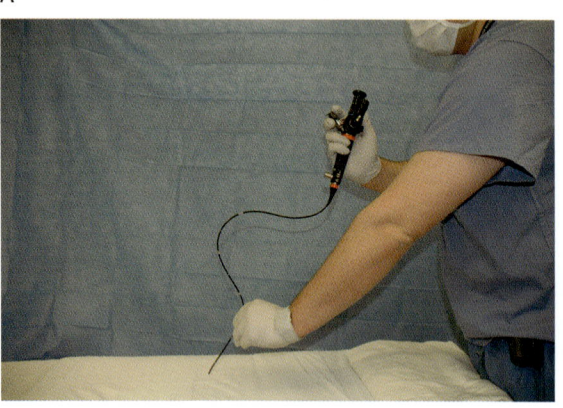

B
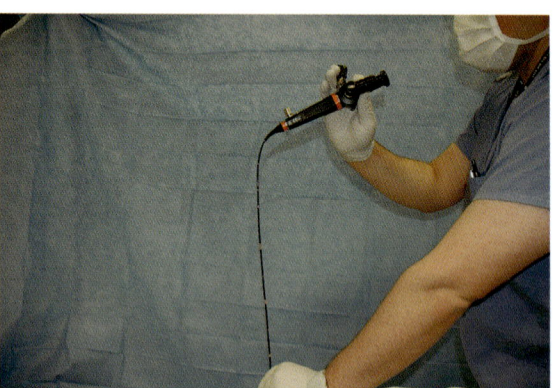

Figure 8.2 Panel A. Fiberoptic Bronchoscope improperly held with slack and a curve in the insertion cord. This hand position may lead to failure of fiberoptic bronchoscopic intubation.
Panel B. The proper technique with the fiberoptic bronchoscope insertion cord held taut.

preteens and teenagers). More often, one is limited by the available scopes, but when feasible, selecting a smaller, tighter-fitting tube for the given scope is prudent to minimize this possibility.

There are a few techniques that may prevent or relieve this problem:

- *Parker Flex-Tip tube:* This tracheal tube has a curved, extended flap over the tip rather than the standard "straight" bevel of standard tubes (Figure 8.3). The curved flap closes/eliminates the angled gap between the bronchoscope and the tube, minimizing hang-up.
- *Hot water soaking of the tracheal tube:* Hot water warms the plastic and dramatically softens it immediately prior to use. Because of the low specific heat of the materials used in tracheal tube construction, there is no risk of burns, even when soaked in very hot water (note: this may not apply for tubes with wire reinforcement). This can be easily tested prior to patient use by feeling the tube after immersion.
- *Bevel orientation:* When advancing the tracheal tube, make sure that the bevel is facing posteriorly, such that when the tube reaches the larynx, the point or apex of the bevel/tube tip is anterior. This keeps any angled gap between the bronchoscope and tracheal tube from getting hung up on laterally positioned laryngeal structures (e.g., arytenoids). If resistance is encountered, the first step is to slightly withdraw the tube to relieve any tension on it, rotate 90 degrees counterclockwise, and reattempt advancement. This may be repeated to test different positions. It is important to release the tension and slightly withdraw the tube prior to

Chapter 8: Flexible Bronchoscopy Techniques: Nasal and Oral Approaches

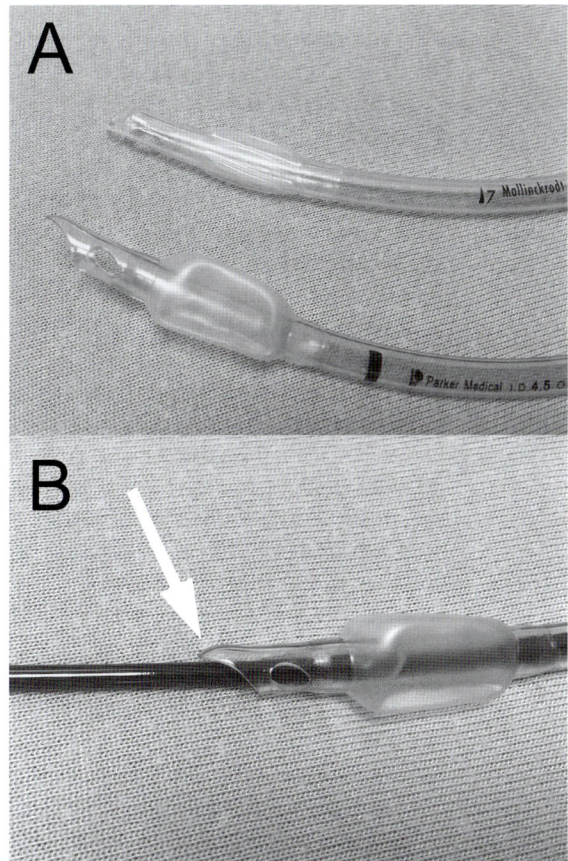

Figure 8.3 Panel A. Standard (top) and Parker Flex-Tip (bottom) tracheal tubes.
Panel B. The curved tip of the Parker Flex-Tip tube more closely articulates with the bronchoscope to prevent laryngeal hang-up during tracheal tube advancement.

each rotation to avoid traumatizing laryngeal structures. Advancing by using tension and a corkscrew-like motion is more likely to cause damage, such as arytenoid dislocation.

- *External laryngeal manipulation* is another technique that can be used. Slight tracheal tube withdrawal, followed by posterior or downward pressure on the larynx, may improve the geometry and facilitate tube passage. If the tube has moved more than previously and resistance is met again, then releasing the external manipulation may be required, particularly in infants as laryngeal compression is more likely.
- *Hybrid techniques:* In patients in whom it is feasible, direct or indirect laryngoscopy can be performed by an assistant (e.g., combination of a GlideScope with fiberoptic bronchoscopy (see Video 9). This may alter the anatomical alignment to facilitate intubation, and may allow the operator to visualize the cause of tube hang-up and determine a solution. Other advantages of this combination technique are the displacement of the tongue, the lifting of the epiglottis, and providing a visual guide for advancement of the scope.

Improving Efficiency of Bronchoscope Navigation and View

A number of techniques can be used to improve laryngeal view, bronchoscope navigation/entry into the larynx and trachea:

- *Upper airway suctioning:* Gentle suctioning of the pharynx and hypopharynx prior to bronchoscope navigation is a simple but important step, which removes secretions that can obscure the lens at the bronchoscope tip, and should be routinely performed.
- *Jaw thrust and tongue pull:* Having an assistant provide anterior jaw thrust/subluxation of the mandible often dramatically increases the size of the upper airway/perilaryngeal space through which to navigate the bronchoscope. Pulling and holding the tongue out of the mouth with dry gauze can achieve a similar effect. At times both maneuvers may be beneficial. A malleable or non-crushing retractor or a tongue stitch may also be used for pulling the tongue and jaw forward. However, using the wrong type of grasper on the tongue or the stitch itself may lead to trauma and bleeding. The stitch may be left in the tongue to use as an airway assist technique post-extubation, if needed.
- *Hand positioning:* Appropriate placement of the user's hands is essential and plays a key role for the oral approach. This is much more important in pediatrics as, when using the ultrathin scopes, they are more prone to drifting laterally with poor hand position, and can build up torque tension if both hands do not rotate the insertion cord and bronchoscope handle in unison. For new users, placing the dominant hand on the insertion cord (i.e., nearest the patient) is recommended as this hand requires the most dexterity (this hand will be referred to as the "insertion hand" and the other the "handle hand").
  - The insertion hand must be stabilized on the patient by placing the fourth and/or fifth finger

directly onto the zygomatic arch. These fingers may be straight or bent, depending on the size of the hand and patient. Presuming that there are no maxillary fractures, this will provide effective and solid positioning of the insertion hand. Placing this hand onto the mandible is counterproductive in that this will push the mandible and tongue toward the larynx, in turn, limiting the perilaryngeal space and directly opposing any tongue pull or jaw thrust.

- The third finger is placed midline at the mouth at the upper maxilla either on the gum line, teeth or, if the patient is awake or sedated, on the bite block. The scope is then placed between the crease of the first and second joint space on the palmer surface of the third finger and the mouth. The third finger maintains a firm, constant pressure on the scope and teeth/gum line to maintain control and keep midline. Since the scope is lubricated, the scope will slide easily between this space and rotation is still allowed. With ultrathin scopes and severe craniofacial abnormalities, the even more exaggerated "S" curve around the base of the tongue, over the arytenoids, and into the subglottis makes it even more difficult to advance these scopes orally. Sliding the scope together with the third finger down the gum line onto the palate while advancing gives the scope better firmness and gives better control for entering the larynx. Adding head extension may also better align the scope's trajectory (i.e., lessen the "S" curve) into the larynx.
- The fist and second finger then "pinch" the scope above the third finger and are used to advance and rotate the scope in conjunction with the handle hand. The insertion hand rotates the scope by rolling the scope between the first and second fingers.
- The handle hand controls the level for flexing the tip of the scope, the "trigger" for suction on the working channel, and advances and rotates the scope together with the insertion hand. Both hands need to rotate the scope together such that there is no tension on the scope otherwise this torque will make it extremely difficult to control the tip in future movements as it flicks back to minimize the torque.
  - Although the nasal approach provides scope stability and prevents lateral drift, using the same hand positioning at the nares to maintain consistency and practice is recommended.

- *"Pink" Screen:* When a screen is pink or reddish, the scope tip is abutting tissue. Withdraw slightly until the path is seen again and advance more slowly to avoid abutting into tissues with the tip.
- *Insertion cord:* Maintaining the insertion cord taut will allow better control and smooth movements of the tip. This can easily be achieved by lowering the operating-room bed, standing on stepstools, and/or thenar flexion of the handle hand wrist. Also, when the insertion cord is straight, rotation results in a simple circular movement of the tip. Once a bend is placed onto the insertion cord as the scope is passed around the base of the tongue, rotation results in an arcing motion of the tip. Thus, precise, directed movements of the scope is preferred to control and appreciate the subtle yet important differences to improve success and TTI.
- *Aim for the anterior commissure:* Given that the pediatric larynx has an anterior laryngeal tilt such that its opening axis points into the base of the tongue, and the anterior insertion of the vocal cords are more inferior (i.e., angled away from the scope), when past the epiglottis and approaching the larynx with the scope, aim for the anterior commissure of the vocal cords and not the middle of the laryngeal inlet. Once at the apex of the anterior commissure, direct the tip of the scope downward and the scope should fall through the cords and into the subglottis.
- *Estimating the distance to the larynx:* Another technique is to hold the bronchoscope next to the patient's mouth/nose (depending which route is chosen) and estimating the distance to the larynx using external landmarks. The bronchoscope is held with the fingers at this point to give the operator an approximation of the required insertion depth, which may help avoid inadequate or excessive insertion of the bronchoscope during navigation. This is more feasible with a nasal approach or when using an intubating oral airway; otherwise, in a straight oral approach, one may drift off midline making success more challenging.

Chapter 8: Flexible Bronchoscopy Techniques: Nasal and Oral Approaches

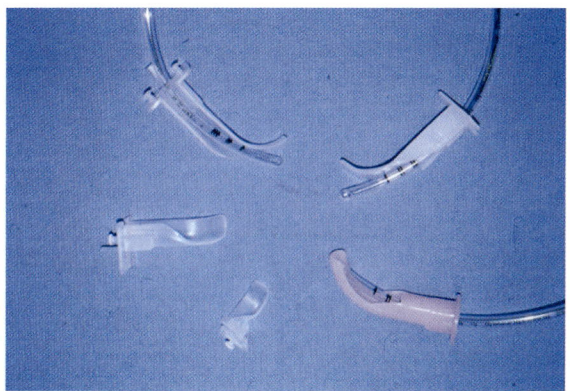

Figure 8.4 A selection of various available intubating oral airways. Intubating oral airways often help keep the fiberoptic bronchoscope midline when passing the base of tongue. Note that very few intubating oral airways are available for use in small children.

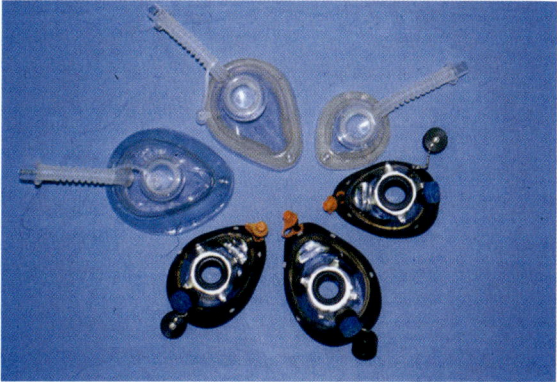

Figure 8.5 Various intubating face masks. These face masks allow the practitioner to continuously ventilate the patient's lungs during fiberoptic bronchoscopy.

- *Modified nasal trumpet technique:* One extremely useful method for facilitating bronchoscopic intubation is to maintain spontaneous ventilation and maintain the anesthesia by delivering volatile anesthetic and oxygen through a modified nasal trumpet. A modified nasal trumpet is a nasopharyngeal airway that either has an appropriately sized 15 mm tracheal tube circuit connector inserted into its external end, or to move the heavy and bulky circuit connection away from the nasal entry, place an appropriately sized uncuffed tracheal tube approximately 2 cm into the external portion of the nasal airway. The anesthesia circuit is then connected to this and the patient breathes the delivered oxygen and volatile anesthetic, while the bronchoscopic intubation is attempted through the opposite nostril or the mouth. This technique is useful because it provides oxygen and anesthesia to the patient, which gives the operator the time and conditions for successful intubation. It is also a "hands-free" technique, in that it frees up the operator's hands to focus on the intubation. Lastly, the shaft of the nasal trumpet usually terminates close to the larynx. Thus, it provides orientation for a parallel path to the airway during scope navigation. Please refer to Chapter 6 for additional techniques of oxygenation such as humidified, high flow oxygenation systems.
- Intubating oral airways are limited for pediatric use both in terms of availability and in benefit (Figure 8.4). In particular, intubating oral airways that are open on the lingual surface provide limited benefit and are best avoided as the tongue's papilla will fill that opening and obscure the scope's view. Jaw thrust, tongue pull, and using hybrid techniques such as combining flexible bronchoscopic intubation with direct laryngoscope, video laryngoscope, or SGA devices are preferable.
- Intubating masks are available and may aid in the case where a nasal approach is required, but the patient also needs CPAP or bilevel positive airway pressure (BiPAP) assistance (Figure 8.5). Using an intubating mask adds time and requires more skill to maneuver the scope as holding the mask to maintain the airway generally impedes the intubation process.
- *Defogging:* Dipping or wiping the tip with a defogging solution or warm saline is always recommended prior to starting. During the intubation, gently touching the tip of the bronchoscope on tissue will help to defog and even clear secretions away. The tissue is analogous to a washcloth wiping the tip. If the bronchoscope has a working channel, then injecting saline, preferably warmed saline, through the channel will also clear away the fog and debris at the tip. Although unlikely, the bronchoscope may need to be removed to manually clear adherent debris.
- Suctioning through the working channel is advocated and is effective in most cases, even with the 2.8 mm bronchoscopes. The technique of insufflating oxygen through the working channel of a bronchoscope to clear the bronchoscope tip of secretions and help maintain oxygenation is

potentially associated with barotrauma including life-threatening pneumothoraces in children. This technique is easily avoided as there are other safer and effective means of providing oxygenation and clearing the bronchoscope tip in these high-risk children, as discussed.
- When advancing the tube, maintain visualization of the carina and verify that the tube is not advancing into the esophagus, which is noted by the bronchoscope being pulled away from the carina. If this occurs, then withdraw the tube, readjust the bronchoscope, and reconsider the following as discussed above: tube size versus bronchoscope size, tube position on the bronchoscope, head and neck position, external laryngeal manipulation, moving to a hybrid technique, or changing intubation techniques. Also reassess for cord closure or laryngospasm.

Nasal Approach

The nasal approach is usually the technique of choice, particularly for awake intubations, since the fiberoptic laryngoscope can avoid the muscular tongue and the biting teeth. Also, flexible bronchoscopic intubation is often easier to accomplish nasally rather than orally. This is partly because of the geometry of a nasal approach: the angles of the curvatures that must be navigated, and the tube advanced over, are less acute. The nasopharynx also provides a good guide to the laryngeal inlet in the majority of cases. In sedated patients, the gag reflex is triggered less by a nasal approach. The principal disadvantage of nasotracheal intubation is the risk of epistaxis, which, if it occurs, can make subsequent visualization and intubation difficult. As described above, preparation of the nasal mucosa with a topical vasoconstrictor may help prevent or lessen epistaxis.

Most pediatric anesthesiologists prefer to navigate the bronchoscope under direct visualization through the nostril, through the nasopharynx, and then into the trachea, followed by advancement of the tracheal tube, as opposed to first inserting the tracheal tube into the nasopharynx followed by the bronchoscope. By inserting and passing the bronchoscope first, the presence of an unobstructed and optimal path to tube advancement is confirmed, and, if epistaxis is created during tube advancement, it is during completion of the intubation and therefore less likely to obfuscate the intubation. This is particularly important in children with craniofacial abnormalities and prior surgeries such as for velopalatine insufficiency.

Orotracheal Intubation

Orotracheal intubation may be required for the procedure being performed, and has the advantage that epistaxis is not a risk. As indicated above, a greater curvature is navigated with orotracheal intubation, and pre-softening the tracheal tube immediately prior to use by soaking the tube in hot water may help facilitate tube passage. Table 8.2 summarizes the differences between different fiberoptic intubation techniques.

Complications

The majority of flexible bronchoscopic intubations proceed without significant complications. However, there are a wide range of potential complications that may occur.[16–18] More common complications result from oversedation and lead to airway obstruction, respiratory depression or failure, and an uncooperative and/or disoriented patient. Additional complications include esophageal intubations, laryngospasm, vagal reactions, barotrauma, damage to the fiberoptic laryngoscope, and mechanical trauma, such as dental damage, laryngeal injury, tongue injury, and epistaxis.[18–27]

Conclusion

The flexible bronchoscope is the most versatile intubation instrument available and is the cornerstone tool of pediatric difficult airway management. Despite the introduction of video laryngoscopy techniques, which simplify airway management in a wide range of clinical scenarios, numerous conditions remain in which the flexible bronchoscope is the only effective intubation tool. As such, acquiring and maintaining the techniques and skills for its use are mandatory for the pediatric anesthesiologist. However, the flexible bronchoscope demands a high degree of experience and skill when dealing with abnormal airways and atypical anatomy. The expertise required is even greater with pediatric ultrathin flexible scopes. The most important use of the flexible scope is in difficult intubations. However, an essential use of the flexible scope is in routine intubations. In the latter setting, the user will

Table 8.2 A Comparison between Different Fiberoptic Intubation Techniques

Route for fiberoptic intubation (FOI)	Advantages	Limitations
Oral	• shorter path to the larynx versus nasal route • avoids shearing of adenoidal tissue and epistaxis	• patient can bite bronchoscope • greater skill required to maneuver the scope
Nasal	• simpler midline placement • relatively straightforward path to larynx • useful in children with extremely limited mouth opening • avoids the risk of the child biting the scope or tracheal tube	• potential risk for epistaxis and/or adenoidal tissue shearing • sinusitis
SGA device-assisted	• provides a hands-free airway • relatively straightforward path to the larynx • ability to overcome upper airway obstruction • can oxygenate and provide inhaled anesthetic during intubation	• modifications of equipment needed for some SGA devices (i.e., LMA Classic), especially when using a cuffed tracheal tube • higher resistance passing the bronchoscope when using polyvinyl chloride (PVC) single-use SGA devices (Ambu, LMA Unique, and Portex) when compared with silicone-based reusable SGA devices

attain and maintain the necessary skills required for success in the difficult airway. Prior to any use of the bronchoscope in patients, one should practice and become proficient on manikins representing various ages. Other common indications in anesthesia include directed endobronchial intubations and verifying the position of double-lumen tubes or bronchial blockers.

Flexible bronchoscopic intubation has greatly facilitated difficult intubations where the laryngeal inlet cannot be seen by conventional means. It can be used alone or in combination with nearly every other advanced airway technique to improve its success. See Video 6 and Video 7 for oral and nasal approaches for performing fiberoptic intubation.

Box 8.1 Top 10 Suggestions to Improve Success when Performing Fiberoptic Bronchoscopy

1. Practice, Practice, Practice
2. Suction prior to intubation
3. Good topical anesthesia
4. Dedicated assistants to provide airway maneuvers
5. Nasal approach
6. Jaw thrust and anterior tongue pull
7. Smallest acceptable ETT to prevent hang-up
8. Taut insertion cord
9. Slow, smooth directed manipulations of the fiberscope
10. Oxygenation of the patient during fiberoptic bronchoscopy

References

1. Murphy P. A Fibre-Optic Endoscope Used for Nasal Intubation. *Anaesthesia* 1967; **22**(3): 489–91.
2. Roth AG, Wheeler M, Stevenson GW, Hall SC. Comparison of a Rigid Laryngoscope with the Ultrathin Fibreoptic Laryngoscope for Tracheal Intubation in Infants. *Canadian Journal of Anesthesia/Journal canadien d'anesthésie* 1994; **41**(11): 1069–73.
3. Finer NN, Muzyka D. Flexible Endoscopic Intubation of the

Section 2: Devices and Techniques to Manage the Abnormal Airway

Neonate. *Pediatric Pulmonology* 1992; **12**(1): 48–51.

4. Kleeman PP, Jantzen JP, Bonfils P. The Ultra-Thin Bronchoscope in Management of the Difficult Paediatric Airway. *Canadian Journal of Anesthesia/Journal canadien d'anesthésie* 1987; **34**(6): 606–8.

5. Monrigal J, Granry J, LeRolle T, Rod B, Bavellar M. Difficult Intubation in Newborns and Infants Using an Ultrathin Fibreoptic Bronchoscope. *Anesthesiology* 1991; 75(A): 1044.

6. Heath ML, Allagain J. Intubation through the Laryngeal Mask. A Technique for Unexpected Difficult Intubation. *Anaesthesia* 1991; **46**(7): 545–8.

7. Tobias R. Increased Success with Retrograde Guide for Endotracheal Intubation. *Anesthesia & Analgesia* 1983; **62**(3): 366–7.

8. Lechman MJ, Donahoo JS, Macvaugh H 3rd. Endotracheal Intubation Using Percutaneous Retrograde Guidewire Insertion Followed by Antegrade Fiberoptic Bronchoscopy. *Critical Care Medicine* 1986; **14**(6): 589–90.

9. Benumof JL. Use of the Laryngeal Mask Airway to Facilitate Fiberscope-Aided Tracheal Intubation. *Anesthesia & Analgesia* 1992; **74**(2): 313–15.

10. Darling JR, Keohane M, Murray JM. A Split Laryngeal Mask as an Aid to Training in Fibreoptic Tracheal Intubation. A Comparison with the Berman II Intubating Airway. *Anaesthesia* 1993; **48**(12): 1079–82.

11. Hasham F, Kumar CM, Lawler PG. The Use of the Laryngeal Mask Airway to Assist Fibreoptic Orotracheal Intubation. *Anaesthesia* 1991; **46**(10): 891.

12. Johnson CM, Sims C. Awake Fibreoptic Intubation via a Laryngeal Mask in an Infant with Goldenhar's Syndrome. *Anaesthesia & Intensive Care* 1994; **22**(2): 194–7.

13. Gupta B, McDonald JS, Brooks JH, Mendenhall J. Oral Fiberoptic Intubation Over a Retrograde Guidewire. *Anesthesia & Analgesia* 1989; **68**(4): 517–19.

14. McGuire B, Dalton AJ. Sugammadex, Airway Obstruction, and Drifting across the Ethical Divide: a Personal Account. *Anaesthesia* 2016; **71**(5): 487–92.

15. Roberts JT. Preparing to Use the Flexible Fiber-Optic Laryngoscope. *Journal of Clinical Anesthesia* 1991; **3**(1): 64–75.

16. Ovassapian A. *Fiberoptic Endoscopy and the Difficult Airway*. Philadelphia: Lippincott-Raven; 1996.

17. Smith M, Calder I, Crockard A, Isert P, Nicol ME. Oxygen Saturation and Cardiovascular Changes during Fibreoptic Intubation under General Anaesthesia. *Anaesthesia* 1992; **47**(2): 158–61.

18. Ovassapian A, Krejcie TC, Yelich SJ, Dykes MH. Awake Fibreoptic Intubation in the Patient at High Risk of Aspiration. *British Journal of Anaesthesia* 1989; **62**(1): 13–16.

19. Hershey MD, Hannenberg AA. Gastric Distention and Rupture from Oxygen Insufflation during Fiberoptic Intubation. *Anesthesiology* 1996; **85**(6): 1479–80.

20. Richardson MG, Dooley JW. Acute Facial, Cervical, and Thoracic Subcutaneous Emphysema: a Complication of Fiberoptic Laryngoscopy. *Anesthesia & Analgesia* 1996; **82**(4): 878–80.

21. Ovassapian A, Yelich SJ, Dykes MH, Brunner EE. Fiberoptic Nasotracheal Intubation – Incidence and Causes of Failure. *Anesthesia & Analgesia* 1983; **62**(7): 692–5.

22. Delaney KA, Hessler R. Emergency Flexible Fiberoptic Nasotracheal Intubation: a Report of 60 Cases. *Annals of Emergency Medicine* 1988; **17**(9): 919–26.

23. Wiles JR, Kelly J, Mostafa SM. Hypotension and Bradycardia Following Superior Laryngeal Nerve Block. *British Journal of Anaesthesia* 1989; **63**(1): 125–7.

24. Moorthy SS, Dierdorf SF. An Unusual Difficulty in Fiberoptic Intubation. *Anesthesiology* 1985; **63**(2): 229.

25. Ovassapian A. Failure to Withdraw Flexible Fiberoptic Laryngoscope after Nasotracheal Intubation. *Anesthesiology* 1985; **63**(1): 124–5.

26. Nichols KP, Zornow MH. A Potential Complication of Fiberoptic Intubation. *Anesthesiology* 1989; **70**(3): 562–3.

27. Siegel M, Coleprate P. Complication of Fiberoptic Bronchoscope. *Anesthesiology* 1984; **61**(2): 214–15.

Section 2 — Devices and Techniques to Manage the Abnormal Airway

Chapter 9

Optical Stylet and Light-Guided Equipment and Techniques

Rajeev Subramanyam and Mohamed Mahmoud

Introduction

Optical stylets are airway tools, which combine features of fiberoptic bronchoscopes and intubation stylets.[1] These devices use fibers to transmit the image to an eyepiece or camera, which can be attached to the eyepiece for viewing on a monitor. Optical stylets are designed to be used independently, with laryngoscopes, or with SGA devices.[2,3] There are wide variations in optical stylet length, malleability, and light sources. The common feature of these devises is their light source, which enables the stylet to be used as a lightwand, while the fiberoptic capability enables visualization of the laryngeal inlet.[4]

The major advantages of optical stylets include maneuverability, the ability to visualize the insertion of the tip of the tracheal tube into the trachea, and lower cost than a fiberoptic bronchoscope. These devices require a mouth opening only as wide as a tracheal tube, and have the capacity for tracheoscopy. Many practitioners find navigation of these relatively rigid stylets more intuitive than the flexible bronchoscope. The rigidity of these devices facilitates control of the stylet tip and allows for the displacement of soft tissue. The learning curve for the proficient use of optical stylets is reported to be 20 uses.[5]

This chapter provides an evidence-based review of the literature regarding current clinical uses of optical stylets. We provide a descriptive account of the evolution, properties, and design variations of optical stylets and the skills required for facilitating intubation. We also discuss their limitations, with a consideration for the future directions of these devices.

History and Development of Optical Stylets

"Optical stylet" is a term first reported in 1979 to describe a straight rigid endoscope (with an optical eyepiece), which was used as a tracheal tube stylet during intubation.[6,7] In general, the optical stylet consists of various components essential to its optimal functioning: stylet, light source, fiber either made of glass or plastic, power source, and viewing mechanism. Incorporating fiberoptic imaging elements in the design of these devices has led to improved function and appeal. Common to all optical stylets is a proximal tube holder compatible with a 15 mm ETT connector. More than a dozen optical stylets have been introduced since 1995.[8] Bonfils[9] modified the early rigid and straight design feature by applying a fixed curve to the distal end. There are various optical stylets and light-guided equipment (Table 9.1): (1) devices that are commercially available, and their use is reported in both adult and pediatric patients, (2) devices that are commercially available, and their use is reported in adult patients, (3) devices that are not commercially available. Specifications of the commercially available individual devices are summarized in Table 9.2.

Devices Reported in Adult and Pediatric Patients

Bonfils Intubation Endoscope

The Bonfils intubation endoscope was named after its designer, Dr. Bonfils from Switzerland. It was introduced into practice in the early 1980s[10] and has been commercially available since 1996. The pediatric version has been available since the late 2000s.

Design and Technical Pearls

The basic design consists of a body (where the light source and the video is attached) and a stylet. Bein and colleagues have described the technique for intubation in children.[11] With the child asleep, the head is placed in neutral position and the Bonfils scope is inserted from the right corner of the mouth. The scope is then advanced until the tip is at

Section 2: Devices and Techniques to Manage the Abnormal Airway

Table 9.1 Examples of Optical Stylets and Light-Guided Equipment

Commercially available, with use reported in both adults and pediatric patients

- Bonfils intubation scope
- Shikani optical stylet

Commercially available, with use reported in adult patients

- Clarus video system (Clarus Medical)
- Levitan scope
- Malleable video stylet (Sharn Anesthesia): no studies reported
- SensaScope (Acutronic Medical Systems)
- StyletScope (Nihon Koden)

Not commercially available

- Aeroview scope system (Imagyn)
- Fiberoptic stylet laryngoscope (American Optical)
- Flexguide (Scientific Sales International)
- Lighted stylets: various brands
- Machida portable stylet fiberscope
- Schroeder stylet (Volpi)

the level of the glottis and the ETT is advanced under direct vision. High-flow oxygen and a jaw thrust were used with success.[11] A slight lift of the tongue with a laryngoscope blade (even if full insertion is not possible) can help with successful intubation.[12] In addition to this conventional intubation, the Bonfils can also be used to perform retromolar intubation and a direct-access intubation with head/neck flexion (Karl Storz endoscope). The technical specifications are provided in the manufacturer brochure (Karl Storz endoscope) and are summarized in Table 9.2.

The Bonfils intubation scope is one of the most widely studied optical stylets, in both adult and pediatric populations. Studies have shown that the Bonfils intubation endoscope is an effective intubation tool in adult patients with normal airways[3] and adult cardiac patients with failed laryngoscopy.[13] For pediatric intubation, the Bonfils scope comes in two sizes: one with an outer diameter of 2 mm (length 22 cm; ETT size up to 3.5 mm internal diameter) and the other with an outer diameter of 3.5 mm (length 35 cm; ETT size > 3.5 mm internal diameter).[11,14]

In a study of 55 children with normal airways and a mean age of 6 years, the pediatric Bonfils fiberscope had high failure rates and increased intubation times. The TTI was a median of 58 seconds with a very wide range of 14–377 seconds.[11] In another study of 50 healthy children aged 2–14 years, the use of the pediatric Bonfils scope was associated with significantly better laryngeal views, but this did not translate into easier intubations.[15] The effectiveness of a standard laryngoscope was compared to a Bonfils scope in a simulated difficult infant airway using manikins with 10 pediatric anesthesiologists and 150 intubations. The Bonfils scope provided a better view than direct laryngoscopy, but the success and TTI were not improved.[16,17]

In a randomized controlled comparison of the Bonfils scope and the GlideScope in 100 children aged < 7 years of age with normal airways, it was found that the intubation times were significantly shorter with a Bonfils scope (mean 36.5 seconds) as compared to GlideScope (mean 48.7 seconds).[14] During a pediatric simulated resuscitation, 126 paramedics participated in a randomized, crossover controlled study comparing Miller laryngoscopy to the Bonfils during resuscitation with and without chest compressions. The TTI was significantly shorter using the Bonfils.[18]

Successful intubation using the Bonfils has been described in a 6-year-old patient with Hurler's syndrome,[16] a 6-year-old with a Pfeiffer syndrome,[19] an 18-month-old with mosaic trisomy 1,[20] a 5-week-old with an unstable airway due to hemorrhagic lymphangiomata compressing the airway,[21] and a full-term 1.5 kg neonate with mandibular hypoplasia.[22] Kaufmann and colleagues compared tracheal intubation with the Bonfils versus fiberoptic scope in 26 children with difficult airways. This study included 46% infants, and mouth opening was restricted in 38%. Both the devices were suitable for pediatric difficult intubation. Intubation with the Bonfils was associated with a significantly shorter TTI and superior ease of intubation as compared to fiberscope.[12]

As seen above, the literature surrounding the use of the Bonfils in pediatrics is controversial. It is our opinion that the Bonfils is an important adjuvant in pediatric difficult intubation and may have a very limited role in normal airway intubations.

Chapter 9: Optical Stylet and Light-Guided Equipment and Techniques

Table 9.2 Specifications of Individual Devices

Device	Specifications	ETT size	Oxygen port	Light source	Type of fibers	Cleaning and sterilization
Bonfils	Outside diameter 3.5 mm and 5 mm; Length 35 cm and 40 cm	4.0–5.5 mm	Yes	LED	Glass	Waterproof; Sterilization up to 60°C; EtO
Adult Shikani optical stylet	Diameter 2.4 mm; Length 39.7 cm	5.5–9.0 mm	Yes	LED		Cidex or sterrad solution (no autoclave)
Pediatric Shikani optical stylet	Diameter 5.1 mm; Length 26.9 cm	2.5–5.0 mm	Yes	LED		Cidex or sterrad solution (no autoclave)
Levitan scope	Approximately 30 cm long; ends at a fitting that accepts the 15 mm connector of a tracheal tube	6.0 mm	Yes	LED		Can be cleaned in a variety of cold sterilization solutions
Malleable video stylet	Information not available					
SensaScope	6.0 mm	≥ 7.0 mm	No	LED	No fibers for image transmission; CMOS imager at distal end; Fibers are only used for illumination to optimize the illuminated field	Soak; EtO; Steris Sterrad 100
Stylet scope	6.0 mm	≥ 7.0 mm	No	Built into stylet handle and powered by 1.5 V alkaline battery	Plastic	Ethylene oxide

Advantages

The Bonfils scope can be used in patients with restricted mouth opening. An advantage is the continuous visualization of the passage of the tube into the trachea and the ability to continuously oxygenate using the side port during intubation.

The Bonfils intubation endoscope is relatively inexpensive and has a shorter preparation time. It is easily portable and can be moved to locations outside the operating room easily.[13] The learning curve is steep after a limited training period.[3]

Limitations

The main limitation is the lack of a suction channel, which can make visualization difficult in the presence of secretions and blood. When combined with a

Section 2: Devices and Techniques to Manage the Abnormal Airway

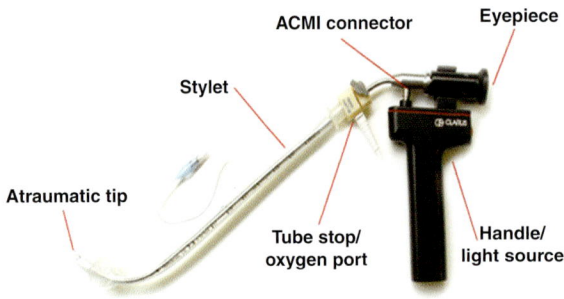

Figure 9.1 The Shikani optical stylet.

conventional laryngoscopy, a second operator is required, which is a major drawback, in emergency situations.[11]

Shikani Optical Stylet

Design

The Shikani optical stylet is a semimalleable stainless steel, J-shaped endoscope with illumination fibers (Figure 9.1). The distal end of this device can be shaped for different applications, including for use with and without a laryngoscope, and insertion through an SGA device. It has a central optical channel that ends in an eyepiece. Glass fiberoptic bundles of 30 000 pixels are used to deliver the image to a fixed focus. The light source of this device is supplied from a standard laryngoscope handle or a battery-powered LED source. The eyepiece can be connected to a video camera system and monitored when teaching and supervision is needed. The Shikani stylet has a proximal tube holder compatible with 15 mm ETT connector. This tube holder is movable by a tube stop adaptor on the stylet shaft, which allows appropriate positioning of the tip of the scope with the ETT. The stylet shaft is 27 cm long with a diameter of 5.0 mm ID range. It is available in a pediatric version compatible with ETTs in the 2.5 mm ID to 5.5 mm ID range.

The company also makes a flexible version of the optical stylet called the *Pocket Scope*. This device is used to confirm placement of a single- or double-lumen tube.

Most of the optical stylets, including Shikani, have a means of insufflating oxygen through the tube to clear secretions from the distal tip. There is debate about how much this is needed and how much oxygen is safe. The author has used low flow rates of 2 L/min. Insufflation should stop once the tip of the device enters the trachea to avoid barotrauma.

In his initial study, Shikani examined the use of the optical stylet in 120 patients: 74 were children, including seven with Cormack–Lehane grade III and IV views. All intubations, including five awake intubations, were successfully performed with the scope: 88% on the first attempt.[1]

A randomized controlled trial examined the Shikani optical stylet as an alternative to the GVL in 60 patients undergoing anesthesia, with a simulated difficult airway. All patients had rigid cervical collars applied to simulate a difficult airway. The study showed that intubation was successful in all patients, with first-attempt success rates of 97% in the GVL group compared with 93% in the Shikani group. The mean (SD) TTI was 64 seconds when using the GVL and 58 seconds in the Shikani group. The results suggest that the Shikani optical stylet provides a clinically comparable TTI with a high success rate, while potentially having lower risks of oral mucosal injury when compared with the GVL, in patients with a simulated difficult airway.[23]

Advantage

The potential benefits of the Shikani scope include improved laryngeal visualization, successful intubation while reducing trauma, improved portability and cost when compared with flexible fiberoptic bronchoscopy, and finally reduction in intubation forces, resulting in less cervical spine movement and hemodynamic stress. The narrow diameter of the stylet facilitates the negotiation of confined spaces, such as around a large epiglottis, and its malleability permits adaptation to unusual anatomical features. Setup times are short, and the appliance is easy to maintain. The Shikani optical stylet can overcome many of the disadvantages of other techniques utilized for difficult intubation like laryngeal-mask airway-guided fiberoptic tracheal intubation, which requires mouth opening sufficient to insert the laryngeal mask.[24,25] The Shikani optical stylet can be a valuable adjunct in this setting. Several authors describe a short learning curve, especially with the Clarus pediatric Shikani when compared with a fiberoptic bronchoscope.[25,26] A further important advantage of the Shikani scope and optical stylet in general is its portability. It could be a valuable aid to intubation in the field or prehospital and ED settings, as well as in the ICU.

Another advantage of the Shikani scope and optic stylets in general over the flexible fiberoptic bronchoscope is its lower cost and its reduced susceptibility to damage. It is a cheaper alternative for difficult intubation in developing countries than flexible fiberoptic technology. It may also be used as a lightwand alone when blood or secretions obscure or temporarily obscure the fiberoptic view.

Limitations

The limitations of the Shikani scope include the short depth of field[26] and poor visibility when the lens is covered in secretions. The short depth of field is not an issue with newer miniature video chip cameras: a wide field of view can be achieved with less noticeable distortion. None of the optical stylets, including Shikani, have a working channel of the type present on flexible fiberoptic bronchoscopes.

The ability to pass the stylet any distance beyond the vocal cords is restricted. Because of the rigidity of the stylets, practitioners should be careful as the ETT is passed into the trachea since the tube tip may impinge on the tracheal rings. To lessen the impaction of the tube on the tracheal rings, the ETT should be rotated clockwise as it is advanced off the stylet. This maneuver will turn the bevel from facing left to facing up, and the leading edge of the tube drops down, disengaging from the tracheal rings. Another important limitation is that it can only be used for oral intubations. Sore throat and minor hoarseness have been reported.[27,28]

Technique Pearls

The operator should optimize the image by adjusting the length and rotation of the ETT prior to use. The optical stylet should not protrude from the ETT and should be protected in the ETT as the distal tip of the stylet will be exposed to secretions and blood, and could injure the airway. The tube holder allows an ideal position for an ETT, which is just overlying (~2–5 mm) the distal tip of the optical stylet. So that the optical element is not exposed, it should not be set too far back, which would compromise the field of view. As with all fiberoptic instruments, insertion of the stylet into the patient's airway may result in an obscured view due to fogging. This can be avoided by applying a commercial antifog solution to the distal lens.

There are two techniques when using this device for intubation: a two-practitioner technique or a single-practitioner technique. For the single-practitioner technique, the Shikani stylet is held in the dominant hand of the operator. The non-dominant hand of the operator is used to provide jaw thrust and the tip of the stylet is placed along the curvature of the tongue in the midline. The Shikani stylet can be placed just past the vocal cords and the tube advanced into the trachea under direct vision. Some practitioners prefer a left-molar approach when using the stylet as a higher success rate with this method has been reported for novice users.[29] It is important to use maneuvers that enlarge the pharyngeal space. A simple maneuver can be the difference between success and failure. Options include a jaw thrust, pulling up on the tongue (using a gauze pad to assist with grip), or using a laryngoscope as a tongue retractor.

The ideal view through the eyepiece should reveal the base of the tongue in the upper half of the image and the space below the tongue in the lower half. If there is no visibility, slowly pull back on the stylet to help obtain a view. Advance the scope through the glottic opening and maintain visual confirmation while twisting the tube off the stylet; then gently remove the stylet by following the curves of the airway.

Devices Reported in the Adult Population
Clarus Video System

Clarus Medical has recently introduced a malleable stylet with an attached video screen (Clarus video system; previously named Trachway).[30] This is a video-based optical stylet with a proximal-mounted video screen, which can be angled by using a thumb control, and comes with a rechargeable battery. This scope has two light sources: two white light LEDs and one red LED, which can be used for anterior neck transillumination. The stylets are of different types and are interchangeable with the length of the ETT.

The advantages of the Clarus video system include direct observation during intubation and easy handling, and it easily overcomes resistance with pharyngeal soft tissues.[30,31] The modified jaw thrust (two-handed, aided by an assistant) is shown to be the most effective way to improve the laryngeal view and shorten intubation time as compared to single-handed chin lift or BURP maneuver.[32]

In a simulated difficult airway scenario with emergency physicians, successful intubation was performed on the first attempt 100% of the time and the Clarus video system was considered to be useful.[34]

In patients with a cervical collar, the Clarus video system had a quicker and easier intubation as compared to the airway scope with a mean intubation time of 19 seconds.[33] The Clarus video system has been successfully used for an awake intubation in an adult patient with halo cervical traction[35] and in another case of a double-lumen ETT intubation in a 54-year-old patient with an epiglottic cyst.[31]

Optiscope

An Optiscope (Pacific Medical) is derived from the Clarus video system and is designed specifically for a double-lumen ETT. This is a rigid video stylet with a malleable tip, a length of 40.5 cm, and an outer diameter of 5 mm. This stylet can accommodate a 35 fr or larger double-lumen ETT.[36] The TTI is a median 15 seconds and was found to be statistically significantly lower than a traditional laryngoscope. The other benefits of Optiscope were better Cormack–Lehane grades, higher first intubation success, and reduced oral mucosal and dental injury.[36] The use of an Optiscope is described in a 57-year-old patient with a difficult airway due to limited mouth opening and head extension.[37]

Levitan Scope

The Levitan scope is a semirigid intubating fiberscope.[38] An online video shows the setup and performance of intubation with the Levitan FPS optical stylet on a manikin and patients, and describes the anatomical landmarks during intubation.[39] The malleable steel surrounding the fiberoptic bundles is shorter than other optical stylets (29 cm). The Levitan scope was designed for use in conjunction with a laryngoscope. It can also be used without a laryngoscope, using a near right-angle bend (~70-degree bend) like the Shikani optical stylet, but its overall shorter length eliminates the height problem for most operators.

Greenland and colleagues compared the Levitan scope with the Portex tracheal introducer in a randomized crossover study of 34 patients. The authors found equal success and a shorter TTI with the tracheal introducer under simulated Cormack–Lehane grade III conditions.[40] However, Kovacs found equivalent success and TTI with the tracheal introducer and the Levitan scope in a manikin with fixed Cormack–Lehane grade III conditions.[41] Evans and colleagues found that the Levitan scope is a better device than the gum elastic bougie in simulated difficult tracheal intubation.[42] Aziz and colleagues examined the use of the Levitan stylet in the operating room as a solo device in 315 consecutive intubations. All intubations except one were successful (99.7%). The mean (SD) intubation times were 23 seconds. Three patients (1%) suffered minor trauma.[43]

Malleable Video Stylet

The malleable video stylet is a rechargeable, reusable, and a latex-free device. It consists of a full-color 1.5″ × 2″ video-display screen with a plug-in video stylet. The reusable stylet is indicated for 100 uses and has a two-hour battery life with USB charging capability. There is no literature describing the use of this stylet at the time of writing this chapter.

SensaScope

Design

The SensaScope (Figure 9.2) was first released in 2006.[44] It is a hybrid intubation device, which combines both the features of a rigid and a flexible scope. Subsequently, a "stand-alone" type of SensaScope was created. This newer version has an endoscope with an inbuilt camera and a light source that is connected to the video monitor via an interface consisting of a small box. The scope has no eyepiece and consists of a thin cable to the video interface, which is produced by a miniature CCD chip at the tip of the device and a tiny LED chip to produce light. The light intensity can be increased or reduced by a control on the handle of the stylet or on the video interface.[45]

At present, there are only a few studies using the SensaScope. Greif and colleagues studied the older

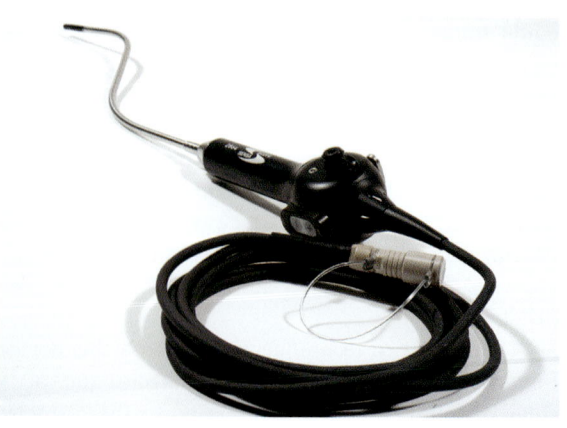

Figure 9.2 The SensaScope.

version of the SensaScope on 13 patients with known or predicted difficult airways. The patients were intubated with airway topicalization and sedation with midazolam or fentanyl with remifentanil infusion. In 9 of the 13 patients, advancement into the trachea was deemed easy, and a minority of patients had difficult visualization due to secretions.[46] In a simulated environment, 24 anesthesiologists were randomized to intubate a manikin with a Macintosh 3 laryngoscope or SensaScope. The SensaScope was beneficial in a difficult anatomy, but was more complicated to use in normal-anatomy manikins.[47]

Advantages

The thin version has increased the maneuverability of the scope and improved the image quality. The image fills up the whole rectangular display screen, unlike some of the older devices, which produce a small circular image at the center of the screen.[45]

Limitations

The SensaScope does not change the way traditional intubation is performed. The proper use of the device requires laryngoscopy and the indication for use in the inventor's institute is an unexpected difficult airway. It is not designed for nasal intubation. The device cannot be used in situations where secretions or blood impair the visualization of airway. The turnover time after use is 45 minutes for disinfection. A waterproof sleeve (SensaSleeve, Acutronic Medical Systems) is available to protect the device.[45] There are no studies to test its utility in rapid-sequence intubations or awake intubations. This device has not been tested in pediatric patients.

Stylet Scope

The fiberoptic stylet scope consists of a plastic fiberoptic imaging system, which is incorporated directly into an ETT stylet and has a diameter of 6.0 mm. The fiberoptic stylet scope can be used for ETT size 7.0 or larger. The basic design and the specifications are summarized in Table 9.2.

The fiberoptic stylet scope was first described in 1999 and is available in Asian markets. In 32 patients with a mean age of 57 years, the rate of successful intubation on the first attempt was 94% with the fiberoptic stylet scope and all others were successfully intubated on the second attempt.[27] In another study, 30 patients with normotension and 30 patients with hypertension were randomly assigned to intubation with a laryngoscope with or without the fiberoptic stylet scope. It was found that the fiberoptic stylet scope attenuated hemodynamic changes and reduced the incidence of sore throat in both normotensive and hypertensive patients.[48] It is not known if a pediatric version of the stylet scope is available. However, a case report describing an unsuccessful intubation with a stylet scope is described in a 35-week fetus during an EXIT procedure, the airway was successfully managed by tracheostomy.[49]

The advantage of this scope is the availability of a lever to manually control the tip. The device can be used successfully even without prior training.[27] The presence of plastic fibers in place of glass makes it resistant to breakage but the image produced is low quality.[8]

Devices Not Available for Commercial Use

Once a prototype device is introduced for commercial use, numerous devices with similar utility start to flow into the market. In 8 years, from 1995 to 2003, 10 new optical stylets were introduced.[8] Various devices have stood the test of time, while others are no longer commercially available (Table 9.1). In general, complexity in the use of the device, cost, and availability of better technology are some of the factors that contributed to commercial failure. Various lighted stylets have been extensively studied and shown to be effective in adults and children.[50] There is currently only a single manufacturer of lighted stylets in the USA.

Summary

Intubation of the difficult airway remains one of the major challenges in anesthesia, and no less so in children, although the incidence is lower. All practitioners are encouraged to explore new devices and techniques that facilitate intubation. The use of optical stylets is a valuable additional aid in pediatric patients with both normal and difficult airways. Data regarding the use of optical stylets in children are promising, but are still limited. Very few rigorous studies have evaluated the efficacy of optical stylets. An in-depth understanding of the device design, technical pearls, and frequent use in patients with normal airways are critical requirements to maximize the safe use of optical stylets in both normal and difficult airway management.

Section 2: Devices and Techniques to Manage the Abnormal Airway

References

1. Shikani AH. New "Seeing" Stylet-Scope and Method for the Management of the Difficult Airway. *Otolaryngology – Head and Neck Surgery* 1999; **120**(1): 113–16.

2. Rudolph C, Schlender M. Clinical Experiences with Fiber Optic Intubation with the Bonfils Intubation Fiberscope. *Anaesthesiologie und Reanimation* 1996; **21**(5): 127–30.

3. Halligan M, Charters P. A Clinical Evaluation of the Bonfils Intubation Fibrescope. *Anaesthesia* 2003; **58**(11): 1087–91.

4. Xue FS, Liu HP, Guo XL. Transillumination-Assisted Endotracheal Intubation with the Bonfils Fiberscope. *European Journal of Anaesthesiology* 2009; **26**(3): 261–2.

5. Gravenstein D, Liem EB, Bjoraker DG. Alternative Management Techniques for the Difficult Airway: Optical Stylets. *Current Opinion in Anaesthesiology* 2004; **17**(6): 495–8.

6. Katz RL, Berci G. The Optical Stylet – a New Intubation Technique for Adults and Children with Specific Reference to Teaching. *Anesthesiology* 1979; **51**(3): 251–4.

7. Berci G, Katz R. Optical Stylet: an Aid to Intubation and Teaching. *Annals of Otology, Rhinology, and Laryngology* 1979; **88**(Pt 1): 828–31.

8. Liem EB, Bjoraker DG, Gravenstein D. New Options for Airway Management: Intubating Fibreoptic Stylets. *British Journal of Anaesthesia* 2003; **91**(3): 408–18.

9. Bonfils P. Difficult Intubation in Pierre-Robin Children, a New Method: the Retromolar Route. *Der Anaesthesist* 1983; **32**(7): 363–7.

10. Bonfils P. Nasal Contralateral Intubation: a New Technique with a Fiberoptic Instrument. *Anaesthesist* 1982; **31**(7): 362–5.

11. Bein B, Wortmann F, Meybohm P, Steinfath M, Scholz J, Dorges V. Evaluation of the Pediatric Bonfils Fiberscope for Elective Endotracheal Intubation. *Paediatric Anaesthesia* 2008; **18**(11): 1040–4.

12. Kaufmann J, Laschat M, Engelhardt T, Hellmich M, Wappler F. Tracheal Intubation with the Bonfils Fiberscope in the Difficult Pediatric Airway: a Comparison with Fiberoptic Intubation. *Paediatric Anaesthesia* 2015; **25**(4): 372–8.

13. Bein B, Yan M, Tonner PH, Scholz J, Steinfath M, Dorges V. Tracheal Intubation Using the Bonfils Intubation Fibrescope after Failed Direct Laryngoscopy. *Anaesthesia* 2004; **59**(12): 1207–9.

14. Kaufmann J, Laschat M, Hellmich M, Wappler F. A Randomized Controlled Comparison of the Bonfils Fiberscope and the GlideScope Cobalt AVL Video Laryngoscope for Visualization of the Larynx and Intubation of the Trachea in Infants and Small Children with Normal Airways. *Paediatric Anaesthesia* 2013; **23**(10): 913–19.

15. Houston G, Bourke P, Wilson G, Engelhardt T. Bonfils Intubating Fibrescope in Normal Paediatric Airways. *British Journal of Anaesthesia* 2010; **105**(4): 546–7.

16. Aucoin S, Vlatten A, Hackmann T. Difficult Airway Management with the Bonfils Fiberscope in a Child with Hurler Syndrome. *Paediatric Anaesthesia* 2009; **19**(4): 421–2.

17. Vlatten A, Aucoin S, Litz S, MacManus B, Soder C. A Comparison of Bonfils Fiberscope-Assisted Laryngoscopy and Standard Direct Laryngoscopy in Simulated Difficult Pediatric Intubation: a Manikin Study. *Paediatric Anaesthesia* 2010; **20**(6): 559–65.

18. Szarpak L, Czyzewski L, Kurowski A. Can BONFILS Intubation Endoscope be an Alternative to Direct Laryngoscopy for Pediatric Tracheal Intubation during Resuscitation? *American Journal of Emergency Medicine* 2015; **33**(2): 293–4.

19. Caruselli M, Giretti R, Pallotto R, Rocchi G, Carboni L. Intubation Using a "Bonfils Fiberscope" in a Patient with Pfeiffer Syndrome. *Journal of Bronchology and Interventional Pulmonology* 2011; **18**(4): 374–5.

20. Laschat M, Kaufmann J, Wappler F. Management of a Difficult Airway in a Child with Partial Trisomy 1 Mosaic Using the Pediatric Bonfils Fiberscope. *Paediatric Anaesthesia* 2010; **20**(2): 199–201.

21. Krishnan PL, Thiessen BH. Use of the Bonfils Intubating Fibrescope in a Baby with a Severely Compromised Airway. *Paediatric Anaesthesia* 2013; **23**(7): 670–2.

22. Caruselli M, Zannini R, Giretti R, Rocchi G, Camilletti G, Bechi P, et al. Difficult Intubation in a Small for Gestational Age Newborn by Bonfils Fiberscope. *Paediatric Anaesthesia* 2008; **18**(10): 990–1.

23. Phua DS, Mah CL, Wang CF. The Shikani Optical Stylet as an Alternative to the GlideScope(R) Videolaryngoscope in Simulated Difficult Intubations – a Randomised Controlled Trial. *Anaesthesia* 2012; **67**(4): 402–6.

24. Jansen AH, Johnston G. The Shikani Optical Stylet: a Useful Adjunct to Airway Management in a Neonate with Popliteal Pterygium Syndrome. *Paediatric Anaesthesia* 2008; **18**(2): 188–90.

25. Pfitzner L, Cooper MG, Ho D. The Shikani Seeing Stylet for Difficult Intubation in Children: Initial Experience. *Anaesthesia and Intensive Care* 2002; **30**(4): 462–6.

26 Shukry M, Hanson RD, Koveleskie JR, Ramadhyani U. Management of the Difficult Pediatric Airway with Shikani Optical Stylet. *Paediatric Anaesthesia* 2005; **15**(4): 342–5.

27 Kitamura T, Yamada Y, Du HL, Hanaoka K. Efficiency of a New Fiberoptic Stylet Scope in Tracheal Intubation. *Anesthesiology* 1999; **91**(6): 1628–32.

28 Gravenstein D, Melker RJ, Lampotang S. Clinical Assessment of a Plastic Optical Fiber Stylet for Human Tracheal Intubation. *Anesthesiology* 1999; **91**(3): 648–53.

29 Yao YT, Jia NG, Li CH, Zhang YJ, Yin YQ. Comparison of Endotracheal Intubation with the Shikani Optical Stylet Using the Left Molar Approach and Direct Laryngoscopy. *Chinese Medical Journal* 2008; **121**(14): 1324–7.

30 Costa F, Mattei A, Massimiliano C, Cataldo R, Agro FE. The Clarus Video System as a Useful Diagnostic Tool. *Anaesthesia* 2011; **66**(2): 135–6.

31 Seo H, Lee G, Ha SI, Song JG. An Awake Double Lumen Endotracheal Tube Intubation Using the Clarus Video System in a Patient with an Epiglottic Cyst: a Case Report. *Korean Journal of Anesthesiology* 2014; **66**(2): 157–9.

32 Lee AR, Yang S, Shin YH, Kim JA, Chung IS, Cho HS, et al. A Comparison of the BURP and Conventional and Modified Jaw Thrust Manoeuvres for Orotracheal Intubation Using the Clarus Video System. *Anaesthesia* 2013; **68**(9): 931–7.

33 Kim JK, Kim JA, Kim CS, Ahn HJ, Yang MK, Choi SJ. Comparison of Tracheal Intubation with the Airway Scope or Clarus Video System in Patients with Cervical Collars. *Anaesthesia* 2011; **66**(8): 694–8.

34 Cooney DR, Cooney NL, Wallus H, Wojcik S. Performance of Emergency Physicians Utilizing a Video-Assisted Semi-Rigid Fiberoptic Stylet for Intubation of a Difficult Airway in a High-Fidelity Simulated Patient: a Pilot Study. *International Journal of Emergency Medicine* 2012; **5**(1): 24.

35 Cheng WC, Lan CH, Lai HY. The Clarus Video System (Trachway) Intubating Stylet for Awake Intubation. *Anaesthesia* 2011; **66**(12): 1178–80.

36 Yang M, Kim JA, Ahn HJ, Choi JW, Kim DK, Cho EA. Double-Lumen Tube Tracheal Intubation Using a Rigid Video-Stylet: a Randomized Controlled Comparison with the Macintosh Laryngoscope. *British Journal of Anaesthesia* 2013; **111**(6): 990–5.

37 Kim YR, Jun BH, Kim JA. The Use of the Clarus Video System for Double-Lumen Endobronchial Tube Intubation in a Patient with a Difficult Airway. *Korean Journal of Anesthesiology* 2013; **65**(1): 85–6.

38 Levitan RM. Design Rationale and Intended Use of a Short Optical Stylet for Routine Fiberoptic Augmentation of Emergency Laryngoscopy. *The American Journal of Emergency Medicine* 2006; **24**(4): 490–5.

39 Airway Cam (24 November 2007). The Levitan FPS Optical Stylet as an Independent Device. Online Video Clip. http://www.youtube.com/watch?v=TyYNstJbImY

40 Greenland KB, Liu G, Tan H, Edwards M, Irwin MG. Comparison of the Levitan FPS Scope and the Single-Use Bougie for Simulated Difficult Intubation in Anaesthetised Patients. *Anaesthesia* 2007; **62**(5): 509–15.

41 Kovacs G, Law JA, McCrossin C, Vu M, Leblanc D, Gao J. A Comparison of a Fiberoptic Stylet and a Bougie as Adjuncts to Direct Laryngoscopy in a Manikin-Simulated Difficult Airway. *Annals of Emergency Medicine* 2007; **50**(6): 676–85.

42 Evans A, Morris S, Petterson J, Hall JE. A Comparison of the Seeing Optical Stylet and the Gum Elastic Bougie in Simulated Difficult Tracheal Intubation: a Manikin Study. *Anaesthesia* 2006; **61**(5): 478–81.

43 Aziz M, Metz S. Clinical Evaluation of the Levitan Optical Stylet. *Anaesthesia* 2011; **66**(7): 579–81.

44 Biro P, Battig U, Henderson J, Seifert B. First Clinical Experience of Tracheal Intubation with the SensaScope, a Novel Steerable Semirigid Video Stylet. *British Journal of Anaesthesia* 2006; **97**(2): 255–61.

45 Biro P. The SensaScope – a New Hybrid Video Intubation Stylet. *Saudi Journal of Anaesthesia* 2011; **5**(4): 411–13.

46 Greif R, Kleine-Brueggeney M, Theiler L. Awake Tracheal Intubation Using the Sensascope in 13 Patients with an Anticipated Difficult Airway. *Anaesthesia* 2010; **65**(5): 525–8.

47 Ludwig AA, Baulig W, Biro P. A Simulated Severe Difficult Airway does Not Alter the Intubation Performance with the SensaScope: a Prospective Randomised Manikin Study. *European Journal of Anaesthesiology* 2011; **28**(6): 449–53.

48 Kimura A, Yamakage M, Chen X, Kamada Y, Namiki A. Use of the Fibreoptic Stylet Scope (Styletscope) Reduces the Hemodynamic Response to Intubation in Normotensive and Hypertensive Patients. *Canadian Journal of Anesthesia/Journal canadien d'anesthésie* 2001; **48**(9): 919–23.

49 Kai T, Ishibe N, Soeda Y, Tanaka M, Hoka S. Two Cases of Fetuses with Difficult Airway that Survived by the EXIT (Ex Utero Intrapartum Treatment) Procedure. *Masui* 2015; **64**(4): 373–8.

50 Davis L, Cook-Sather SD, Schreiner MS. Lighted Stylet Tracheal Intubation: a Review. *Anesthesia & Analgesia* 2000; **90**(3): 745–56.

Rigid Bronchoscopy Equipment and Techniques

Jessica M. Van Beek-King and Jeffrey C. Rastatter

Introduction

Rigid bronchoscopy is an important procedure practiced primarily by otolaryngologists and thoracic surgeons, which allows visualization of the trachea and proximal bronchi. The bronchoscope was introduced in 1806 by Bozzini.[1] Its first successful reported use was in 1897 when Gustav Killian retrieved an aspirated pork bone from the right mainstem bronchus, avoiding a tracheostomy.[2,3] Around the same period, Chevalier Jackson created his own illuminated endoscopes, and in 1907 published his findings in his landmark book, *Tracheobronchoscopy, Esophagoscopy and Bronchoscopy*.[3,4]

The modern bronchoscope has undergone several modifications, including the addition of the rod-lens telescope by Harold Hopkins and the cold illumination source by Karl Storz in the 1950s to allow for improved visualization.[3] In addition, the introduction of optical grasping forceps has improved therapeutic application, particularly with foreign-body retrieval.[3]

Performing bronchoscopy requires surgical skill, an experienced anesthesiologist, attentive support staff, and good communication and coordination among all team members.

Indications

In the pediatric population today, rigid bronchoscopy is used for the diagnosis and treatment of a variety of airway pathologies from the larynx to the proximal bronchi. For examination of the bronchial tree beyond the main bronchi, flexible bronchoscopy becomes a better tool. Indications include, but are not limited to, patients with stridor, unresolving and recurring pneumonitis, persistent atelectasis, persistent cough, tracheoesophageal fistula, airway trauma and tumor, and suspicion of foreign body.[1]

The ventilating bronchoscope allows for unhindered ventilation through the bronchoscope when the Hopkins telescope is removed. This feature allows for longer procedures in patients subject to hypoxia, and permits the rigid bronchoscope to be used to secure and ventilate a difficult airway. Furthermore, a child with a difficult airway may be intubated by placing an ETT directly over the Hopkins rod using the Seldinger technique.[1,5]

Therapeutic interventions are possible using rigid bronchoscopy. These include dilation of stenosis or scars, marsupialization or debulking of cysts or tumors (cold, cautery, laser, or other techniques), biopsy of lesions, brushing for cytology/bronchoalveolar lavage specimens, stent placement, and retrieval of foreign bodies. Visualization during foreign-body retrieval is greatly facilitated by using optical grasping forceps with an appropriate Hopkins rod.[1,6]

Necessary Equipment

1. **Rigid bronchoscope** (Figure 10.1)
   The rigid bronchoscope is available in several brands and sizes, but its general construction is

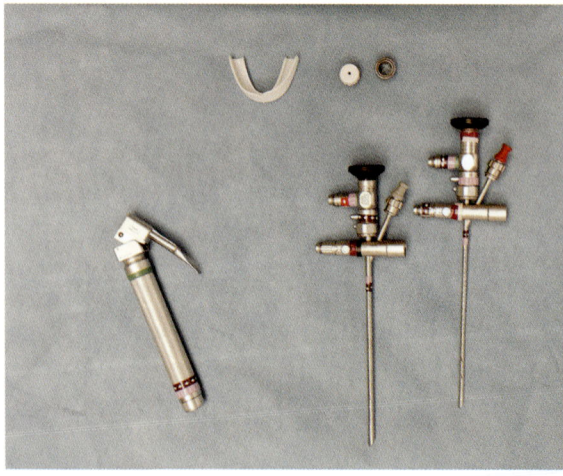

Figure 10.1 Rigid bronchoscope setup: rigid bronchoscopes fitted with appropriate Hopkins telescopes, solid prism light source, and covered side port. Also visualized is an intubating laryngoscope, tooth guard, glass eye, and rubber cover.

Table. 10.1 Approximate Karl Storz Rigid Bronchoscope Sizes Based on Age

For premature infants and children with other medical comorbidities known to potentially affect the structure or caliber of the airway, bronchoscope sizes should be adjusted appropriately.

Age	Bronchoscope size (Karl Storz)	
	Size	Outer diameter (mm)
Premature infant	2.5	3.7
Term newborn (newborn to 3 months)	3.0	5.0
6 months	3.5	5.7
18 months	3.7	6.3
3 years	4	6.7
5 years	5	7.8
10 years	6	8.2

similar. It consists of a solid metal tube, open on each end, and containing multiple ports.[6] The pediatric rigid bronchoscope is shorter and has a smaller diameter than those used in adults. The length is between 16 cm and 30 cm with an internal diameter from 3.2 mm to 7 mm.[7] The thickness of the tube itself measures 2 mm to 3 mm, which must be added to obtain the external diameter.[7] The Storz pediatric bronchoscope sizes range from a 2.5 to a 6. The 2.5 has an external diameter of 4.2 mm whereas the 6 is 8.2 mm.[8] It is important to choose the appropriately sized bronchoscope for a patient based on age and size to minimize airway trauma (Table 10.1). In addition, alternative sizes of bronchoscopes (a size up and down) should also be available if needed.

a. The tip of the bronchoscope is beveled to allow for careful maneuvering and to facilitate improved visualization. The distal third contains lateral ventilating holes: critical when working in the main bronchi to allow for ventilation of the contralateral lung.[6,8]

b. The proximal bronchoscope working port is grooved and connects to an adaptor used to secure the Hopkins telescope and allow for ventilation. On most bronchoscope models, there are three ports. One port connects to the ventilator circuit. An accordion extension is often useful to decrease tension by the circuit on the bronchoscope. A second port of entry allows passage of flexible suction, cautery, or laser devices. The third port accepts a solid prism light source. This is important to allow for visualization of the airway when the Hopkins rod is removed.[6]

2. **Hopkins telescope** (Figure 10.1)
The Hopkins telescope may be used by itself to visualize the airway. This is the preferred method by many surgeons for diagnostic bronchoscopy when the airway is easily exposed and the risk of oxygen desaturations during the procedure is low. When the Hopkins telescope is used in conjunction with the bronchoscope, it attaches via an adapter to the working port. Using this gasket creates a seal to allow continuous ventilation during the procedure.[6] The Hopkins rod comes in multiple lengths and diameters. It is important to select a Hopkins telescope of the appropriate length and diameter to properly fit each bronchoscope. The appropriately sized telescope should sit just proximal to the beveled tip of the bronchoscope. In addition, there should be adequate space around the rod to allow for ventilation and passage of flexible suction or other necessary devices. It is important to note that narrower diameter telescopes have an increased propensity to bend and fracture the optics. The telescope itself attaches to a light cord and source. In addition, the proximal telescope may be attached to a camera to allow for better visualization.

3. **Laryngoscope(s)** (Figure 10.1)
Laryngoscopes come in various styles and sizes (e.g., Macintosh, Miller, Parsons, Phillips). The laryngoscope is important to allow for visualization of the larynx to facilitate atraumatic intubation of the airway with the bronchoscope. In some difficult airway situations, visualization of the larynx may not be possible with a laryngoscope. In this case, the bronchoscope may be used to access the airway without prior laryngeal exposure by the laryngoscope.

Light Source and Cord

Each rigid bronchoscopy setup should contain two light sources and two light cords. One cord attaches via a prism to the bronchoscope itself. The second light source connects to the Hopkins telescope. It is imperative to have the second source attached to the bronchoscope to visualize the airway when the Hopkins rod is removed.

Monitoring Screens

Ideally, two video screens are available for the procedure. One screen is positioned straight on over the patient and is a view from the camera connected to the bronchoscope. The patient's vitals are placed on the second monitor. In this way, the surgeon is constantly aware of the state of the patient.

Tooth Guard

A rubber tooth guard or saline-soaked gauze (for edentulous children) should be used to protect the teeth and gingiva during bronchoscopy. In patients who undergo frequent bronchoscopy, consideration may be made to have a custom tooth guard fashioned. Although the bronchoscope should rest on the surgeon's finger and not on the patient's teeth, there is still a risk of damage to the teeth, which increases with difficulty of the airway.

Topical Anesthesia

Spontaneous breathing throughout the procedure is preferred during pediatric bronchoscopy. Therefore, patients typically do not receive neuromuscular blocking drugs, which increases the risk of laryngospasm. To decrease this risk, topical anesthesia is applied to the vocal cords via an atomizer prior to insertion of the bronchoscope. This is often facilitated with 1–4% topical lidocaine spray. The potency of lidocaine is dictated by weight of the child and the toxic dose.[7]

Suction and Tubing

An assortment of rigid large-bore suctions and flexible suctions that fit through the side port of the bronchoscope should be available. In addition, there should be functional suction with adequate length suction tubing.

Optical Grasping Forceps (Figure 10.2)

There are a variety of optical forceps available to the surgeon. These include up-and-straight cups, alligator forceps, biopsy forceps, and peanut graspers. A Hopkins rod fits within the forceps for improved visualization. The unit as a whole slides into the main channel of a size 3.5 Storz bronchoscope or larger. These are especially useful for retrieval of foreign bodies.[9]

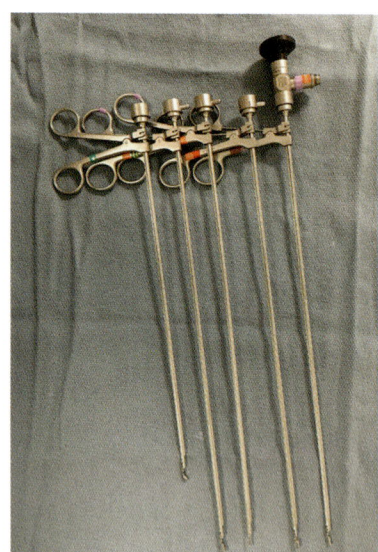

Figure 10.2 Variety of optical forceps equipped with appropriately fitting Hopkins telescope. The optical forceps fit into a size 3.5 Storz bronchoscope or larger.

Glass Eye

A glass viewing eye can be placed on the proximal end of the bronchoscope with the Hopkins telescope removed. This allows for a seal and improved ventilation of the patient while still being able to visualize the airway.

Accessory Equipment

Other equipment may be necessary in certain situations for endoscopic intervention. These can be passed through the working or accessory ports.

- **Balloons**
  Balloons can be useful to dilate areas of stenosis.[6]
- **Bugby catheters**
  The bugby catheter is useful for marsupialization of subglottic or other airway cysts, and for hemostasis.
- **Flexible lasers**
  Flexible lasers are often useful for dilation of stenosis or excision of granulation tissue, and other masses or lesions.[6]

Chapter 10: Rigid Bronchoscopy Equipment and Techniques

Technique

Prior to every bronchoscopy, it is imperative to ensure all equipment is present, functional, and well organized. The surgeon and operating-room staff should be familiar with all equipment. In addition, a discussion should be held with anesthesia and support staff to optimize preparation for each case.

Anesthetic Induction

Anesthesia places the patient under general anesthesia while ideally still spontaneously breathing. This plane of anesthesia can be obtained by administering a volatile anesthetic agent, such as sevoflurane supplemented with intravenous propofol, once an intravenous line is secured. Alternatively, total intravenous anesthesia can be used by administering propofol and opioids such as remifentanil.

Ability to bag-mask-ventilate the patient is confirmed by the anesthesiologist. If there is resistance, an oral airway with jaw thrust are often beneficial.[1,10]

Patient Positioning (Figure 10.3)

The head of bed is turned 90 degrees toward the surgeon. The surgeon confirms continued ability to bag-mask-ventilate. The patient is kept in the supine position with the head at the top edge of the bed. The chest is exposed to visualize chest rise. The height of the bed is adjusted to approximately the xyphoid process of the surgeon in the seated position. An upper tooth guard or saline-soaked gauze is placed to protect the upper dentition or gingiva. The head of the patient is placed in slight extension with the non-dominant hand to expose the glottic plane.[3,7]

Monitor Positioning

Two monitors should be used for the procedure. The first should be positioned straight on from the surgeon over the patient and shows the bronchoscopy itself. The second should be positioned in the surgeon's indirect line of sight and display the patient's vitals. The bronchoscopy equipment should all be easily accessible and tension free at operating length.

Laryngeal Exposure

The preferred laryngoscope of the surgeon is used to expose the glottis. Excessive secretions are suctioned, as necessary, being careful not to trigger laryngospasm. The vocal cords are sprayed with topical anesthetic via an atomizer. The patient is mask-ventilated to allow the anesthetic agent to take effect. Once appropriate time has passed, the larynx is re-exposed. Good exposure of the larynx may often require external laryngeal manipulation and/or cricoid pressure.

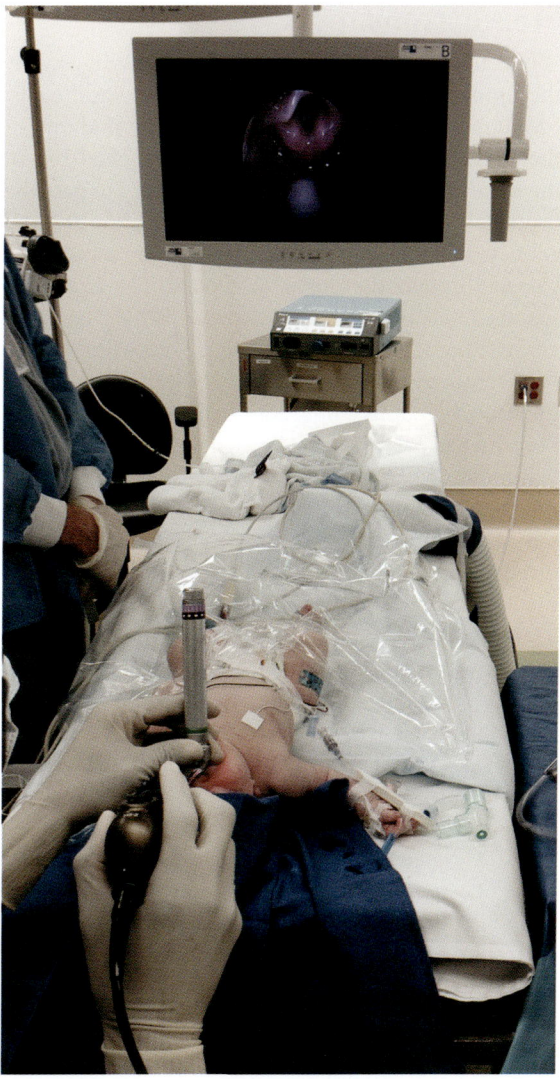

Figure 10.3 Optimum patient positioning for rigid bronchoscopy and airway evaluation in a neonatal patient.

Laryngoscopy

The Hopkins telescope alone or the bronchoscope is passed through the oral cavity to visualize the larynx. The larynx is inspected for any abnormalities. Mobility of the vocal folds is assessed.

Bronchoscopy

While the larynx is exposed with the laryngoscope, the bronchoscope is passed through the vocal folds. Ideally, the scope is passed when the vocal folds are in the abducted position. If the vocal folds are fixed in the medialized position, or if it is necessary to pass the bronchoscope while the vocal folds are in the adducted position, the bronchoscope should be passed through the posterior glottis. The bronchoscope should be rotated 90 degrees to help facilitate an atraumatic entry. The laryngoscope is then carefully removed from the mouth. The middle finger of the bronchoscopist's non-dominant hand is placed in the patient's palate for the bronchoscope to rest on. It is important that downward torque is not applied to the teeth when moving the rigid scope. The palm of the non-dominant hand is rested on the patient's forehead to help control the head and allow for easier maneuvering of the bronchoscope.[3,6,7]

If exposure is not able to be attained with the laryngoscope, the bronchoscope may be passed without direct visualization of the larynx. In this event, the non-dominant hand is positioned as above to extend the patient's head and protect the teeth. The bronchoscope is inserted into the right side of the mouth and passed along the right glossotonsillar sulcus. The tongue is gently elevated to view the epiglottis. The scope is placed posteriorly along the posterior pharyngeal wall and under the epiglottis. The epiglottis is carefully lifted to expose the glottis. At this point, the bronchoscope is turned 90 degrees to traverse the cords.

The bronchoscope is connected to the anesthesia circuit to allow for ventilation. An accordion connector may be useful to decrease tension from the circuit. The bronchoscope is rotated back to the usual orientation. The immediate subglottis is inspected. The bronchoscope is then passed distally to visualize the trachea, carina, and bronchi. To view the left bronchi, the patient's head should be turned to the right and opposite for the right bronchi. If any resistance is encountered during the procedure, consideration should be made to use a smaller bronchoscope.[3,6]

Secretions may be suctioned with a rigid suction by removing the Hopkins rod. The second light source allows the surgeon to visualize the distal airway and suction with the naked eye. Alternatively, a flexible suction catheter (generally 4–6 fr) can be passed through the accessory port along the Hopkins telescope. Should the patient become hypoxic, the Hopkins rod can be removed and the end of the bronchoscope blocked off with a finger or glass eye to allow for immediate oxygenation/ventilation.[3]

Therapeutic Interventions

During bronchoscopy, therapeutic interventions may be undertaken to address pathology. These include bronchoalveolar lavage or brushing for cytology, balloon and rigid dilation of stenosis, biopsy, debulking of cysts or tumors, stent placement, and retrieval of foreign bodies. For retrieval of foreign bodies, the optical grasping forceps are invaluable. There are a variety of optical forceps. If the object is known, the grasper that would most likely provide the best chance of retrieval is selected, with alternative graspers available.[3]

Post-Bronchoscopy Management

For routine bronchoscopy, antibiotics are generally not indicated. However, in the event of a postobstructive pneumonia they may be necessary.[7] Steroids may be given to decrease edema at the discretion of the surgeon. Chest films may be needed following therapeutic intervention to ensure a pneumothorax is not present.[8]

Most patients can be monitored in the postanesthesia care unit and discharged on the same day following a diagnostic or only minimal intervention bronchoscopy. Little-to-no analgesia is required. Humidified air or oxygen may be useful to help the patient clear any excessive secretions.[7]

If the patient undergoes a more invasive intervention, remains intubated, there is concern of airway obstruction or edema, or there are significant other medical comorbidities, then monitoring the patient on the inpatient ward or ICU may be necessary.

Complications

Risk of complication varies based on underlying airway pathology, type and difficulty of therapeutic intervention, experience of the surgeon, and the patient's medical comorbidities.[7]

The most common complications are related to oxygenation and ventilation. Frequently, patients may become hypoxic or hypercapnic, which may lead to bradycardia, cardiac arrhythmias, and arrest. Barotrauma can occur (e.g., pneumothorax, pneumomediastinum) from inadequate egress of air from insufflation of oxygen during bronchoscopy.[6,7]

Introduction of the laryngoscope, the Hopkins telescope, or bronchoscope can damage the teeth, gingiva, or surrounding soft tissue. It is important to be aware of the bronchoscope position with regards to the lips and teeth to avoid pinching the lip with the scope or against the teeth. In addition, downward force should not be placed onto the maxillary teeth with the bronchoscope. The tooth guard or saline-soaked gauze and adequate hand positioning can help minimize this risk. If dentition is damaged, a dental consult should be acquired.[6,7]

When passing the bronchoscope, gentle maneuvering around the soft tissue of the posterior pharyngeal wall and epiglottis is important to avoid laceration and/or laryngeal fracture. In addition, there may be damage to the arytenoids or vocal folds when traversing this area. Ensuring that the bronchoscope passes through abducted vocal cords, posteriorly and at a 90-degree angle can help to minimize laryngeal trauma. Furthermore, placing the bronchoscope into the subglottic region and trachea can trigger a vagotonic response and bradycardia, which is typically more pronounced in children < 6 months of age.[7,8]

Significant trauma from the bronchoscope itself or from the therapeutic intervention could potentially induce a pneumothorax. If a pneumothorax is suspected, all operating-room staff should be made aware of the situation, a chest film obtained immediately and appropriate surgical team consulted for chest tube placement.[6]

References

1. Basu A. Pediatric Airway Endoscopy. *Journal of Indian Association of Pediatric Surgeons* 2016; **21**(1): 6–7.
2. Zollner F. Gustav Killian: Father of Bronchoscopy. *Archives of Otlaryngology* 1965; **82**: 656–9.
3. Nicastri D, Weiser T. Rigid Bronchoscopy: Indications and Techniques. *Operative Techniques in Thoracic and Cardiovascular Surgery* 2012; **17**(1): 44–51.
4. Boyd A. Chevalier Jackson: The Father of American Bronchoesophagoscopy. *Annals of Thoracic Surgery* 1994; **57**: 502–5.
5. Wilkinson S, Sudarashn P, Smyth A, et al. The Role of Airway Endoscopy in Children. *Paediatrics and Child Health* 2015; **25**(4): 182–6.
6. Petrella F, Borri A, Casiraghi M, et al. Operative Rigid Bronchoscopy: Indications, Basic Techniques and Results. *Multimedia Manual of Cardio-Thoracic Surgery* 2014; 1–6.
7. Perez-Frias J, Galdo A, Ruiz E, et al. Pediatric Bronchoscopy Guidelines. *Archivos de Bronconeumología* 2011; **47**(7): 350–60.
8. Nicolai T. The Role of Rigid and Flexible Bronchoscopy in Children. *Paediatric Respiratory Reviews* 2011; **12**: 190–5.
9. Ganie A, Ahangar G, Lone, et al. The Efficacy of Rigid Bronchoscopy for Foreign Body Aspiration. *Bulletin of Emergency and Trauma* 2014; **2**(1): 52–4.
10. Malherbe S, Whyte S, Singh P, et al. Total Intravenous Anaesthesia and Spontaneous Respiration for Airway Endoscopy in Children – a Prospective Evaluation. *Paediatric Anaesthesia* 2010; **20**: 434–8.

Section 2 Devices and Techniques to Manage the Abnormal Airway

Chapter 11

Hybrid Approaches to the Difficult Pediatric Airway

Patrick N. Olomu, Grace Hsu, and Justin L. Lockman

Despite advances in equipment for difficult airway management, no individual device or technique has a 100% success rate: every device and technique has known limitations.[1] In recent years, hybrid techniques have been increasingly recognized as important difficult airway management options.[2] Hybrid techniques involve the simultaneous use of at least two different modalities for management of the difficult airway. The goal of these techniques is to take advantage of the best features of each device, while minimizing disadvantages.

The goal of this chapter is to review some of the more common hybrid approaches to the pediatric difficult airway. The following hybrid techniques will be discussed in this chapter:

- fiberoptic tracheal intubation through a supraglottic airway
- video laryngoscopy-assisted fiberoptic intubation (VLAFOI)
- retrograde-assisted fiberoptic intubation (RAFOI)

Fiberoptic Tracheal Intubation Through the SGA Device

Dr. Archie Brain first invented the LMA in 1983 and then introduced it into clinical practice in 1988. Since then, the SGA device has been commonly used for elective anesthetic care and has also filled a critical role in the management of failed ventilation in difficult airway algorithms for both adults and children.[3,4] In difficult airway management, an SGA device can provide oxygenation and ventilation for a patient who is difficult to mask-ventilate, and may also provide a conduit for tracheal intubation in a patient who is difficult to tracheally intubate. There are several advantages to using the SGA device to assist in tracheal intubation in difficult airway management. First, the SGA device can be placed awake in select children with severe upper airway obstruction and then used to induce inhalational general anesthesia; this technique provides a continual means to overcome airway obstruction, provide oxygenation, and maintain positive-pressure ventilation during general anesthesia. Additionally, the SGA device often aligns the airway to provide an effective oropharyngeal conduit for FOI in patients who are otherwise difficult to intubate fiberoptically. Similarly, in children with unanticipated difficult airways, the SGA device serves as both a rescue ventilation and oxygenation device, and also the very conduit through which a patient may ultimately be tracheally intubated.

The LMA

The use of the LMA Classic as a conduit for fiberoptic-guided tracheal intubation was described by Heard and colleagues.[5] However, given that it was not designed for this purpose, there are several limitations.[6] The LMA airway tube and tracheal tubes are often similar in length, making it challenging to remove the LMA without dislodging the tracheal tube. A number of techniques have been described to mitigate this problem. One solution is to use a longer-than-standard tracheal tube.[7] Some providers have advocated a temporary increase in the length of the tracheal tube by telescoping a second uncuffed tracheal tube of the same size or smaller into the proximal end of the desired cuffed tracheal tube.[8,9] This double tracheal tube assembly allows the clinician to hold the distal tracheal tube in place while removing the LMA from the mouth, but does include a risk of tracheal tube disconnection. Another technique is to stabilize the tracheal tube with microlaryngeal forceps while removing the LMA. In some situations, the LMA may remain in place during a procedure, but this leads to difficulty in securing the tracheal tube and is generally not a good long-term solution for patients who remain intubated following surgery.[10] Additionally, one may cut and shorten the

LMA airway tube prior to removal; the disadvantage of this technique is that one then destroys the ability to further use the LMA for oxygenation or ventilation.[11]

Another limitation of the LMA as a conduit for intubation is that it has aperture bars designed to prevent the epiglottis from occluding the distal end of the shaft. The bars narrow the conduit and must be cut and removed for the LMA to accommodate a cuffed tracheal tube and its pilot balloon; thereby removing the protective design feature. Third, the aperture of the airway connector on an LMA is not wide enough to accommodate the pilot balloon of a cuffed tracheal tube: the pilot balloon must be cut to allow the tracheal tube to pass through the shaft during LMA removal. While a severed pilot balloon may be repaired, the extra time and steps may delay necessary positive-pressure ventilation. Repairing the pilot balloon involves insertion of a 22-gauge angiocatheter into the inflation line tubing and needleless attachment of a one-way valve to the proximal end of the angiocatheter. The cuff may subsequently be inflated to the desired pressure using the needleless one-way valve.[12]

air-Q

Several intubating SGA devices have been developed: the most well studied is the air-Q intubating laryngeal airway.[13,14] The air-Q has an oval-shaped mask with a short and wide shaft. It has a number of unique features that are useful in SGA device-assisted tracheal intubation. First, the mask is oval-shaped and has ridges; improving the seal of the cuff against the oropharynx. Second, the air-Q has an easily removable 15 mm circuit adapter. This feature eliminates one of the narrowest portions of the air-Q and potential areas where a tracheal tube pilot balloon can become lodged during SGA device removal after tracheal intubation.[13] Third, the air-Q has a raised mask heel near the ventilating orifice of the shaft, designed to prevent epiglottic obstruction of the airway tube. As such, the air-Q does not have aperture bars, and thus does not need to be modified to use as a conduit for tracheal intubation with cuffed tracheal tubes. Additionally, the air-Q has a wide shaft, able to accommodate a tracheal tube that is larger than typically necessary for a patient of a given weight. Air-Q sizing is demonstrated in Table 11.1, and should be based on the patient's ideal

Table 11.1 Air-Q Available Sizes and Sizing Recommendations

Size	Ideal body weight	Maximum TT
0.5	< 4 kg	4.0 mm
1.0	4–7 kg	4.5 mm
1.5	7–17 kg	5.0 mm
2.0	17–30 kg	5.5 mm
2.5	30–50 kg	6.5 mm
3.5	50–70 kg	7.5 mm
4.5	70–100 kg	8.5 mm

body weight. The wide shaft is helpful in the circumstance a patient has limited mouth opening and can only accommodate a smaller-than-standard SGA device, but still needs an appropriately sized cuffed tracheal tube.[15]

Finally, the air-Q has a shaft that is 2–3 cm shorter than the shaft of the LMA Classic. This improves ease of removal of the SGA device after tracheal intubation as the proximal end of the tracheal tube is generally well above the shaft of the air-Q. Cookgas also produces a removal stylet for stabilization of the tracheal tube during SGA device removal. Successful removal of the air-Q with or without the removal stylet has been well described.[14,16] Another device that has been used in a similar fashion with comparable results is the Ambu Aura-i.[13]

Technique for Fiberoptic-Guided Tracheal Intubation Through a Supraglottic Airway Device (Video 3 and Video 4)

Placing the SGA Device

Consider deepening anesthesia while preserving spontaneous ventilation by slowly administering 0.5–1 mcg/kg dexmedetomidine intravenously. Open the patient's mouth and elevate the tongue either via a mandibular lift or a tongue blade at the base of the tongue. Place the device in the mouth and advance it into the oropharynx, applying gentle downward and inward pressure, following the curvature of the mask and shaft. Advance until resistance to forward motion is felt. Once the SGA device is in its final position, air may be added or removed from the mask to obtain an optimal seal.

Fiberoptic Tracheal Intubation Through an SGA Device

Disconnect the anesthesia circuit from the device and remove the 15 mm circuit adapter, being careful not to misplace it. The air-Q includes a connector to prevent loss of this device. Place the fiberoptic bronchoscope through a cuff-deflated tracheal tube and insert the fiberoptic bronchoscope into the shaft of the SGA device. Advance the fiberoptic bronchoscope through the SGA device. In general, a well-seated SGA device will allow for easy visualization of the glottis at the aperture, whereas a poor view may mean the SGA device is improperly seated in the airway. Consider application of topical lidocaine to the vocal cords. Advance the fiberoptic bronchoscope past the vocal cords and visualize the tracheal carina. While maintaining fiberoptic bronchoscope visualization of the carina, advance the tracheal tube over the fiberoptic bronchoscope and confirm tracheal tube placement via bronchoscopy, exhaled carbon dioxide, and auscultation. If there is difficulty advancing the tracheal tube past the vocal cords, externally manipulate the glottis toward the direction of the tracheal tube.

Removal of the SGA Device Over the Tracheal Tube

To remove the SGA device after tracheal intubation, disconnect the tracheal tube from the anesthesia circuit. Remove the tracheal tube (not the SGA device) 15 mm adapter. For air-Q SGA devices, the disposable air-Q removal stylet may be inserted into the proximal end of the tracheal tube and used for stabilization of the tracheal tube during withdrawal of the air-Q over the tracheal tube and removal stylet. Remove the stylet. Reinsert the tracheal tube 15 mm adapter, reconnect the tracheal tube to the anesthesia circuit, and reconfirm acceptable tracheal tube position. For other SGA devices (or as an alternative technique for air-Q SGA devices), laryngeal forceps, the fiberoptic bronchoscope, an airway exchange catheter, or a second tracheal tube may be used to stabilize the tracheal tube during removal of the SGA device (Figure 11.1 and Figure 11.2).

Technique Modification: Fiberoptic Tracheal Intubation Through an SGA Device with Continuous Ventilation (Video 4)

For select patients, it may be desirable to avoid the apneic period required to perform fiberoptic intubation through the SGA device as described above. In these situations, a modification of the technique allows tracheal intubation through an SGA device while also providing continuous positive-pressure ventilation. Doing so requires preparation of an SGA device and tracheal tube apparatus by removal of the 15 mm circuit adapter from the SGA device and partial insertion of a lubricated, cuffed tracheal tube into the shaft of the SGA device. Inflation of the tracheal tube cuff creates a seal, allowing for ventilation through the apparatus when a circuit is attached to the 15 mm adapter of the tracheal tube. By attaching a bronchoscope swivel adapter to the proximal

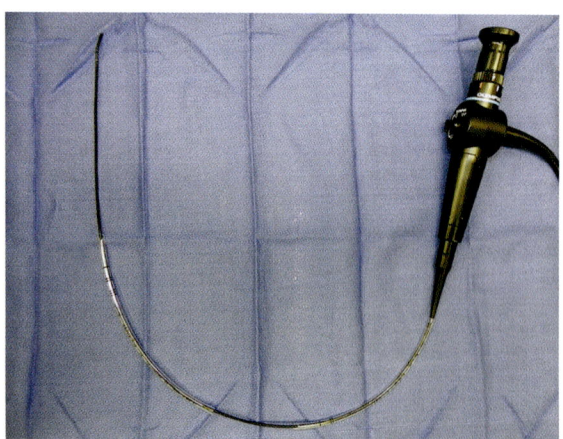

Figure 11.1 Fiberoptic bronchoscope with two tracheal tubes of the same size. The proximal tracheal tube will telescope into the distal tracheal tube to hold it in place during removal of the SGA device.

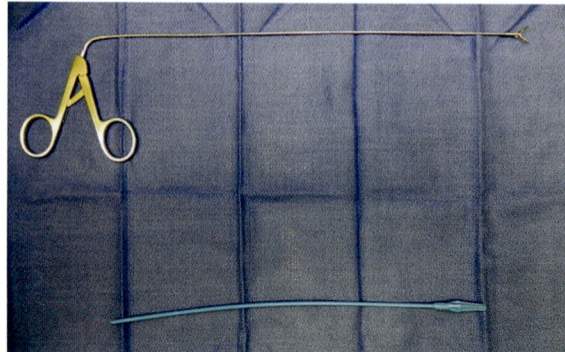

Figure 11.2 Laryngeal forceps and the air-Q removal stylet to aid in holding the tracheal tube in place while removing the SGA device.

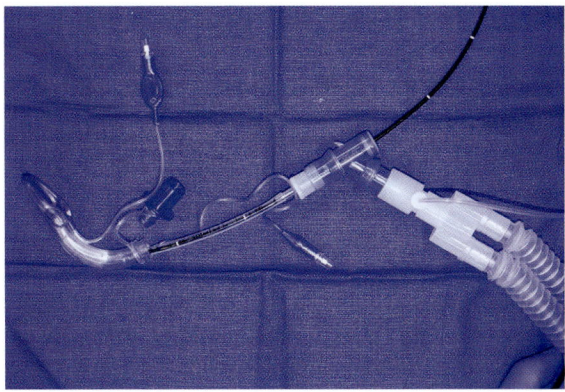

Figure 11.3 SGA device and tracheal tube apparatus for continuous ventilation. A bronchoscopic swivel adaptor is attached to the end of the tracheal tube and to the anesthesia circuit. The tracheal tube is inserted into the SGA device, and the cuff of the tracheal tube inflated.

end of the tracheal tube, fiberoptic intubation and visualization of the tracheal carina may be performed through the swivel adapter, the tracheal tube, and the SGA device (in series) while ventilation is maintained (Figure 11.3). Next, the provider deflates the tracheal tube cuff and advances the tracheal tube over the fiberoptic bronchoscope and into the trachea, often still without interrupting ventilation. Once tracheal tube position has been confirmed, the SGA device may be removed as described above: this is the only time during the procedure when ventilation must be stopped briefly.

Indications

There are special circumstances in which the SGA device is particularly useful as a conduit for tracheal intubation in the child with a difficult airway. One of these circumstances is after placement of the SGA device in the awake infant. A neonate who has severe upper airway obstruction and cannot tolerate being supine, such as one with Pierre Robin sequence, can have the SGA device placed while he is awake and prone. With the patient breathing spontaneously, anesthesia can then be induced with sevoflurane.[17] In the older infant who has an intact gag reflex, after appropriate local anesthetic topicalization of the oropharynx, an SGA device may also be inserted while the patient is awake. With a gloved finger, one can swab the infant's posterior oropharynx with 2% lidocaine gel. Local anesthetic can also be delivered to the oropharynx via a pacifier with multiple perforations.[18] Additionally, the SGA device can be inserted in an awake infant if it is lubricated with viscous lidocaine.[16] In some patients who undergo awake SGA device placement, awake fiberoptic intubation via an SGA device may also be beneficial; in others, induction of anesthesia proceeds smoothly after adequate ventilation via an SGA device is established.

Although controversial, some experts have recommended using the SGA device as a conduit for tracheal intubation during rapid-sequence induction of a child with an anticipated difficult airway, history of severe upper airway obstruction, and an increased risk for aspiration, such as an infant with Pierre Robin sequence and comorbid severe gastroesophageal reflux.[19] A suggested induction sequence would be as follows: Obtain intravenous access before induction. Decompress the stomach by placing a nasogastric tube and suctioning repeatedly (in different patient positions) until no fluid returns. Remove the nasogastric tube. Topicalize the airway with local anesthetic. Place the SGA device into the pharynx. Remove the 15 mm SGA device circuit adapter. Preload a fiberoptic bronchoscope with an appropriately sized and lubricated cuffed tracheal tube. Place the fiberoptic bronchoscope through the SGA device until a view of the larynx is obtained. While viewing the larynx with the fiberoptic bronchoscope, administer intravenous medications (i.e., propofol and succinylcholine). When the patient is paralyzed, advance the fiberoptic bronchoscope into the trachea, and thread the tracheal tube over the fiberoptic bronchoscope. When tracheal intubation is confirmed, remove the SGA.

Contraindications

There are relative contraindications to using an SGA device as a conduit for tracheal intubation. These include when the patient has limited mouth opening, has restricted head and neck movement, or when their oropharyngeal anatomy is distorted and malaligned.[20]

Tips for Success

Simple techniques can increase the likelihood of successful tracheal intubation through an SGA device. An important consideration is using an appropriately sized fiberoptic bronchoscope for the tracheal tube. Using a fiberoptic bronchoscope that is too thin for a tracheal tube increases the likelihood of the tracheal tube veering off midline and catching on the posterior arytenoids when attempting to thread the tracheal tube into the trachea.

When a fiberoptic view of the larynx is not optimal, one can perform these maneuvers to improve the view: jaw thrust, head and neck extension, advancing the SGA device, or withdrawing the SGA device without completely removing it.[21]

Complications

Blind intubation through an SGA device is not recommended in children as there is a high percentage of epiglottic downfolding, even when an SGA device has a good pharyngeal seal and ventilation is normal. Jagannathan and colleagues found that epiglottic downfolding occurred in 17/60 (28%) intubation attempts when an air-Q was used, and 12/60 (20%) times when an Aura-i was used. In these instances, the operator was still able to obtain a full view of the vocal cords by guiding the fiberoptic bronchoscope beneath the epiglottis.[13]

Another potential complication in tracheal intubation through an SGA is tracheal tube dislodgement during removal of the SGA device. Galgon and colleagues reported inadvertent extubation in 3/100 (3%) instances during air-Q removal over a tracheal tube.[22] Wong and colleagues reported a similar rate of tracheal tube dislodgement at 6/291.[23]

VLAFOI

Combination techniques, such as direct laryngoscopy with FOI, have previously been described; in these techniques, direct laryngoscopy is used to elevate the tongue and surrounding tissues, providing a path for the fiberoptic bronchoscope.[2]

The last decade has seen an explosion of devices utilizing video technology for airway management. Commonly used video laryngoscopes include GlideScope, C-MAC, Truview PCD, King Vision (Ambu), and McGrath MAC. Some devices have a guiding channel to direct the tracheal tube toward the glottis, including Airtraq, Pentax airway scope, and the King Vision.[24]

Most video laryngoscopes and optical stylets have the advantage of a wide angle of view (40–80 degrees), provision of a magnified and indirect image of the glottis, an antifogging mechanism, and a form of recording capability. Because of the curvature of most video laryngoscope blades, a stylet is usually required to guide the tracheal tube along the blade. Some devices such as the C-MAC and channeled devices such as the McGrath MAC may be used without a stylet.

Introduced in 2001, the GlideScope is the prototype video laryngoscope and one of the most extensively studied video laryngoscopes. Despite a very high intubation success rate, Cooper and colleagues reported a failure rate of 3.7% in intubation with the GlideScope in normal adults.[25] Similarly, Aziz and colleagues found a 3% failure rate in adults.[1] Despite improvement in the Cormack–Lehane grade in video laryngoscopy when compared to direct laryngoscopy, intubation attempts may still result in failure in difficult cases. Combination techniques using another modality, such as the fiberoptic bronchoscope, can improve the intubation success rate in difficult airway management.[26] The ability to use the fiberoptic bronchoscope as a controllable and maneuverable stylet becomes an important technique to achieve successful intubation in video laryngoscopy. FOI also has its own limitations. There is a steep learning curve to mastering the fiberoptic bronchoscope. The scope provides only a narrow-angle view of the airway, and fogging, secretions, and blood can render it unusable. Oropharyngeal soft tissue and anatomical distortion may make it challenging to maintain the fiberoptic bronchoscope in a midline position, and thus also cause difficulty in advancing the scope. Combining both the video laryngoscope and fiberoptic bronchoscope has the potential to maximize the advantages of both devices, and to overcome their individual limitations.

Much of the reported uses of VLAFOI has been case reports or case series.[27-30] Lenhardt and colleagues compared VLAFOI with video laryngoscopy only and found VLAFOI to be a feasible alternative to video laryngoscopy-only intubations in adult patients with predicted or known difficult airways.[26] The largest case collection of VLAFOI in pediatrics can be found in the PeDI Registry. Of the 71 reported cases of VLAFOI in the PeDI Registry, 56 (79%) were successful. Patient ages ranged from 0.5 to 310 months and weights ranged from 2.2 to 106 kg (unpublished report).

Practical Technique of VLAFOI (Figures 11.4–10 and Video 9)

Prior to performing VLAFOI, it is important to enlist the help of another clinician who is familiar with both

Chapter 11: Hybrid Approaches to the Difficult Pediatric Airway

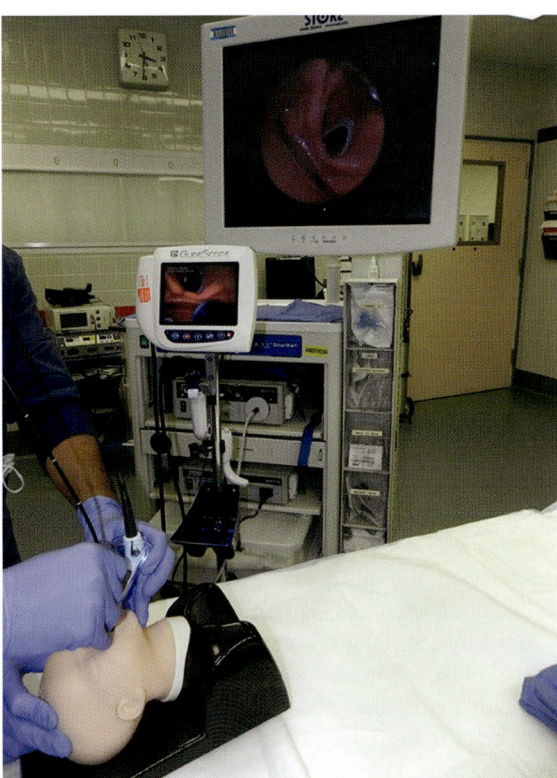

Figure 11.4 Fiberoptic tower and video laryngoscope arrangement in VLAFOI.

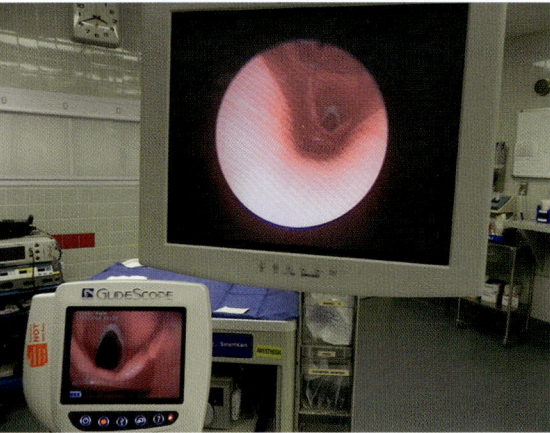

Figure 11.5 Video laryngoscopic and fiberoptic views of the glottis.

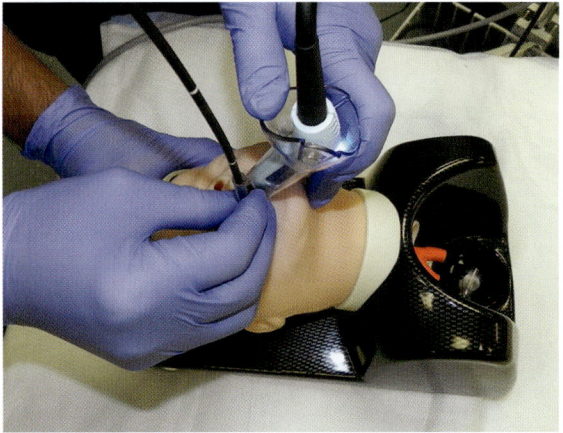

Figure 11.7 Proper positioning of video laryngoscope blade and fiberoptic scope in manikin (note, two operators).

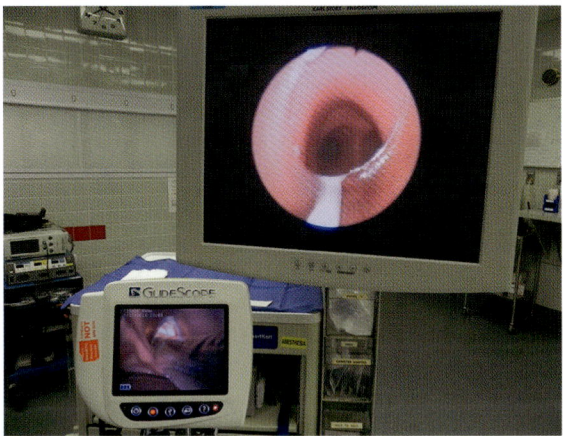

Figure 11.6 Fiberoptic view of carina and ETT advancement under video laryngoscope visualization.

the video laryngoscope and the fiberoptic bronchoscope to be used: this assistant will be operating one of the devices. Preload the fiberoptic bronchoscope with the desired tracheal tube. Select the appropriate video laryngoscope blade based on patient size; having multiple blade sizes readily available is advisable, particularly for patients with limited mouth opening. Induce anesthesia and perform gentle video laryngoscopy, being careful to avoid airway trauma or bleeding. In patients in whom there is suspected difficult ventilation, consider moderate-to-deep sedation with airway topicalization. When the best view of the glottis is obtained, tilt the video laryngoscope blade slightly to the left of midline, to open a midline path for the fiberoptic bronchoscope. Advance the fiberoptic bronchoscope toward the glottic opening. If the glottic view is a grade 1 or 2, continue to advance the fiberoptic bronchoscope, using it as a controllable stylet. If the glottic view is a Cormack–Lehane grade 3 or 4, maneuver the fiberoptic bronchoscope until

123

Section 2: Devices and Techniques to Manage the Abnormal Airway

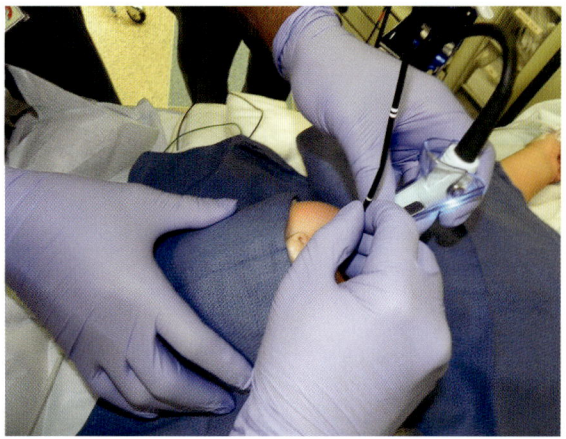

Figure 11.8 Proper positioning of video laryngoscope blade and fiberoptic scope in an infant.

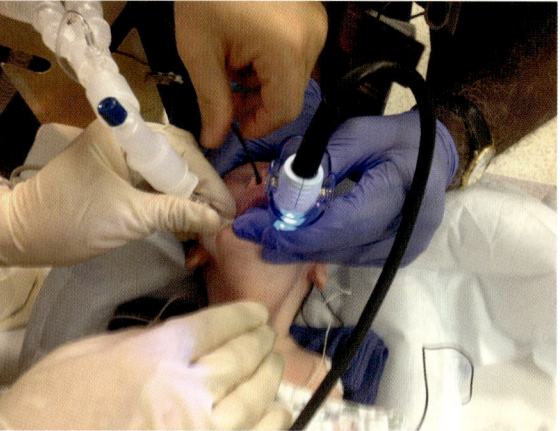

Figure 11.9 Use of VLAFOI for orotracheal to nasotracheal tube exchange.

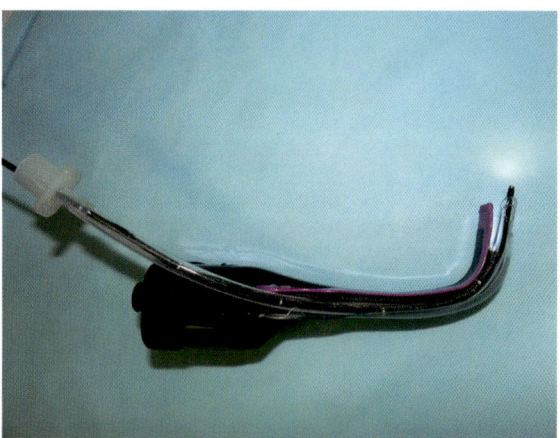

Figure 11.10 Pediatric Airtraq optical laryngoscope loaded with a fiberoptic bronchoscope and ETT.

the view of the laryngeal inlet is improved. Advance the fiberoptic bronchoscope past the vocal cords, into the trachea and to the carina. Advance the tracheal tube into the trachea under video laryngoscopic guidance and confirm final tracheal tube position with the fiberoptic bronchoscope.

Indications

There are specific circumstances where VLAFOI is particularly useful, including when rescuing a failed intubation when using a video laryngoscope or fiberoptic bronchoscope alone. Video laryngoscopy may provide an excellent glottic view, but a clinician may have difficulty maneuvering the tracheal tube with a rigid stylet; the fiberoptic bronchoscope acts as a moldable stylet. VLAFOI is also useful in a child with a fixed or unstable cervical spine – an assistant must hold the unstable cervical spine in-line as the clinician places the video laryngoscope. VLAFOI is also helpful in tracheal intubation with a double-lumen tube in a patient with a difficult airway. In this situation, the video laryngoscope provides a glottic view and oropharyngeal pathway for the double-lumen tube to pass, and the fiberoptic bronchoscope helps advance the double-lumen tube through the vocal cords, into the trachea, and into the desired mainstem bronchus. Similarly, VLAFOI is helpful in tracheal tube exchange in a patient with a known difficult airway: the video laryngoscopy provides a view of the tracheal tube, placement of the airway exchange catheter, removal of the initial tracheal tube, and then placement of the desired tracheal tube. This technique may also be used to change out an oral tracheal tube for a nasal tracheal tube in difficult airway patients. Finally, VLAFOI is a useful technique to teach proper fiberoptic-scope maneuvers to novices. The video laryngoscopy gives the trainer the advantage of a view of the oropharynx and location of the fiberoptic bronchoscope, allowing accurate direction and correction of trainee fiberoptic-bronchoscope movements.

Contraindications

VLAFOI is relatively contraindicated in patients with limited mouth opening because visualization via video laryngoscopy may be difficult. However, newer low-profile devices may lessen this problem. Additionally, oropharyngeal trauma or pathology with active bleeding into the oropharynx is a relative contraindication, as bloody secretions can obscure the airway view with both the video laryngoscope and fiberoptic bronchoscope.

Advantages

There are several advantages to VLAFOI in the management of the difficult pediatric airway. First, the video laryngoscope maintains an oropharyngeal pathway for fiberoptic bronchoscope advancement by displacing soft tissue. Additionally, the clinician has two views of the location of the fiberoptic bronchoscope: the fiberoptic bronchoscope itself and a simultaneous view of the fiberoptic bronchoscope with the video laryngoscope. This may improve guidance of the scope through the oropharynx and reduce the likelihood of unwanted fiberoptic bronchoscope and tracheal tube movements off the midline and thus can reduce upper airway trauma. Finally, the clinician has the advantage of visualizing the tracheal tube passing through the oropharynx and into the trachea via the video laryngoscope, allowing the ability to correct the tracheal tube position if it catches on the arytenoids.

Disadvantages

A major disadvantage of this technique is that it requires two skilled clinicians: one to operate the video laryngoscope and the other to operate the fiberoptic bronchoscope. Additionally, the fiberoptic-bronchoscope images are prone to deterioration due to excessive lighting. Reducing the brightness of the fiberoptic bronchoscope or video laryngoscope (if this function is available) will mitigate this problem.

Tips for Success

It is important to optimize lighting and bronchoscope brightness to minimize excessive glare. For nasotracheal intubation, the fiberoptic bronchoscope light is used to advance through the nasal passage and may be dimmed or turned off once the tip is visualized in the VL monitor. Alternatively, the brightness of the VL may be dimmed, if this feature is available. On entering the subglottis, the fiberoptic bronchoscope light is turned back on or the brightness increased for optimal tracheal imaging. The fiberscope should never be advanced blindly as this may cause severe airway trauma.

Retrograde-Assisted Fiberoptic Intubation (RAFOI)

Although retrograde intubation techniques are well established in adult difficult airway management, only few pediatric cases using this technique have been reported. Of the 30 cases reported in the literature, Audenaert and colleagues reported on the largest series of 20 cases.[31] Patients in the series ranged from 1 day to 17 years old, and weighed between 2.9 kg and 74 kg. They show that retrograde intubation can be successfully performed in both anticipated and unanticipated pediatric difficult airways.

The anatomical differences between adult and pediatric patients add to the difficulty in performing retrograde intubation, especially in neonates and infants. In our smallest patients, landmarks are difficult to palpate, the cricothyroid membrane is very small, and the larynx is located more cephalad when compared to adults.

Several techniques for retrograde intubation have been described in adult patients, including the classic technique (utilizing an epidural catheter), the guidewire technique, and the fiberoptic-assisted technique. The RAFOI technique is the preferred technique in pediatric patients and is the technique Audenaert and colleagues described.[31]

Technique for RAFOI
Anesthetic Goal

The overall anesthetic goal for the RAFOI is to provide sedation, local anesthetic airway topicalization, airway drying, and vasoconstriction of nasal passages in nasotracheal intubation. If local anesthetic airway topicalization is performed, one must remain vigilant to administer less than the maximum recommended dose for the pediatric patient.

Technique

RAFOI is best performed with a skilled assistant. Preload a fiberoptic bronchoscope with the appropriate-sized tracheal tube. Perform cricothyroid puncture with either a 22 gauge angiocatheter or a Tuohy needle. Consider identifying the cricothyroid membrane with an ultrasound in neonates or infants. Aseptically, insert a guidewire via the cricothyroid membrane using a 0.018″-diameter wire; for infants, the wire should be at least 100 cm in length. Advance the fiberoptic bronchoscope over the guidewire using a Seldinger technique though the suction port. When

Section 2: Devices and Techniques to Manage the Abnormal Airway

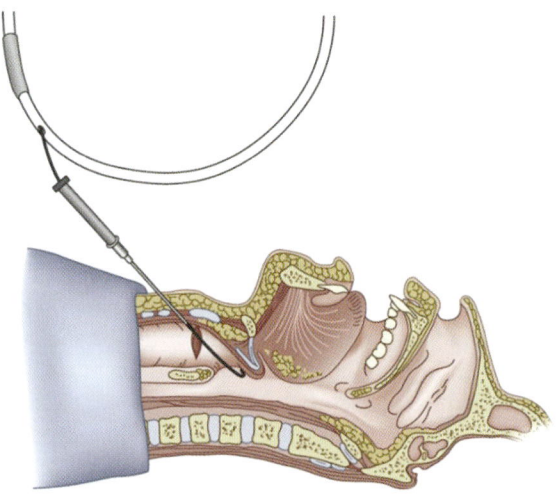

Figure 11.11 Advance guidewire through angiocatheter. (From *Benumof and Hagberg's Airway Management*, Philadelphia, 2013, with permission.)

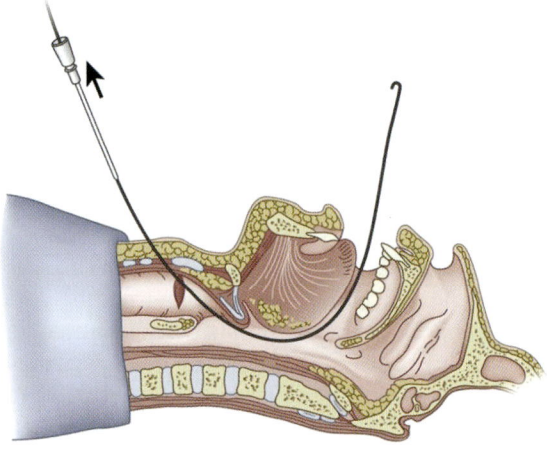

Figure 11.12 Retrieve guidewire from the mouth and remove angiocatheter. (From *Benumof and Hagberg's Airway Management*, Philadelphia, 2013, with permission.)

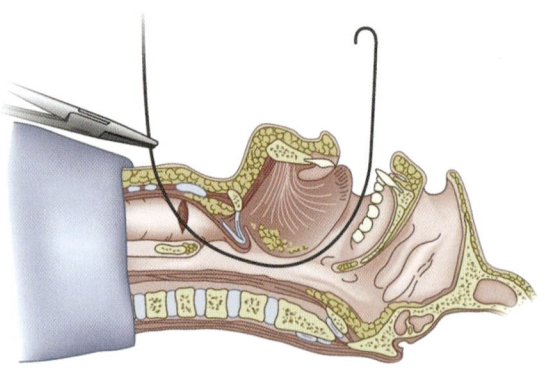

Figure 11.13 Pull out guidewire to appropriate length to fit length of fiberoptic bronchoscope and secure with a hemostat. (From *Benumof and Hagberg's Airway Management*, Philadelphia, 2013, with permission.)

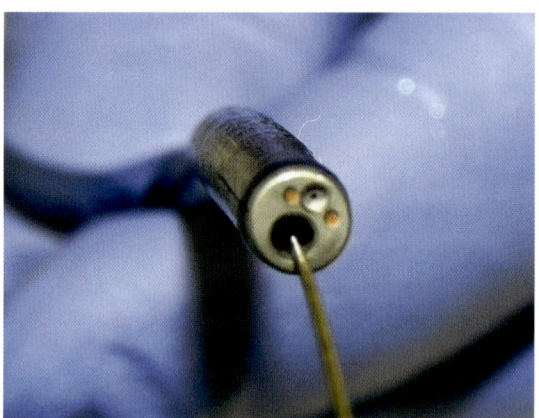

Figure 11.14 Feed guidewire into working port of fiberoptic bronchoscope.

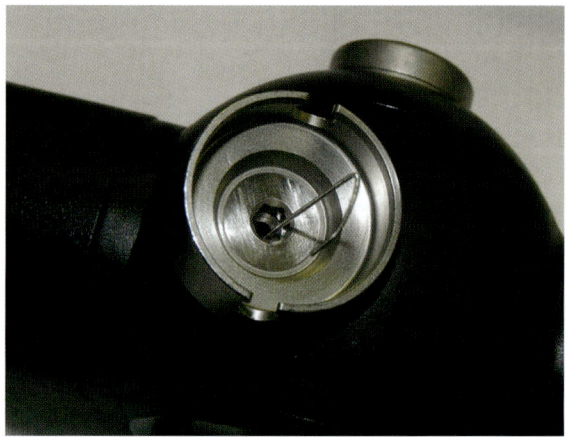

Figure 11.15 Retrieve guidewire from handle of fiberoptic bronchoscope.

the tip of the fiberoptic bronchoscope has passed the vocal cords, advance the tracheal tube into the trachea. A visual demonstration of this technique is shown in Figures 11.11–17.

Advantages

RAFOI allows the ability to secure the airway while the patient is awake and breathing spontaneously. Additionally, having a guidewire in the trachea allows for the clinician to rapidly find a view of the glottis with the fiberoptic bronchoscope with minimal maneuvering in the oropharynx. The fiberoptic bronchoscope also provides a conduit by which to insufflate

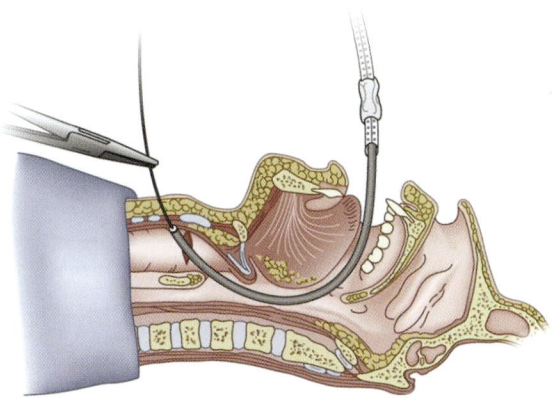

Figure 11.16 Advance preloaded fiberoptic bronchoscope to the cricothyroid membrane. (From *Benumof and Hagberg's Airway Management*, Philadelphia, 2013, with permission.)

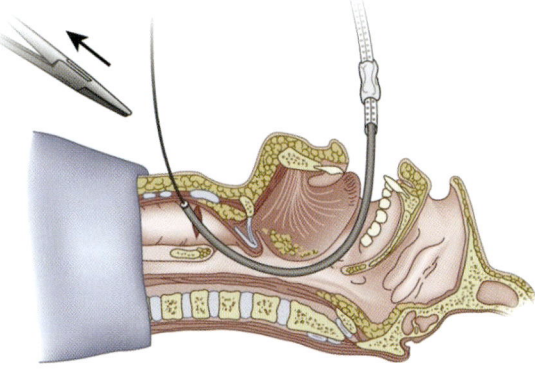

Figure 11.17 Remove hemostat (by an assistant), advance fiberoptic bronchoscope into trachea and complete intubation as with standard fiberoptic intubation. (From *Benumof and Hagberg's Airway Management*, Philadelphia, 2013, with permission.)

oxygen. In the series by Audenaert and colleagues, RAFOI was found to have a higher success rate compared to the use of either retrograde intubation or fiberoptic intubation alone.[31]

Complications

Potential serious complications associated with RAFOI are bleeding and subcutaneous emphysema. Other potential complications include cricothyroid needle or guidewire breakage, esophageal injury, tracheal and pretracheal infections, pneumothorax, and pneumomediastinum.

Summary

This chapter has reviewed a subset of hybrid approaches to management of the difficult pediatric airway. There are countless variations on these techniques, as well as hybrid approaches involving instruments not discussed here. Regardless of which techniques are used, the guiding principle should remain the same: to minimize complications by combining the advantages of multiple devices. To be successful at these techniques, the clinician caring for the pediatric patient must have baseline mastery of the individual techniques as described elsewhere in this text.

Acknowledgments

Special thanks to Ferenc Kupovics (Biomedical Photographer), Douglas Preuss (Biomedical Photographer), and Tanveer Khan (Lead Anesthesia Technician), Children's Health System of Texas at Dallas, for the outstanding pictures and videos.

References

1. Aziz MP, Heal D, Kheterpal S, et al. Routine Clinical Practice Effectiveness of the Glidescope in Difficult Airway Management: an Analysis of 2004 Glidescope Intubations, Complications, and Failures from Two Institutions. *Anesthesiology* 2011; **114**: 34–41.
2. Gil KSL, Diemunsch PA. Fiberoptic and Flexible Endoscopic-Aided Techniques. In Hagberg C., 3rd ed. *Benumof and Hagberg's Airway Management*. Philadelphia: Elsevier; 2013: 389–94.
3. Practice Guidelines for Management of the Difficult Airway. An Updated Report by the American Society of Anesthesiologists Task Force on Management of the Difficult Airway. *Anesthesiology* 2013; **118**: 251–70.
4. Weiss M, Engelhardt T. Proposal for the Management of the Unexpected Difficult Pediatric Airway. *Pediatric Anaesthesia* 2010; **20**: 454–64.
5. Heard C, Caldicott L, Fletcher J, et al. Fiberoptic-Guided Endotracheal Intubation via the Laryngeal Mask Airway in Pediatric Patients: a Report of a Series of Cases. *Anesthesia & Analgesia* 1996; **82**: 1287–9.
6. Rabb M, Minkowitz H, Hagberg C. Blind Intubation through the Laryngeal Mask Airway for Management of the Difficult Airway in Infants. *Anesthesiology* 1996; **84**: 1510–11.
7. Preis CA, Preis IS. Oversize Endotracheal Tubes and Intubation

Section 2: Devices and Techniques to Manage the Abnormal Airway

via Laryngeal Mask Airway. *Anesthesiology* 1997; **87**: 187.

8   Chadd GD, Walford AJ, Crane DL. The 3.5/4.5 Modification for Fiberscope-Guided Tracheal Intubation Using the Laryngeal Mask Airway. *Anesthesia & Analgesia* 1992; **72**: 307–8.

9   Theroux MC, Kettrick RG, Khine HH. Laryngeal Mask Airway and Fiberoptic Endoscopy in an Infant with Schwartz-Jampel Syndrome. *Anesthesiology* 1995; **82**: 605.

10 Benumof JL. Use of the Laryngeal Mask Airway to Facilitate Fiberscope-Aided Tracheal Intubation. *Anesthesia & Analgesia* 1992; **74**: 313–15.

11 Osborn IP, Soper R. It's a Disposable LMA, Just Cut it Shorter – for Fiberoptic Intubation. *Anesthesia & Analgesia* 2003; **97**: 299–300.

12 Kovatsis PG, Fiadjoe JE, Stricker PA. Simple, Reliable Replacement of Pilot Balloons for a Variety of Clinical Situations. *Pediatric Anesthesia* 2010; **20**: 490–4.

13 Jagannathan N, Sohn LE, Sawardekar A, et al. A Randomized Trial Comparing the Ambu Aura-i with the air-Q Intubating Laryngeal Airway as Conduits for Tracheal Intubation in Children. *Pediatric Anesthesia* 2012; **22**: 1197–204.

14 Whyte SD, Cook E, Malherbe S. Usability and Performance Characteristics of the Pediatric air-Q Intubating Laryngeal Airway. *Canadian Journal of Anesthesia/Journal canadien d'anesthésie* 2013; **60**: 557–63.

15 Jagannathan N, Roth AG, Sohn LE, et al. The New air-Q Intubating Laryngeal Airway for Tracheal Intubation in Children with Anticipated Difficult Airway: a Case Series. *Pediatric Anesthesia* 2009; **19**: 618–22.

16 Fiadjoe JE, Stricker PA, Kovatsis PG, et al. Initial Experience with the air-Q as a Conduit for Fiberoptic Tracheal Intubation in Infants. *Pediatric Anesthesia* 2010; **20**: 195–207.

17 Jagannathan N, Jagannathan R. Prone Insertion of a Size 0.5 Intubating Laryngeal Airway Overcomes Severe Upper Airway Obstruction in an Awake Neonate with Pierre Robin Syndrome. *Canadian Journal of Anesthesia/Journal canadien d'anesthésie* 2012; **59**: 1001–2.

18 Jagannathan N, Truong CA. Simple Method to Deliver Pharyngeal Anesthesia in Syndromic Infants Prior to Awake Insertion of the Intubating Laryngeal Airway. *Canadian Journal of Anesthesia/Journal canadien d'anesthésie* 2010; **57**: 1138–9.

19 Jagannathan N, Sohn LE, Eidem JM. Use of the air-Q Intubating Laryngeal Airway for Rapid-Sequence Intubation in Infants with Severe Airway Obstruction: a Case Series. *Anesthesia* 2013; **68**: 636–8.

20 Asai T. Is it Safe to Use Supraglottic Airway in Children with Difficult Airways? *British Journal of Anaesthesia* 2014; **112**: 620–2.

21 Reber A, Paganoni R, Frei FJ. Effect of Common Airway Manoeuvres on Upper Airway Dimensions and Clinical Signs in Anaesthetized, Spontaneously Breathing Children. *British Journal of Anaesthesia* 2001; **86**: 217–22.

22 Galgon RE, Schroeder KM, Schmidt CS, et al. Fiberoptic-Guided Tracheal Tube Placement through the air-Q Intubating Laryngeal Airway: a Performance Study in a Manikin. *Journal of Anesthesia* 2011; **25**: 721–6.

23 Wong D, Apichatibutra N, Arora G, et al. Repeated Attempts Improve Tracheal Tube Insertion Time Using the Intubating Laryngeal Airway in a Mannequin. *Journal of Clinical Anesthesia* 2010; **22**: 619–24.

24 Cavus E, Dorges V. Video Laryngoscopes. In Hagberg C., 3rd ed. *Benumof and Hagberg's Airway Management*. Philadelphia: Elsevier; 2013: 544–5.

25 Cooper RM, Pacey JA, Bishop MJ, et al. Early Clinical Experience with a New Videolaryngoscope (Glidescope) in 728 Patients. *Canadian Journal of Anesthesia/Journal canadien d'anesthésie* 2005; **52**: 191–8.

26 Lenhardt R, Burkhart MT, Brock GN, et al. Is Video Laryngoscope-Assisted Flexible Tracheoscope Intubation Feasible for Patients with Predicted Difficult Airway? A Prospective, Randomized Clinical Trial. *Anesthesia & Analgesia* 2014; **118**: 1259–65.

27 Blasius K, Gooden C. A Pediatric Difficult Airway Managed with a Glidescope-Assisted Fiberoptic Intubation. *Pediatric Anesthesiology* 2011 (Abstract) CSF141.

28 Moore MS, Wong AB. Glidescope Intubation Assisted by Fiberoptic Scope. *Anesthesiology* 2007; **106**: 885.

29 Doyle JD. Glidescope-Assisted Fiberoptic Intubation: a New Airway Teaching Method. *Anesthesiology* 2004; **101**: 1252.

30 Sukernik MR, Bezinover D, Stahlman B, et al. (January 2009). Combination of Glidescope with Fiberoptic Bronchoscope for Optimization of Difficult Endotracheal Intubation. A Case Series of Three Patients. Glidescope and Bronchoscope article. Website. http://www.priory.com/medicine/Glidescope_bronchoscope.htm

31 Audenaert SM, Montgomery CL, Stone B, et al. Retrograde-Assisted Fiberoptic Tracheal Intubation in Children with Difficult Airways. *Anesthesia & Analgesia* 1991; **73**: 660–4.

Section 2 **Devices and Techniques to Manage the Abnormal Airway**

Chapter 12

Muscle Relaxants

Annery Garcia-Marcinkiewicz and John E. Fiadjoe

In the territory between the Amazon and Orinoco rivers in the late sixteenth century, Sir Walter Raleigh observed natives use arrows with a "poison" so strong that its victims died, not by direct physical injury, but rather by the perishing effect of its poison.[1] Curiosity in this substance by European explorers helped transform curare from an arrow poison to a surgical relaxant.[2] The introduction of muscle relaxants revolutionized anesthetic practice as it allowed for improved surgical conditions, lower levels of volatile anesthetics, and improved tracheal intubation conditions.[2]

Since the early twentieth century, muscle relaxants have been shown to be beneficial, safe, and generally well tolerated by children.[3] Advances in modern anesthesia practice, including new anesthetic techniques, ventilators, airway equipment such as the LMA, and surgical techniques have certainly influenced when muscle relaxants are used.[4] Tracheal intubation without using neuromuscular blocking agents in children is common practice, particularly when managing difficult airways. When managing a difficult airway, the anesthesia clinician is often faced with a crucial decision: "to paralyze or not to paralyze?"

As part of traditional anesthesiology training, emphasis is placed on maintaining spontaneous ventilation during tracheal intubation of a challenging airway to use this as a fail-safe mechanism should the elimination of muscle tone prove to be detrimental. But the potential for functional airway obstruction due to patient coughing, bronchospasm, and laryngospasm can convert an airway, which would have otherwise been easily managed, into a challenging airway. To avoid such events, muscle relaxants are typically administered by many clinicians after confirming easy face-mask ventilation. Data from the PeDI Registry were analyzed in three groups. Patients managed with spontaneous ventilation, controlled ventilation with neuromuscular blocking drugs, and controlled ventilation without neuromuscular blocking drugs. Analysis revealed more non-severe complications in the spontaneous ventilation group. However complications were similar in the two controlled ventilation groups, which suggests that anesthetic depth may play a role in the increased complications in the spontaneous group.

It is well known that manipulation of the airway at an insufficient depth of anesthesia is a major cause of laryngospasm and other adverse airway events.[5] A single-center study of healthy pediatric patients found a strong association between spontaneous ventilation and poor intubation conditions.[6] Due to the strength of that association, the authors suggest that, when utilizing their technique (8% dialed sevoflurane and 60% N_2O preceded by 0.6 mg/kg of midazolam with no muscle relaxant), if the patient continues to breathe spontaneously, intubation should not be attempted until ventilation can be controlled.

The anesthetic strategy for difficult pediatric airways requires meticulous planning. There are clinical situations in which muscle relaxants are contraindicated, such as in patients with mediastinal tumors, airway masses, and poor tissue compliance. It is important to remember that the "difficulty" of each airway can be due to a variety of problems (e.g., craniofacial dysmorphism versus severe airway reactivity) or reside in a different anatomical location (e.g., limited mouth opening versus severe tonsillar hypertrophy, subglottic stenosis, or a mediastinal tumor). Furthermore, clinical circumstances are continually changing, which means there cannot be a standard anesthetic approach for all difficult airways. When considering whether or not to use a muscle relaxant in an otherwise healthy child, it is crucial to quickly distinguish between anatomical and mechanical airway obstruction versus functional airway obstruction.[7] In a prospective study looking at perioperative adverse respiratory events (PRAE) during elective pediatric surgery, Mamie and colleagues[8] found that the risk of PRAE was significantly lower when the anesthetic technique included tracheal intubation using neuromuscular blocking drugs (OR = 0.6, 95% CI 0.45–0.95). A recent meta-analysis of 34 randomized control trials by Lundstrom and colleagues[9] involving 3565 participants aged 14 years or older found that avoidance of neuromuscular-blocking drugs is associated with both an increased risk of difficult tracheal intubation and an increased risk of upper airway discomfort or injury. The risk of difficult tracheal intubation increases 13-fold (RR = 13.27, 95% CI 8.19–21.49, $p < 0.00001$), and the risk of airway discomfort or injury 1.4-fold (RR = 1.37, 95% CI 1.09 – 1.74, $p = 0.008$) when neuromuscular-blocking drugs are not used. The authors conclude that the use of neuromuscular-blocking drugs may create better conditions for tracheal intubation in clinical practice. Most of these studies examined patients with normal airways, and, traditionally, patients with difficult airways have been categorized differently because of concerns for the "cannot intubate cannot ventilate scenario". Anticipated difficult airways should be managed similarly. If the patient is experiencing airway obstruction due to an anatomical or mechanical problem, then this should be resolved accordingly (repositioning, use of oral or nasopharyngeal airways, clearance of secretions). If the patient is experiencing a functional airway obstruction, unless there is clear judgment that loss-of-airway tone will be even more detrimental, the problem should be corrected according to the primary cause of the functional issue: insufficient anesthetic depth should be deepened, muscle relaxants should be considered for laryngospasm and opioid-induced muscle rigidity, and epinephrine for severe bronchospasm. In healthy children, functional airway obstruction remains the leading cause of adverse events,[10] with laryngospasm remaining the leading cause of an adverse airway event in these patients[11,12] and a leading complication in children with difficult tracheal intubation in the PeDI Registry.[13]

Recent guidelines published by the Difficult Airway Society recommend that, if an airway is difficult, further attempts should not proceed without full neuromuscular block to optimize intubating conditions prior to performing a surgical airway.[14] With increased consideration of the use of neuromuscular blockers in overcoming functional airway obstruction in both anticipated and unanticipated difficult airways, sugammadex may play a role in adding safety to this approach. Sugammadex is a novel drug that may offer a potential rapid "rescue" from neuromuscular blockade. There are limited data regarding its administration in pediatric patients.[15] Sugammadex can reverse neuromuscular blockade with a mechanism different than acetylcholinesterase inhibitors. It encapsulates rocuronium or vecuronium, even with a profound block, reducing its effective concentration at the neuromuscular junction.[16,17] There has been favorable experience with the use of sugammadex in children, including in neuromyopathic disorders, myasthenia gravis, Duchenne muscular dystrophy, and even in a few neonatal cases, with rapid reversal of neuromuscular blockade with little adverse effect.[15] Dosing is based on the train of four (TOF) response with 2 mg/kg when there are ≥ 2 twitches on TOF, 4 mg/kg if there are 1–2 post-tetanic twitches, and maximum dose of 16 mg/kg for reversal immediately following an intubating dose of rocuronium. The reported adverse effect profile of sugammadex has generally been limited to nausea, vomiting, pain, and hypotension. Preclinical trials reported bradycardia and anaphylactoid reactions.[15] The point of understanding where the cause of the "difficulty" of a difficult airway lies is again emphasized: sugammadex can be relied on to completely reverse a rocuronium-induced neuromuscular block, but it may not necessarily establish airway patency as was described in the "can't intubate, can't oxygenate" case report of a patient with airway edema resulting from multiple intubation attempts.[18] Management of a difficult airway involves meticulous attention to the balance of two crucial components: (1) the airway management technique itself; that is, selecting the right device for the right patient and performing this technique appropriately with limited attempts while providing passive oxygenation, and (2) ensuring the right anesthetic depth and the right timing with each patient. Airway manipulation should never proceed in children until anesthetic depth is adequate. The Larson Maneuver is a simple manuever that applies pressure to the body of the mandible anterior to the mastoid process. Lack of physical response (body movement) to this maneuver has been shown to predict adequate conditions for laryngeal mask placement in adults. The Larson Maneuver may be a useful technique to assess anesthetic adequacy for airway manipulation in children.

Use of neuromuscular blocking drugs in children with difficult airways is controversial. A dogmatic practice of avoiding neuromuscular blocking drugs in this population may result in patient harm. Most children can be intubated without neuromuscular blocking drugs, but meticulous attention should be paid to assuring an adequate plane of anesthesia prior to intubation attempts. Clinicians should have a low threshold for using neuromuscular blocking drugs if there are signs of functional airway obstruction.

References

1. Gray, TC. The Use of D-Tubocuranine Chloride in Anaesthesia. *Annals of the Royal College of Surgeons in England* 1947; **1**(4): 191–203.
2. Foldes, FF. Anesthesia before and after Curare. *Anaesthesiology and Reanimation* 1993; **18**(5): 128–31.
3. Bush GH. The Use of Muscle Relaxants in Infants and Children. *British Journal of Anaesthesia* 1963; **35**: 552.
4. Fisher DM. Neuromuscular Blocking Agents in Paediatric Anaesthesia. *British Journal of Anaesthesia* 1999; **83**: 58–64.
5. Orliaguet GA, Olivier G, Savoldelli G, et al. Case Scenario: Perianesthetic Management of Laryngospasm in Children. *Anesthesiology* 2012; **116**: 458–71.
6. Politis GD. Frankland MJ. James RL. Reville et al. Factors Associated with Successful Tracheal Intubation of Children with Sevoflurane and No Muscle Relaxant. *Anesthesia & Analgesia* 2002; **95**: 615–20.
7. Weiss M. Engelhardt T. Cannot Ventilate – Paralyze! *Pediatric Anesthesia* 2012; **22**: 1147–9.
8. Mamie C, Habre W, Delhumeau C, et al. Incidence and Risk Factors of Perioperative Respiratory Adverse Airway Events in Children Undergoing Elective Surgery. *Paediatric Anesthesia* 2004: **14**: 218–24.
9. Lundstrøm LH, Duez CHV, Nørskov AK, et al. Use of Neuromuscular Blocking Agent for Improving Conditions during Tracheal Intubation. A Cochrane Systematic Review. *British Journal of Anaesthesia* 2018; **120**(6): 1381–93.
10. Bhananker SM, Ramamoorthy C, Geiduschk JM, et al. Anesthesia-Related Cardiac Arrest in Children: Update from the Pediatric Perioperative Cardiac Arrest Registry. *Anesthesia & Analgesia* 2007; **105**: 344–50.
11. Cook TM, Woodall N, Harper J, et al. Major Complications of Airway Management in the UK: Results of the Fourth National Audit Project of the Royal College of Anaesthetists and the Difficult Airway Society. *British Journal of Anaesthesia* 2011; **106**: 632–42.
12. Von Ungern-Sternberg BS, Boda K, Chambers NA, et al. Risk Assessment for Respiratory Complications in Paediatric Anaesthesia: a Prospective Cohort Study. *The Lancet* 2010; **376**: 773–83.
13. Fiadjoe JE, Nishisaki A, Jagannathan N, et al. Airway Management Complications in Children with Difficult Tracheal Intubation from the Pediatric Difficult Intubation (PeDI) Registry. A Prospective Cohort Analysis. *The Lancet Respiratory Medicine* 2016; **4**: 37–48.
14. Frerk C, Mitchell VS, McNarry AF, et al. Difficult Airway Society 2015 Guidelines for Management of Unanticipated Difficult Intubation in Adults. *British Journal of Anaesthesia* 2015; **115**(6): 827–48.
15. Tobias JD. Current Evidence for the Use of Sugammadex in Children. *Pediatric Anesthesia* 2017; **27**: 118–25.
16. Naguib M. Sugammadex: Another Milestone in the Clinical Neuromuscular Pharmacology. *Anesthesia & Analgesia* 2007; **104**: 575–81.
17. Chamber D, Paylden M, Paton I, et al. Sugammadex for Reversal of Neuromuscular Block after Rapid Sequence Intubation: a Systematic Review and Economic Assessment. *British Journal of Anaesthesia* 2010; **105**: 568–75.
18. Curtis R, Lomax S, Patel B. Use of Sugammadex in a "Can't Intubate, Can't Ventilate" Situation. *British Journal of Anaesthesia* 2012; **108**(4): 612–14.

Section 2 Devices and Techniques to Manage the Abnormal Airway

Chapter 13
Management of the "Can't Intubate, Can't Oxygenate" Scenario

Vivian Man-ying Yuen, Stefano Sabato, and Birgitta Wong

The "Can't Intubate, Can't Oxygenate" Scenario

When oxygenation is difficult or impossible, critical decision-making and immediate management to correct hypoxemia is of the utmost importance to avoid major morbidity and mortality. Failure to oxygenate in children most commonly results from functional airway obstruction. Functional airway obstruction can occur in many different areas of the pediatric airway. Upper airway obstruction in babies is often due to a blocked nose and having the tongue stuck to the hard palate. Bronchospasm in asthmatics and tracheomalacia in children with previous tracheoesophageal fistulae are examples of lower airway obstruction. However, laryngospasm is by far the most common functional airway problem. Laryngospasm is easily managed by deepening anesthesia and/or administering succinylcholine. If management is delayed, severe hypoxia, bradycardia, and even cardiac arrest may occur. Invasive airway access through the front of the neck directly into the trachea is not indicated in these situations. This chapter will focus on the "can't intubate, can't oxygenate" (CICO) emergency caused by anatomical or pathological causes that necessitate invasive access through the front of the neck. Anatomical upper airway obstruction may be caused by congenital abnormalities, infection, swelling, and malignant or non-malignant growths of the upper airway. In the Fourth National Audit Project of the Royal College of Anaesthetists and the Difficult Airway Society (NAP4), 75% of cases (43 out of 58) who required emergency invasive airway were patients with head and neck pathologies.[1] Children presenting with severe upper airway obstruction secondary to anatomical or pathological conditions almost always have significant past medical histories. Therefore, their presentation should be easily distinguished from children with functional upper airway obstruction. Children with anatomical or pathological upper airway abnormalities may deteriorate gradually over time, or suddenly when their upper airway obstruction is aggravated by secondary infection or simple upper respiratory tract infection. Use of neuromuscular blockade or deepening anesthesia to manage anatomical or pathological obstruction could be detrimental in these deteriorating children as cessation of spontaneous ventilation could result in oxygenation failure. It is of utmost importance in these cases that spontaneous ventilation is maintained while securing the airway.

Invasive airway access is required when it is confirmed that oxygenation is impossible or difficult via the oral and nasal route. Guidelines from the Difficult Airway Society and the Association of Paediatric Anaesthetists of Great Britain and Ireland[2] recommend rescue techniques and establishment of an invasive airway when the oxygen saturation is less than 80% and continues to fall, and/or with the onset of bradycardia. However, oxygen saturation serves as an arbitrary guide only, and the patient's clinical condition should be taken into consideration when the decision to achieve an invasive airway is made. When attempts to relieve severe hypoxemia by tracheal intubation, face-mask ventilation, and insertion of an SGA device have failed, immediate invasive airway access is indicated.[3] This could be an extremely difficult clinical decision as the incidence of CICO is very rare in children, and experience in managing these challenging conditions is limited. Fixation error can also lead to a delay in declaring a CICO emergency. According to the NAP4 report, "the decision to perform an emergency surgical airway was commonly inappropriately delayed,"[1] despite the fact that invasive airway access could be lifesaving.

Chapter 13: Management of the "Can't Intubate, Can't Oxygenate" Scenario

Case 1

A 3-year-old 14 kg girl with a history of respiratory tract papilloma presented to the ED with increasing respiratory distress. The papilloma had been resected 6 months prior, and she had been asymptomatic until the onset of a viral upper respiratory tract infection 5 days prior to her presentation. The patient was scheduled for microlaryngoscopy and further resection of papillomatosis. She had a documented grade 1 laryngoscopy from her previous anesthetic. After ensuring the surgeon was scrubbed and had a rigid ventilating bronchoscope prepared, the patient was induced with sevoflurane in 100% oxygen. After intravenous access was secured, and the patient was judged to be adequately anesthetized, direct laryngoscopy and intubation was attempted. The vocal cords could not be visualized as the entire glottis was covered by papilloma (Figure 13.1), and an attempt at intubation was unsuccessful. Subsequently, the airway obstruction became more severe, and the oxygen saturation dropped below 80%. A 20 G needle was inserted into the trachea via the cricothyroid membrane, but oxygenation of the patient was not achieved as the correct equipment to oxygenate via a cannula was not pre-prepared and immediately available. The patient continued to desaturate further, and bradycardia developed. A second attempt at direct laryngoscopy was performed, and the child was successfully intubated with a size 2 ETT by following the air bubbles as the patient was spontaneously breathing. The papilloma was resected, and the child had an uneventful recovery.

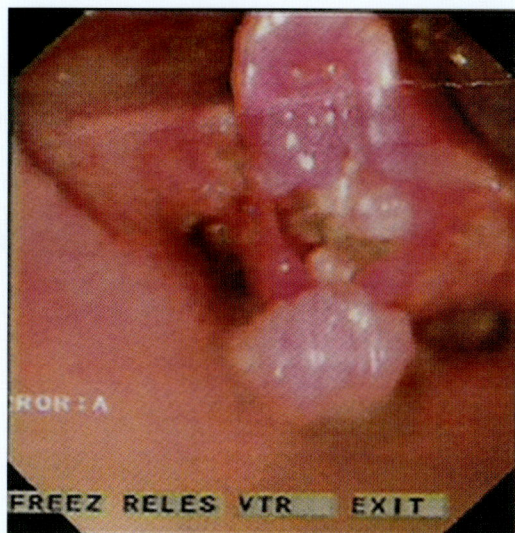

Figure 13.1 Severe upper airway obstruction from papilloma.

Case 2

An 8-month-old 7 kg girl with a past history of a tracheoesophageal fistula repair had a known subglottic stenosis from her prolonged intubation as a neonate (Figure 13.2). The child had previously been treated with multiple resections by CO_2 LASER to relieve the stenosis. When well, she required nocturnal CPAP and minimal oxygen therapy in the ICU. After her previous resections, a size 2 ETT would fit through the stenosis. Unfortunately, granulomatous inflammatory tissue repeatedly accumulated at the surgical site, and, after developing an upper respiratory tract infection, she developed respiratory distress unrelieved by CPAP. The child was brought to the operating theater for emergency endoscopic surgery and surgical tracheostomy. After sevoflurane induction in 100% inspired oxygen, endoscopic assessment by a pediatric otolaryngologist revealed a very tight subglottic stenosis that did not allow the passage of size 2 ETT. Spontaneous ventilation was maintained and CPAP was administered with T-piece circuit and a face mask. The patient was immediately positioned for surgical tracheostomy. The pediatric otolaryngologist managed to complete the tracheostomy procedure within 10 minutes, and the anesthesiologist managed to maintain oxygen saturations above 80% until the airway was secured.

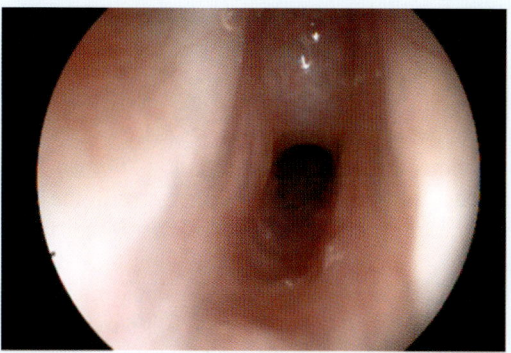

Figure 13.2 Subglottic stenosis.

Both these emergencies occurred in known high-risk patients where difficulty in managing the airway was anticipated. Both patients had chronic airway problems that worsened, acutely highlighting the need to be prepared at all times. Preparation includes systems to avoid human errors such as fixation error that could prevent acknowledgment that a CICO emergency has occurred. Preparation also includes having the technical skill to perform an invasive airway technique, and having the correct equipment immediately available. Although functional airway problems are relieved by muscle paralysis, the maintenance of spontaneous ventilation in these patients was important in ensuring their survival. This chapter expands on these learning points and provides an update on the literature.

Institutional and Multidisciplinary Approach to Management of CICO

The invention and use of various supraglottic devices has transformed difficult airway management, and therefore CICO situations in children have become exceedingly rare.[4] Preparation, planning, team training, and preprepared equipment are important to successful management of rare emergencies. There are many controversies in management of CICO in adults, and even more so in the management of CICO in young children, infants, and neonates. There is not enough published research to inform anesthesiologists as to the best technique to achieve invasive airway access via the front of the neck. Moreover, there are many different commercial and self-assembled types of equipment available for airway access and for emergency oxygenation. Therefore, it is important that each institution develops a protocol that creates a uniform approach to preparation, training, technique, and equipment. Regular technical skill acquisition and maintenance workshops are necessary to be able to perform the technique. However, it is also important to conduct team training exercises in scenario-based simulations to improve non-technical "human factor" skills such as declaring a CICO emergency at the correct time, and improving the ability to carry out the invasive access in simulated stressful situations. A dedicated CICO pack/box, or a dedicated compartment of the difficult airway cart (DAC), should be prepared to guide and assist management of CICO conditions in all anesthesia locations including the intensive care and EDs. Equipment to perform oxygenation via a cannula tracheotomy or cricothyrotomy is also important if a cannula technique is performed. The lack of appropriate equipment to oxygenate the patient contributed to a delay in oxygenation in example case one.

Anatomy of the Cricothyroid Membrane and Surrounding Structures

The cricothyroid membrane is the quickest, safest, and easiest invasive route to obtain an airway in the CICO emergency. The cricothyroid membrane is trapezoid in shape and extends from the inferior border of the thyroid cartilage to the superior border of the cricoid cartilage.[5] The cricothyroid membrane is superficial, and is only covered by skin and thin layers of fascia. In adults, the thyroid cartilage is readily identified and therefore the cricothyroid membrane may be palpated as the first indentation immediately caudad to the thyroid cartilage. In small children, the thyroid cartilage is difficult to palpate, and the most prominent structures are the hyoid bone and the cricoid cartilage.[6] The prominent hyoid may be mistaken as a thyroid cartilage resulting in a FONA attempt through the thyrohyoid space. The thyroid cartilage and the cricothyroid membrane are more cephalad, and access to the membrane may be hindered by the overlying mandible. Important structures close to the cricothyroid membrane include the common carotid artery, the internal and external jugular veins, the esophagus, and the thyroid gland and thyroid vessels. Importantly, the isthmus of the thyroid gland crosses the midline immediately caudad to the cricothyroid membrane and is supplied by the superior thyroid artery.

Despite the more obvious surface landmark in adults, the central point of the cricothyroid membrane was only accurately identified by 30% of anesthetists when the central points of the membrane were first located by ultrasound.[7] Correct identification of the cricothyroid membrane would be even more unreliable in children.

The average dimensions of the cricothyroid membrane estimated from adult cadavers were greater than 8 mm and 10 mm in height and width respectively.[8,9] The dimensions were consistently smaller in female adults. Based on these studies, it was recommended that the outer diameter of the ETT should not exceed 8 mm for adults. In a study of 27 neonatal cadavers in a neutral head and neck position, the mean height and width of cricothyroid membrane was 2.61 +/− 0.71 mm and 3.03 mm +/− 0.63 mm respectively.[10]

Position for Invasive Access to Airway

Infants and small children have relatively large heads compared with adults, resulting in neck flexion when lying supine without a pillow. While this position is ideal for endotracheal intubation, head and neck extension is required to maximize the length of the cricothyroid membrane and allow access to it without

Chapter 13: Management of the "Can't Intubate, Can't Oxygenate" Scenario

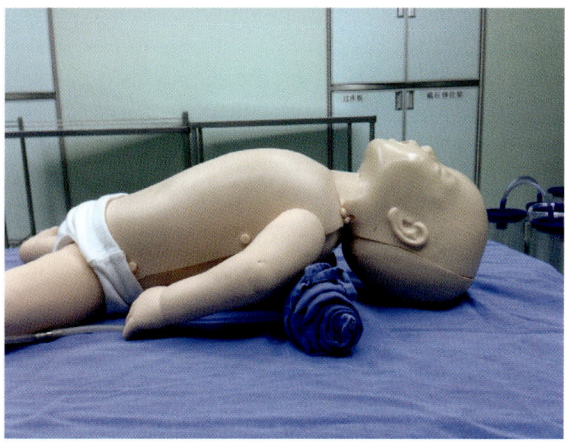

Figure 13.3 Demonstration of cricothyrotomy on self-made model and use of Enk OFM for oxygenation.

the approach being blocked by the mandible. Both cannula and scalpel FONA techniques require maximal head and neck extension by placing a roll under the shoulders. With proper neck extension, the cricoid ring may become palpable and obvious even in small infants and children (Figure 13.3).

Invasive Airway Access

Invasive airway access via the front of the neck includes formal surgical tracheostomy by an otolaryngologist, cannula/scalpel cricothyrotomy or tracheotomy by anesthesiologists or other critical care physicians, and access to the trachea using proprietary purpose-built kits that allow percutaneous access, or use a Seldinger technique. Access to the trachea via the cricothyroid membrane is more successful than access further caudad along the trachea,[11] and this is the preferred anatomical location to perform FONA in a true CICO emergency. However, it may not be possible to accurately determine the location of the cricothyroid membrane, or approach it with a flat-enough angle to avoid posterior tracheal wall puncture. Therefore, a tracheotomy may need to be performed. When an otolaryngologist is available, the best option is a formal surgical tracheostomy or rigid bronchoscopy. However, if severe upper airway swelling, bleeding, or anatomical distortion are present, rigid bronchoscopy may not be possible. Also, even otolaryngologists may experience difficulty in performing an emergent surgical tracheostomy in infants and neonates with acute airway obstruction because the tracheal is small, compressible, and laterally displaced easily. It is extremely challenging to perform surgical tracheostomy in small critically ill children under time pressure. Despite this, a senior experienced otolaryngologist is the best person to perform emergency FONA if immediately available as was described in the second example case.

If a senior otolaryngologist, with the necessary equipment prepared, is not present, invasive airway access must be achieved by the treating clinician (anesthesiologist, emergency physician, or intensive care physician). Cannula cricothyrotomy or scalpel cricothyrotomy are options in this situation. While cricothyrotomy refers to the access of airway via the cricothyroid membrane, it may also be called cricotomy, cricothyroidotomy, or thyrocricotomy. The choice between a cannula or a scalpel is controversial. This controversy creates significant logistical issues for hospitals to prepare and train for the CICO emergency.[12] Both procedures are potentially lifesaving, but difficult to perform and associated with significant risks, especially in infants with a cricothyroid space of 2 mm. Complications, such as fracture of the cricoid ring, trauma to posterior trachea wall, and future permanent subglottic stenosis could occur.

Cannula Cricothyrotomy

Cannula cricothyrotomy is invasive airway access via the front of the neck with an intravenous cannula or specific cannulas designed for invasive airway access such as the Ravussin catheter and jet ventilation catheter. As with scalpel techniques and proprietary kits, head-and-neck extension is required to allow palpation and identification of the cricothyroid membrane. This is a relatively less traumatic and less technically demanding procedure. When surveyed, anesthesiologists' preferred first choice to perform invasive airway access is narrow-bore cannula cricothyrotomy.[13,14] All anesthesiologists are familiar with needle cannulation. When correctly inserted, a narrow-bore cannula may be used as means of oxygenation. Alternatively, it can be used to pass a guidewire in Seldinger techniques for percutaneous cricothyrotomy. The steps of cannula cricothyrotomy are illustrated in Table 13.3 and the *Cannula Insertion* video.[15] Aspiration of air from the cannula has a 97% positive predictive value of correct placement of the cannula in the trachea.[16] Based on the limited evidence available, an 18 G intravenous cannula should be used in neonates, and a 16 G in infants and larger.[12,17]

Scalpel Cricothyrotomy

By scalpel cricothyrotomy, the authors refer to invasive access to the trachea via the front of the neck using a scalpel to allow passage of an appropriately sized endotracheal or tracheostomy tube. Placement of an ETT allows oxygenation *and ventilation* using ordinary reservoir bags and anesthetic circuits. Scalpel cricothyrotomy may be achieved by performing the scalpel-bougie technique[18] or by using a vertical skin incision and then the finger to locate the underlying trachea. Table 13.1 reveals the step-by-step procedure for surgical cricothyrotomy in teenage pediatric patients. It is noteworthy that the initial skin incision is midline and vertical so as to avoid injuries to important blood vessels. Once the subcutaneous tissue is dissected and the cricothyroid membrane is identified, a horizontal incision is made into the membrane and access to the trachea is obtained with scalpel and/or bougie, followed by an appropriately sized ETT.

Percutaneous Cricothyrotomy and Seldinger Sets

Commercial percutaneous cricothyrotomy sets are available to gain access to the trachea via the cricothyroid membrane. Sets that use the Seldinger technique involve cannulating the trachea and placing a guidwire into the airway. A dilator is then introduced into the trachea over the wire to open a stoma, and the definitive airway catheter is placed in situ. This catheter allows for ventilation and oxygenation as it is a wide-bore catheter. The advantage of a Seldinger technique is that it can be performed over a narrow-bore cannula, causing less tracheal compression, and reduces the chance of posterior tracheal wall puncture.[19] However, the Seldinger techniques require multiple steps in a time-critical CICO emergency, and inserting the catheter into the airway is not always successful. Percutaneous cricothyrotomy sets involve a direct puncture into the trachea with a wide-bore trocar over which the definitive airway catheter is inserted. These sets involve only one step, but require the use of a wider bore trocar. Commonly available proprietary CICO sets are listed in Table 13.2. The details and steps for each device are not discussed since they all follow the same principle with slight variations. Evidence on the efficacy and safety of percutaneous cricothyrotomy in young children is limited.[6] Clinicians who keep these cricothyrotomy sets in their difficult intubation cart should be familiar with the steps involved in using these sets. As with all techniques, regular and repeated training should be performed to maintain the skill of the clinicians.

Table 13.1 Surgical Cricothyrotomy

1. *Position patient* in optimal position with neck extension and shoulder elevation to facilitate identification of landmarks and performance of the procedures.
2. *Identify the landmarks*: palpate with non-dominant hand for the thyroid and cricoid cartilage. Feel for the indentation between the cartilages.
3. *Immobilize larynx* with non-dominant hand.
4. *Make vertical skin incision in midline* from thyroid cartilage to just below the cricoid cartilage. Perform blunt dissection of subcutaneous tissue with scalpel handle or scissors down to the cricothyroid membrane.
5. *Incise the cricothyroid membrane* transversely using the same scalpel. Use speculum, scalpel handle or bougie to assist insertion of ETT.
6. *Insert appropriately sized endotracheal or tracheostomy tube.*

Table 13.2 Commercial Cricothyrotomy Kits

Trade name	ID (mm)	Insertion method	Cuff/ uncuff
Melker	3.5, 4.0, 5.0, 6.0	Seldinger techniques	5.0 with cuff, others uncuff
Quicktrach	1.5, 2.0, 4.0	Trocar curved needle with stopper	Cuff
Pedia-Trake	3.0, 4.0, 5.0	Large tapered needle and dilator	Uncuff
Pertrach	3	Split needle with introducer	Uncuff
Nu-Trake	4.5, 6.0, 7.2	Large tapered needle and dilator	Uncuff

Table 13.3 Cannula Cricothyrotomy

1. *Position patient* in optimal position with neck extension and shoulder elevation to facilitate identification of landmarks and performing the procedures.
2. *Identify the landmarks*: palpate with non-dominant hand for the thyroid and cricoid cartilage. Feel for the indentation between the cartilages.
3. *Immobilize larynx* with non-dominant hand.
4. Insert cannula with needle in caudal direction via the cricothyroid membrane. Stop when a "give" is felt and air is aspirated with 3 ml syringe.
5. Thread cannula over needle; remove needle.
6. *Confirm position* of cannula by *positive air aspiration*.
7. Do not use cannula if air cannot be aspirated from cannula. Either reposition the cannula by gradual withdrawal under continuous aspiration or repeat the whole procedure with a new cannula.

Evidence and Complications for Each Technique

Currently there is insufficient evidence to determine the best approach to emergency FONA to the airway in children and infants. Although cannula cricothyrotomy is the first choice and preferred approach by most anesthesiologists,[13,14] the failure rate was reported to be 63% (12 out of 19) in the NAP4 audit.[1] This has led to a change in recommendations in the latest iteration of the Difficult Airway Society guidelines for management of the CICO emergency in adults.[3] However, closer inspection of the NAP4 data showed that the overall success rate for anesthetists using either scalpel or cannula techniques was extremely poor. The success rate of scalpel techniques in the NAP4 audit was higher than that of cannula techniques, but most of these were performed by head-and-neck surgeons in semi-controlled circumstances while the anesthetist maintained oxygenation.[20] The high failure rate may also reflect a lack of training in the cannula cricothyrotomy technique. Safe oxygenation with a cannula cricothyrotomy requires both successful cannulation of the trachea and safe "jet" oxygenation. Both aspects of the technique are challenging and require training. Repeated cannula tracheostomies were tested in postmortem rabbits by anesthetists experienced with all types of invasive airway.[16] The rabbit trachea is of a similar dimension to the human infant trachea. The overall success rate was 60% with 14 G and 16 G intravenous cannula, and there was no difference in the rate of kinking between the two sizes of cannulas. There were no successful attempts with the Quicktrach child device in this study.[16] In two other studies using a postmortem piglet model, success rates were better when the transtracheal cannulation was performed by anesthesiologists compared with physicians.[21,22] In both these studies, the participants had received a lecture and presentation as to how to perform the technique, but were not considered experienced in CICO techniques. The success rates by anesthesiologists were 65.6% and 68.8% with a jet ventilation catheter (VBM Medizintechnik) and intravenous cannula (BD Venflon Pro Safety [14 gauge]) respectively.[21] When the procedure was performed by a group of physicians, the success rate was only 26.7% with a 16 G or 18 G intravenous cannula.[22] It should be noted that, in these two studies on piglets, the success rate of tracheotomy was higher than the cannula cricothyrotomy. However, the time to establish a tracheotomy was significantly longer than the time taken to perform a cannula technique. A tracheotomy was considered successful if completed within 4 minutes.

In these studies, the procedures were observed with endoscopy or fiberoptic bronchoscopy.[16,21,22] There was a 40–50% incidence of posterior tracheal wall perforation, which was the commonest reason for failure. Kinking of the cannula was another frequent complication. Nevertheless, gradual withdrawal under continuous aspiration enabled eventual correct position of the cannula.[16] It was uncertain if the posterior tracheal wall injuries would lead to further complications when high-pressure ventilation was carried in the presence of such injuries. With better needle and cannula design, complications associated with cannula cricothyrotomy may decrease.[23]

Provision of safe "jet" oxygenation is the second challenge of the cannula technique. As illustrated by the case described, a lack of appropriate purpose-built equipment can lead to delays in oxygenation, and could lead to barotrauma and volutrauma if the anesthetist is not properly trained in their use. Methods of providing effective and safe oxygenation with narrow-bore cannula are discussed later. While narrow-bore cannulas allow oxygenation with a high-pressure oxygen supply, it does not allow effective ventilation.

It is only a temporary measure to increase oxygen reserve so that definitive airway access can be achieved.

In many studies comparing the effectiveness and safety of different methods of cricothyrotomy, the success rate of formal surgical tracheostomy and scalpel cricothyrotomy is higher than that of cannula cricothyrotomy.[21,22,24,25] However, these studies are limited by the lack of bleeding in cadavers, and the use of adult models. Moreover, the compliance of the trachea in cadaveric models is different from that of young children and infants.

A study comparing the Melker cricothyrotomy with scalpel-bougie technique in 4 kg postmortem rabbits demonstrated a 100% success rate when the procedures were performed at the most proximal tracheal ring. Success rates decreased as the attempts were made at more caudad level of trachea.[11] In this study, invasive airway access was obtained by two proceduralists experienced in emergency airway management. Both techniques were associated with significant complication rates including lateral and posterior wall injury. Posterior tracheal wall injury was as high as 50% with both techniques. Since the procedures were performed in postmortem animals, it is not certain if the associated injuries would lead to short-term or long-term consequences.

Other complications of cricothyrotomy include unrecognized misplacement in the pretracheal or paratracheal space that would lead to ineffective ventilation. Moreover, secondary complications from attempted ventilation or oxygenation would cause more injuries, including subcutaneous emphysema, which in turn may increase difficulty of subsequent attempts. Fracture of the cricoid cartilage and thyroid cartilages, puncture and injuries to posterior wall of larynx or trachea, injuries to the thyroid gland and vocal cords, and injury to the carotid artery leading to massive bleeding and subglottic stenosis are other possible complications.[24,25] Previous investigation revealed that the force of insertion was proportional to the diameter of device, which in turn is associated with a greater incidence of complications.[26] Apart from familiarity of the device, appropriate choice of and size of the device is also an important factor to reduce complications associated with cricothyrotomy.[6]

The Difficult Airway Society 2015 guidelines for management of the unanticipated difficult intubation in adults recommends scalpel cricothyrotomy as the rescue technique as this is the fastest and most reliable method of securing the airway in the emergency setting, with the advantage of protection from aspiration when a cuffed tube is used.[3] This would certainly apply to adult patients and to clinicians with training and skill in scalpel cricothyrotomy procedure. The small dimensions of the neonatal and infant cricothyroid membrane have led authors to caution against passing ETTs or large-bore catheters through the membrane and into the trachea due to concerns about causing severe damage to the larynx and trachea.[10] The APLS guidelines recommend 12 years as the safe age for consideration of "surgical" cricothyrotomy.[27] The recommendation on age is arbitrary as there is no supporting evidence for a safe age limit for scalpel cricothyrotomy.

The challenges and difficulties with FONA in children and infants are presented. Understanding these challenges should help anesthesiologists to prepare for the CICO situation in children. According to the guidelines from the Difficult Airway Society and the Association of Paediatric Anaesthetists of Great Britain,[2] emergency FONA should be achieved by cannula cricothyrotomy when otolaryngologists are not immediately available. However, if cannula cricothyrotomy is unsuccessful, a scalpel-based technique must be immediately employed.

Oxygenation via Narrow-Bore Cannula

Effective and safe oxygenation is a vital component of a cannula cricothyrotomy.[28] It is important to be aware of the principles of safe high-pressure insufflation, and the impact of a potentially closed glottis or upper airway. If the glottis is closed, then expiration of insufflated oxygen is limited, and barotrauma and volutrauma can ensue, leading to tension pneumothoraces, pneumomediastinum, and cardiovascular arrest. In a true CICO scenario, a partially or completely closed glottis or upper airway is likely to be present. Several devices are available for oxygenation via a cannula: the Manujet ventilator, the Enk OFM, the Meditech System Rapid O_2 insufflator, and the Ventrain. The Manujet and the Enk OFM have been studied in anesthetized rabbit models of the infant lung and trachea[29] and the Enk OFM flow rates have also been studied in a bench test.[17] These devices connect to the Luer of the cannula without the need for an adaptor, thereby protecting against inadvertent disconnection during the emergency.

The Manujet is a hand-triggered jet injector, which allows regulation of both pressure and flow. Flow is controlled by manually depressing the trigger to a greater or lesser extent, and pressure is adjusted by turning the pressure regulator on the side of the device. The Manujet has the ability to generate very high pressures and flows, which can be useful in adults with patent upper airways and an effective means of oxygenation.[30] However, it has no mechanism to allow expiration via the device, and therefore there is no means for expiration when the glottis and upper airway are closed. Although the Manujet has been used successfully in piglet[31,32] and rabbit models with patent upper airways,[29] the risk of barotrauma is considerable.[33] In another study using live rabbit models with severe upper airway obstruction, the Manujet ventilation invariably resulted in barotrauma and mortality, even when the driving pressure was set at the lowest with slow respiratory frequency and long inspiratory and expiratory ratio.[34] Therefore, the use of Manujet or jet ventilator in small children with upper airway obstruction should be discouraged.

The Enk OFM and insufflator are similar devices in principle. Both attach to a wall-mounted oxygen flowmeter, and oxygenation is achieved by occluding holes (five small holes in the Enk OFM, and one large single hole in the insufflator) to force oxygen down the cannula. When the holes are not occluded, no further oxygen is insufflated into the trachea because there is a low resistance pathway to the external environment. During this "non-oxygenation" phase of the resuscitation with the Enk OFM/insufflator, egress of insufflated oxygen via the device is possible. Therefore, these devices offer more protection against barotrauma and volutrauma. Animal studies of the Enk OFM suggest that it has an improved safety profile compared with the Manujet.[35,36] The Enk OFM effectively oxygenated 3–5 kg rabbits[29] as well as moderate-sized piglets over 30 kg.[32] During the author's research,[29] the Enk OFM was observed to be a more forgiving device as no rabbit experienced barotrauma even with upper airway obstruction, high-flow oxygen rates (15 L/min), and high respiratory frequency of 100/min (unpublished data). It was noted that a flow rate as low as 3 L/min with respiratory rate of 15/min was adequate in maintaining oxygenation for 5 minutes in these rabbits. A bench test of the Enk OFM suggests starting at a flow rate of 1 L/(kg min) flow rate with Enk OFM in small children and infants, and then titrating the flow up to achieve the desired effect.[17] There is less published research for the Rapid O_2 insufflator. Both are compact, easy to handle, and provide tactile feedback to the digits occluding the hole(s) in the event of cannula blockage or kinking.

The Ventrain is a new "ventilatory" device, which receives oxygen from a flowmeter and attaches to a Luer connector. It delivers oxygen when the trigger is manually depressed and assists expiration (when the trigger is released) by jet flow generated suction using the Bernoulli principle.[37] It has been tested in animal models with upper airway obstruction.[38] It has also been reported to be used successfully in adult[39] and infant[40] patients in CICO situations. This is a relatively new and promising insufflation device, but still requires familiarity and training in its use. It is still unproven in children and, in theory, may not generate enough suction for active expiration at the lower oxygen flow rates recommended in infants. The amount of suction generated at the lower oxygen flow rates used in infants and small children needs to be further explored.

It is important to maintain upper airway patency during oxygenation via cannula cricothyrotomy to allow egress of insufflated oxygenation. Maneuvers such as jaw thrust and insertion of an oropharyngeal airway should be continued to avoid buildup of intrathoracic pressure. The lowest driving pressure or flow rate should be used to provide oxygenation, and, once chest excursion is observed, insufflation should be stopped to allow adequate time for expiration to occur. In an emergency, there may be a tendency for some clinicians to use rapid respiratory rates during insufflation, as is common when using high-frequency jet ventilation for elective airway procedures. However, instead of rapid respiratory frequency, a slow rate of oxygenation should be employed. Once the chest has risen during insufflation, oxygenation should cease. The time for the initial insufflation will vary with the size of the child. There will be a delay in the rise of the oxygen saturations due to the fact that most oximeters average the saturations over a 15–30-second time period, but the color of the patient's lips and skin should improve rapidly, provided there is adequate cardiac output. The second insufflation should not begin until the chest has fallen and the oxygen saturation begins to

Section 2: Devices and Techniques to Manage the Abnormal Airway

Key points

1. The CICO emergency is even more challenging in children than adults; although, thankfully, it is extremely rare.
2. Debate remains as to the best technique to perform and achieve FONA to the trachea. The authors recommend a cannula technique as the first approach. However, airway doctors also need to be proficient in scalpel-based techniques if cannula oxygenation is unsuccessful.
3. Avoid delaying in the initiation of rescue technique.
   - Consider the use of a checklist or cognitive aids in difficult airway management to address human factor errors.
4. Develop an institutional approach:
   - Have equipment and oxygenation strategies in place.
   - Ensure regular skills training.
   - Hold multidisciplinary drills or simulation training.
5. Effective oxygenation via narrow-bore cannula may be safely performed with the correct technique:
   - Ensure the cannula is in the trachea by positive air aspiration.
   - Oxygenation is the goal, not ventilation.
   - Use the lowest deliverable driving pressure or flow rate.
   - Insufflation of oxygenation should be brief and should cease when the chest has risen. Do not repeat insufflation until the chest has fallen and the oxygen saturations fall.
   - Maintain upper airway patency during transtracheal oxygenation to aid expiration.

decline. In a bench study, it was revealed that high respiratory rate and high pressure is associated with increase in peak and mean pressure.[35] In another experiment on live rabbit models with upper airway obstruction, it was noted that faster respiratory rate and higher pressure or flow rate was associated with buildup of intrathoracic pressure when Manujet or Enk OFM were used as the rescue oxygenation devices.[34] In summary, oxygenation, but not ventilation, is the goal and this temporary measure should allow the surgeon to achieve definitive surgical airway in a controlled manner.

The use of self-assembled devices using oxygen tubing and three-way stopcocks is no longer recommended as the single small orifice does not offer a low resistance path to the environment. Therefore, when the small orifice is not occluded, oxygen will still be insufflated into the trachea, leading to barotrauma. When a three-way stopcock was connected to an oxygen source and the side port was used for pressure release, pressure higher than 70 cmH$_2$O was detected at the catheter tip, even when the side port was left open.[36] Adequate pressure release was only possible when the flow from the oxygen source was lower than 6 L/min, which may be an inadequate flow rate except in small children and infants. Previous reports have described the use of the adaptor of a 3 mm ETT to connect the cannula to a self-inflating bag, or a barrel of 3 ml syringe with an 8 mm ETT adaptor to a self-inflating bag.[41] However, it was noted in a benchtop study that the minute ventilation delivered by a self-inflating bag using various cannula sizes was not detectable.[30] Also, self-assembled devices require time to prepare and are prone to falling apart during stressful emergencies.

References

1 Cook TM, Woodall N, Frerk C. Fourth National Audit P: Major Complications of Airway Management in the UK: Results of the Fourth National Audit Project of the Royal College of Anaesthetists and the Difficult Airway Society. Part 1: Anaesthesia. *British Journal of Anaesthesia* 2011; **106**: 617–31.

2 Paediatric Difficult Airway Guidelines. The Difficult Airway Society and the Association of Paediatric Anaesthetists of Great Britain and Ireland. Website. https://www.das.uk.com/guidelines/paediatric-difficult-airway-guidelines

3 Frerk C, Mitchell VS, McNarry AF, Mendonca C, Bhagrath R, Patel A, O'Sullivan EP, Woodall NM, Ahmad I. Difficult Airway

Society 2015 Guidelines for Management of Unanticipated Difficult Intubation in Adults. *British Journal of Anaesthesia* 2015; **115**: 827–48.

4. Jagannathan N, Ramsey MA, White MC, Sohn L. An Update on Newer Pediatric Supraglottic Airways with Recommendations for Clinical Use. *Paediatric Anaesthesia* 2015; **25**: 334–45.

5. Boon JM, Abrahams PH, Meiring JH, Welch T. Cricothyroidotomy: a Clinical Anatomy Review. *Clinical Anatomy* 2004; **17**: 478–86.

6. Cote CJ, Hartnick CJ. Pediatric Transtracheal and Cricothyrotomy Airway Devices for Emergency Use: which are Appropriate for Infants and Children? *Paediatric Anaesthesia* 2009; **19**(Suppl. 1): 66–76.

7. Elliott DS, Baker PA, Scott MR, Birch CW, Thompson JM. Accuracy of Surface Landmark Identification for Cannula Cricothyroidotomy. *Anaesthesia* 2010; **65**: 889–94.

8. Bennett JD, Guha SC, Sankar AB. Cricothyrotomy: the Anatomical Basis. *Journal of the Royal College of Surgeons of Edinburgh* 1996; **41**: 57–60.

9. Dover K, Howdieshell TR, Colborn GL. The Dimensions and Vascular Anatomy of the Cricothyroid Membrane: Relevance to Emergent Surgical Airway Access. *Clinical Anatomy* 1996; **9**: 291–5.

10. Navsa N, Tossel G, Boon JM. Dimensions of the Neonatal Cricothyroid Membrane – How Feasible is a Surgical Cricothyroidotomy? *Paediatric Anaesthesia* 2005; **15**: 402–6.

11. Prunty SL, Aranda-Palacios A, Heard AM, Chapman G, Ramgolam A, Hegarty M, Vijayasekaran S, von Ungern-Sternberg BS. The "Can't Intubate Can't Oxygenate" Scenario in Pediatric Anesthesia: a Comparison of the Melker Cricothyroidotomy Kit with a Scalpel Bougie Technique. *Paediatric Anaesthesia* 2015; **25**: 400–4.

12. Sabato SC, Long E. An Institutional Approach to the Management of the "Can't Intubate, Can't Oxygenate" Emergency in Children. *Paediatric Anaesthesia* 2016; **26**: 784–93.

13. Ezri T, Szmuk P, Warters RD, Katz J, Hagberg CA. Difficult Airway Management Practice Patterns among Anesthesiologists Practicing in the United States: Have We Made any Progress? *Journal of Clinical Anesthesia* 2003; **15**: 418–22.

14. Wong DT, Lai K, Chung FF, Ho RY. Cannot Intubate–Cannot Ventilate and Difficult Intubation Strategies: Results of a Canadian National Survey. *Anesthesia & Analgesia* 2005; **100**: 1439–46.

15. DrAMBHeardAirway (2013). Heard A: 01 Cannula Insertion. Online Video Clip. https://www.youtube.com/watch?v=6LDEMmOcSB8&feature=player_embedded

16. Stacey J, Heard AM, Chapman G, Wallace CJ, Hegarty M, Vijayasekaran S, von Ungern-Sternberg BS. The "Can't Intubate Can't Oxygenate" Scenario in Pediatric Anesthesia: a Comparison of Different Devices for Needle Cricothyroidotomy. *Paediatric Anaesthesia* 2012; **22**: 1155–8.

17. Baker PA, Brown AJ. Experimental Adaptation of the Enk Oxygen Flow Modulator for Potential Pediatric Use. *Paediatric Anaesthesia* 2009; **19**: 458–63.

18. DrAMBHeardAirway (2013). Heard A: 02 Scalpel Bougie. Online Video Clip. https://www.youtube.com/watch?v=SbhEyGIf9Y4

19. Heard A, Dinsmore J, Douglas S, Lacquiere D. Plan D: Cannula First, or Scalpel Only? *British Journal of Anaesthesia* 2016; **117**: 533–5.

20. Heard AM. Can't Oxygenate Scenario (CICO): Implications of the National Audit Project (NAP4) of the Royal College of Anaesthetists. *ANZCA Bulletin* 2011.

21. Holm-Knudsen RJ, Rasmussen LS, Charabi B, Bottger M, Kristensen MS. Emergency Airway Access in Children – Transtracheal Cannulas and Tracheotomy Assessed in a Porcine Model. *Paediatric Anaesthesia* 2012; **22**: 1159–65.

22. Johansen K, Holm-Knudsen RJ, Charabi B, Kristensen MS, Rasmussen LS. Cannot Ventilate–Cannot Intubate an Infant: Surgical Tracheotomy or Transtracheal Cannula? *Paediatric Anaesthesia* 2010; **20**: 987–93.

23. Hebbard PD, Ul Hassan I, Bourke EK. Cricothyroidotomy Catheters: an Investigation of Mechanisms of Failure and the Effect of a Novel Intracatheter Stylet. *Anaesthesia* 2016; **71**: 39–43.

24. Chan TC, Vilke GM, Bramwell KJ, Davis DP, Hamilton RS, Rosen P. Comparison of Wire-Guided Cricothyrotomy versus Standard Surgical Cricothyrotomy Technique. *Journal of Emergency Medicine* 1999; **17**: 957–62.

25. Schober P, Hegemann MC, Schwarte LA, Loer SA, Noetges P. Emergency Cricothyrotomy – a Comparative Study of Different Techniques in Human Cadavers. *Resuscitation* 2009; **80**: 204–9.

26. Abbrecht PH, Kyle RR, Reams WH, Brunette J. Insertion Forces and Risk of Complications during Cricothyroid Cannulation. *Journal of Emergency Medicine* 1992; **10**: 417–26.

27. Practical Procedures: Airway and Breathing. In Samuels M,

Wieteska S, eds. *Advanced Paediatric Life Support: the Practical Approach*. 5th ed. West Sussex, UK: Wiley-Blackwell, BMJ Publishing; 2012: 201–16.

28 Bould MD, Bearfield P. Techniques for Emergency Ventilation through a Needle Cricothyroidotomy. *Anaesthesia* 2008; **63**: 535–9.

29 Wong CF, Yuen VM, Wong GT, To J, Irwin MG. Time to Adequate Oxygenation Following Ventilation Using the Enk Oxygen Flow Modulator versus a jet Ventilator via Needle Cricothyrotomy in Rabbits. *Paediatric Anaesthesia* 2014; **24**: 208–13.

30 Flint NJ, Russell WC, Thompson JP. Comparison of Different Methods of Ventilation via Cannula Cricothyroidotomy in a Trachea-Lung Model. *British Journal of Anaesthesia* 2009; **103**: 891–5.

31 Preussler NP, Schreiber T, Huter L, Gottschall R, Schubert H, Rek H, Karzai W, Schwarzkopf K. Percutaneous Transtracheal Ventilation: Effects of a New Oxygen Flow Modulator on Oxygenation and Ventilation in Pigs Compared with a Hand Triggered Emergency Jet Injector. *Resuscitation* 2003; **56**: 329–33.

32 Yildiz Y, Preussler NP, Schreiber T, Hueter L, Gaser E, Schubert H, Gottschall R, Schwarzkopf K. Percutaneous Transtracheal Emergency Ventilation during Respiratory Arrest: Comparison of the Oxygen Flow Modulator with a Hand-Triggered Emergency Jet Injector in an Animal Model. *The American Journal of Emergency Medicine* 2006; **24**: 455–9.

33 Depierraz B, Ravussin P, Brossard E, Monnier P. Percutaneous Transtracheal Jet Ventilation for Paediatric Endoscopic Laser Treatment of Laryngeal and Subglottic Lesions. *Canadian Journal of Anesthesia/Journal canadien d'anesthésie* 1994; **41**: 1200–7.

34 Yuen VMY, Wong CHP, Wong SSC, Wong GTC. Rescue Oxygenation in Small Infants. *Anaesthesia* 2017; **72**: 1564–5.

35 Lenfant F, Pean D, Brisard L, Freysz M, Lejus C. Oxygen Delivery during Transtracheal Oxygenation: a Comparison of Two Manual Devices. *Anesthesia & Analgesia* 2010; **111**: 922–4.

36 Hamaekers A, Borg P, Enk D. The Importance of Flow and Pressure Release in Emergency Jet Ventilation Devices. *Paediatric Anaesthesia* 2009; **19**: 452–7.

37 Hamaekers AE, Borg PA, Enk D. Ventrain: an Ejector Ventilator for Emergency Use. *British Journal of Anaesthesia* 2012; **108**: 1017–21.

38 Paxian M, Preussler NP, Reinz T, Schlueter A, Gottschall R. Transtracheal Ventilation with a Novel Ejector-Based Device (Ventrain) in Open, Partly Obstructed, or Totally Closed Upper Airways in Pigs. *British Journal of Anaesthesia* 2015; **115**: 308–16.

39 Borg PA, Hamaekers AE, Lacko M, Jansen J, Enk D. Ventrain for Ventilation of the Lungs. *British Journal of Anaesthesia* 2012; **109**: 833–4.

40 Willemsen MG, Noppens R, Mulder AL, Enk D. Ventilation with the Ventrain through a Small Lumen Catheter in the Failed Paediatric Airway: Two Case Reports. *British Journal of Anaesthesia* 2014; **112**: 946–7.

41 Wheeler M, Cote CJ, Todres ID. The Pediatric Airway. In Cote CJ, Lerman J, Todres ID, eds. *A Practice of Anesthesia for Infants and Children*. 4th ed. Philadelphia: Saunders Elsevier; 2009: 237–78.

Section 2 Devices and Techniques to Manage the Abnormal Airway

Chapter 14

Ultrasonography for Airway Management

Michael S. Kristensen, Wendy H. Teoh, and Thomas Engelhardt

Introduction

Airway ultrasonography is becoming an integrated part of management of the pediatric airway. In this chapter we will:

- describe the equipment needed for pediatric airway ultrasonography
- describe the typical features of airway ultrasonography, including the tissue/air border
- show how the airway appears on ultrasonography from the tip of the tongue to the pleura
- list the most useful clinical indications for airway ultrasonography and provide detailed instructions of these techniques

Equipment Required for Airway Ultrasonography

There is no single ultrasound probe available that allows visualization of all airway structures in children of all ages. In larger children above approximately 8 years of age, the linear medium-to-high frequency (5–14 MHz) transducer is suitable for imaging superficial airway structures (within 0–5 cm beneath the skin surface).[1] The curved low-frequency transducer (~4.0 MHz) is most suitable for obtaining sagittal and parasagittal views of the tongue and structures in the submandibular and supraglottic regions, mainly because of its wider field of view. Linear transducers, which are used for assessment of the upper airways, provide excellent images of superficial structures, such as ribs and the pleura, but deeper structures can be difficult to assess. A micro-convex transducer (~8.0 MHz) is a good all-round transducer for focused ultrasonographic examination of the lungs, since most micro-convex transducers have an acceptable image quality of both superficial (pleura) and deeper structures (e.g., lung consolidation, atelectasis). Furthermore, micro-convex transducers are often small, which makes it easier to access the posterior thoracic wall, when the patient can only be examined in the supine position. An alternative to the micro-convex transducer for examination of the lungs is the curved low-frequency transducer (~4.0 MHz), which also has an acceptable image quality of both superficial and deeper structures. Since visualization of superficial and deep structures is needed, it is important to continuously optimize transducer frequency to obtain the best possible images. The presence or absence of artifacts are an important part of lung ultrasonography; hence, one should be mindful to deactivate any image optimization software that is inherently built into newer ultrasound machines as this would remove or diminish the presence of these useful artifacts when performing lung ultrasonography.

In small children, a smaller linear hockey-stick high-frequency (4–15 MHz) probe is suitable and produces a smaller linear image. This probe has similar imaging characteristics to the standard linear transducer, but the smaller footprint allows better access into the necks of younger children who have shorter necks rich in subcutaneous fat. A small footprint, micro-convex probe is particularly useful in imaging the chest, allowing visualization through the intercostal spaces when required. Three-dimensional ultrasonography is a promising modality for airway imaging[2] and is especially suitable for prenatal diagnosis of airway abnormalities.

The Typical Features of Airway Ultrasonography, Including the Tissue/Air Border

Reflected energy arriving back to the transducer is used to construct the images with the intensity of the received echoes projected at different gray levels. The result is that different anatomical structures in the body are portrayed at a different echogenicity, ranging from completely black (anechoic/echolucent), dark appearances (hypoechoic), spanning up to very bright and white appearances (hyperechoic) on the ultrasound screen.

- *B-mode scanning* (B: brightness mode): These are two-dimensional standard ultrasound images with structural information in the images obtained with multiple scan lines of different brightness of gray refreshed at different frequencies per second. The lower the frequency utilized, the deeper the penetration and information obtained, but this will result in the images of deeper structures becoming less detailed.
- *M-mode scanning* (M: motion mode): The information that creates the image comes from one single scan line placed over the area of interest with a graphical movement of the structures along this scan line projected as depth versus time. A classic example where such M-mode is useful is in assessing the movement of the pleural layers sliding against each other.

Appearances of the Anatomical Airway Structures

It is important to be consistent with the imaging parameters and settings to be able to develop a "mental database" of normal appearances. Below are the expected echogenic appearances of different anatomical structures when scanned at higher frequencies (as one would expect to utilize in children when imaging superficial structures).

- *Air:* Air is a very poor conductor of ultrasound.[3] Hence, an interface between the ultrasound probe and the skin excluding air is required for successful transmission of the ultrasound energy provided by the use of ultrasound gel.

   As soon as the ultrasound beam reaches air, a strong echo (= a strong white line) will appear. This is the tissue/air border and everything beyond that line is only artifact. This means that we can visualize the tissue from the skin and until the anterior part of the airway as, for example, the posterior surface of the tongue, the mucosal lining of the anterior trachea, and the pleura. Intraluminal air will thus prevent visualization of structures such as the posterior pharynx, posterior commissure, and posterior wall of the trachea.

- *Air bubbles:* Air bubbles result in tiny hyperechoic (bright) foci: these often have a "ring-down artifact." This is a characteristic appearance resulting in a "comet-tail appearance" secondary to resonance phenomenon by the air bubbles. When a whole interface of air is encountered (for example, at the lung surface), this appears hyperechoic with similar artifacts seen deep to the superficial surface.
- *Fat:* Fat appears hyperechoic (bright). Such appearances can be consistently seen in the subcutaneous fat, but also in between structures in the neck.
- *Muscle:* Muscular structures are generally of lower echogenicity (= dark) on ultrasound. Within these, one can see hyperechoic linearity from the connective tissue supporting the muscular fibers. On transverse imaging, these can be seen as brighter dots while they appear more linear when the muscle group is imaged in the longitudinal plane. Hyperechogenicity may be appreciated around the muscles from the supporting tissue.
- *Bone:* Ultrasound travels very poorly through bone. Bony structures result in a very bright line/interface at the surface of the bone with a significant posterior acoustic shadowing. This is limiting, or even eliminating, the information that can be obtained behind the bony structures. An alternative window should be attempted if possible to study such structures.
- *Cartilage:* Appearances of cartilaginous structures can be variable depending on the density and how much calcification is present within. However, as a general rule, cartilage appears hypoechoic (low echogenicity/dark) when compared to fat around it.
- *Fluid:* The echogenic appearances of fluids are variable and depend on the consistency and density of the material in question. Clear fluid (such as urine in the bladder) appears anechoic (black). Similar appearances are seen in cysts containing clear fluid that can be encountered in the neck (such as cystic hygroma or a simple thyroid cyst; blood in vessels appear dark).
- *Vascular structures:* These appear as hypoechoic, round or oval structures in the transverse plane, and linear tube-like structures in the longitudinal plane. Flow is identified if interrogated with Doppler ultrasound.

- *Glandular structures:* The major glandular structures such as the thyroid gland or submandibular or parotid gland appear mildly hyperechoic.

The Sonographic Appearance of the Airway, from the Tongue to the Pleura

The normal airway from the tongue to the pleura is depicted in Figures 14.1–10.

Clinical Indications for Airway Ultrasonography and Detailed Instructions of these Techniques

There are numerous indications for the use of ultrasonography in pediatric airway management. The currently most useful applications are:

- qualifying and quantifying airway pathology or deviations from normal anatomy

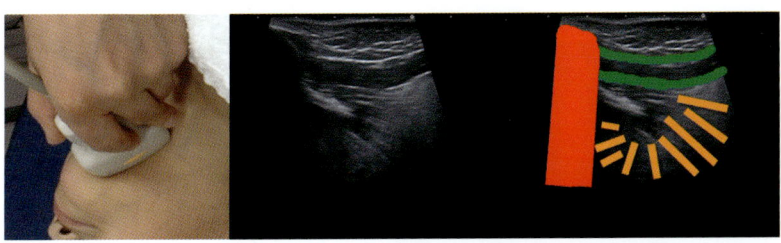

Figure 14.1 Tongue longitudinal. Left: the position of the transducer. Middle: the scanning image, showing B-mode scanning. Right: the linear transducer positioned in the midline of the submental region. The following structures are identified: the mentum of the mandible and the shadow it forms (red), tongue (orange), and muscles of the floor of the mouth (green).

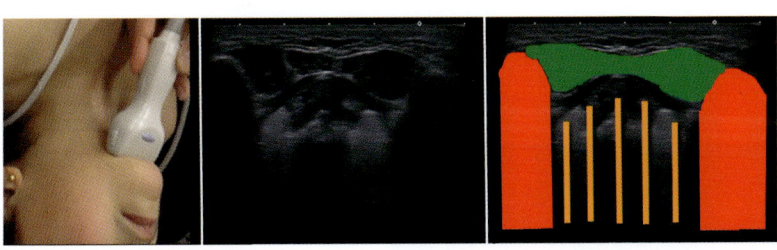

Figure 14.2 Tongue transverse. Left: the patient is positioned supine. A planar linear high-frequency transducer is placed horizontally and transversely in the submental region. Middle: the scanning image, showing B-mode scanning. Right: tongue (orange), muscles of the floor of the mouth (green). The mandible and the shadow from the mandible (red).

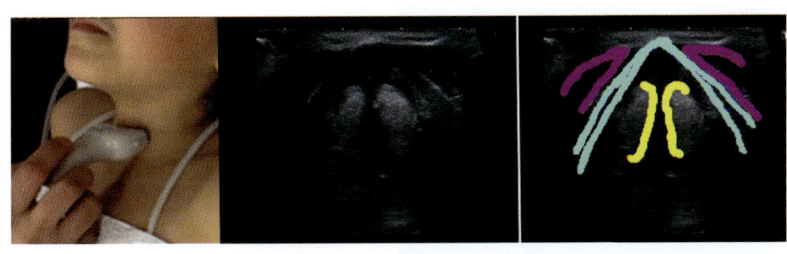

Figure 14.3 Larynx with false cords. Left: the position of the transducer. Middle: the scanning image, showing B-mode scanning.
Transverse image at the level of the upper larynx. Right: the strap muscles are hypoechoic (purple), thyroid cartilage (light blue), and the echogenic false vocal cords (yellow).

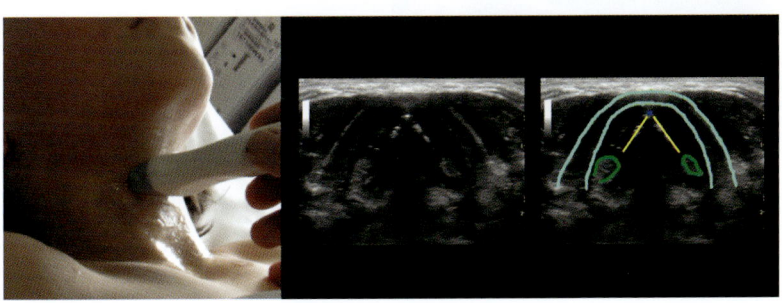

Figure 14.4 Larynx with vocal cords. Left: the position of the transducer. Middle: the scanning image, showing B-mode scanning. Right: thyroid cartilage (light blue), the free edge of the vocal cords (yellow), anterior commissure (blue), and the arytenoid cartilages (green).

Section 2: Devices and Techniques to Manage the Abnormal Airway

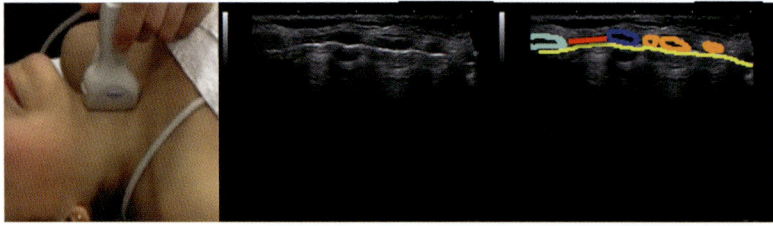

Figure 14.5 Lower larynx and upper part of the trachea.
Left: the position of the transducer. Middle: the scanning image, showing B-mode scanning. Right: midline longitudinal view. Thyroid cartilage (light blue), cricothyroid membrane (red), anterior part of the cricoid cartilage (dark blue), anterior part of tracheal rings (orange), and the tissue/air border at the mucosal lining inside the airway (yellow).

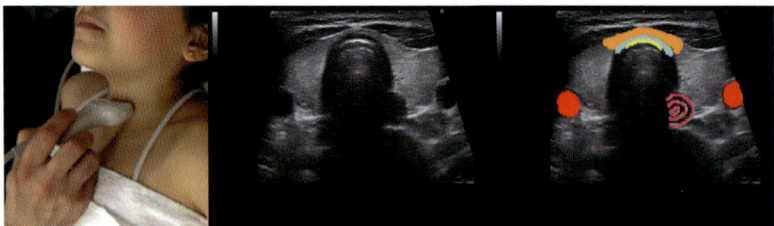

Figure 14.6 Transverse scan of middle/upper part of the trachea.
Left: the position of the transducer. Middle: the scanning image, showing B-mode scanning. Right: isthmus of the thyroid gland (orange), anterior part of tracheal ring (light blue), the tissue/air border of the anterior luminal side of the trachea (yellow), and the carotid arteries (red). The esophagus posteromedial to the trachea on the left is seen as a multilayered structure (purple).

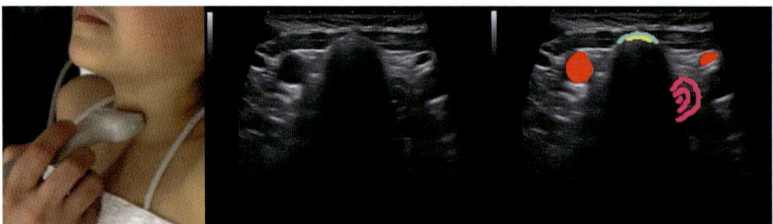

Figure 14.7 Transverse scan of the trachea just cephalic to the suprasternal notch.
Left: the position of the transducer. Middle: the scanning image, showing B-mode scanning. Right: anterior part of tracheal ring (light blue), the tissue/air border of the anterior luminal side of the trachea (yellow), the carotid arteries (red). The esophagus posteromedial to the trachea on the left is seen as a multilayered structure (purple).

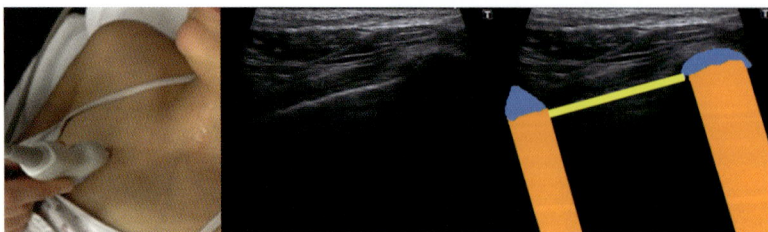

Figure 14.8 Ribs and pleural line.
Left: the position of the transducer, the probe placed transversely to the orientation of the ribs. Middle: the scanning image, showing B-mode scanning. Right: both ribs can be seen as a hyperechoic structure (blue) with associated posterior acoustic shadowing (orange). The pleura (combined visceral and parietal) is seen as an echogenic bright white line (yellow) deep to this level. This echogenic line is seen to move slightly with ventilation (lung sliding). The picture is from an older child. In very young children, the pleural line may be seen on the pleural side of the rib.

Chapter 14: Ultrasonography for Airway Management

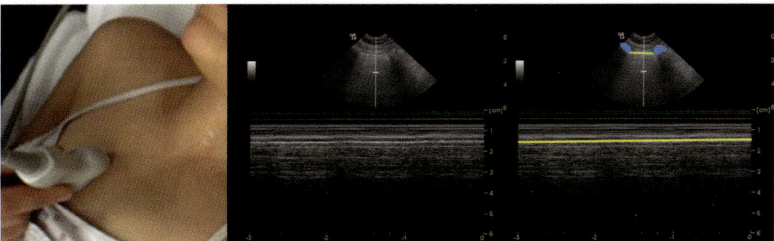

Figure 14.9 Sliding lung sign.
Lung sliding. Left: the transducer is placed over an interspace between two ribs during normal ventilation. Middle: the scanning image, showing B-mode scanning above and M-mode scanning below. Right: the pleural line is marked in yellow and the ribs in blue (the curved lines at each end of the straight line). In the M-mode image, it is easy to distinguish the nonmoving tissue above the pleural line from the artifact caused by respiratory movement of the visceral pleura relative to the parietal pleura. This is called the "seashore sign" or the "sandy beach sign" because the nonmoving part resembles waves and the artifact pattern below resembles a sandy beach.

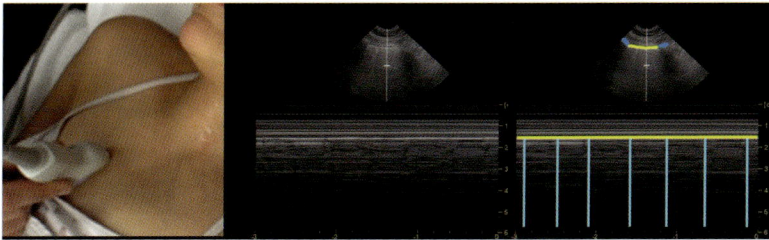

Figure 14.10 Lung pulse.
Left: placement of the transducer. Middle: the scanning image, showing B-mode scanning above and M-mode scanning below. In this non-ventilated lung, the only movement is that caused by the heartbeat, which creates a subtle movement of the lungs and the pleura. This movement is visualized in the M-mode image synchronous with the heartbeat and is called the "lung pulse." Right: the pleural line is marked in yellow and the ribs in blue. The light blue lines indicate the lung pulse.

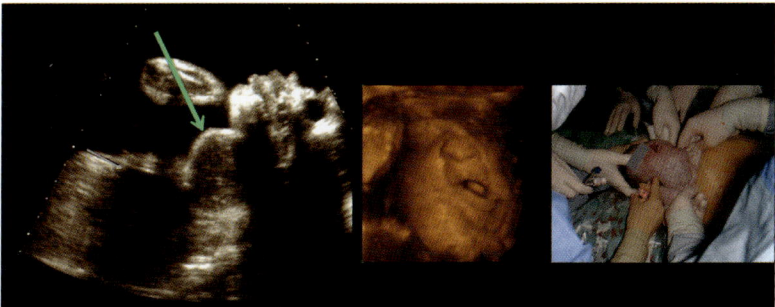

Figure 14.11 Fetal airway ultrasonography.
Left: a large tumor is seen on the neck of the fetus (green arrow). Middle: 3D ultrasonographic image. Right: the head is delivered and the airway is managed while the fetal circulation is still intact. (Courtesy of Connie Jørgensen. MD Rigshospitalet, University Hospital of Copenhagen.)

- identification of the trachea and the cricothyroid membrane prior to airway management in a known or suspected difficult airway before induction of anesthesia
- prediction of the optimal tracheal tube diameter
- correct tracheal tube placement
- confirmation or exclusion of an intraoperative pneumothorax

Qualifying and Quantifying Airway Pathology and Foreign Bodies

Fetal ultrasound screening can reveal fetal airway abnormalities.[4] The EXIT procedure permits a controlled partial delivery of a fetus with prenatally diagnosed airway obstruction, allowing continued placental function while the fetal airway is secured (Figure 14.11).

Advances in ultrasound technology now enable three- and four-dimensional imaging, providing additional detail and three-dimensional renderings of the fetal anatomy. The abnormalities detected and treated include teratoma (cervical, pharyngeal, epignathus), lymphatic/vascular malformation, congenital giant ranula, and severe micrognathia.

There are several ultrasound-guided screening procedures that have been demonstrated to predict difficult direct laryngoscopy in subgroups of adult patients, but none of these have yet demonstrated their value as a screening tool in the general[3] or in the pediatric population. A foreign body can be visualized as long as it is in contact with the superficial part of the natural orifice in which it is lodged (mouth, pharynx, trachea, esophagus). Ultrasonography may be useful in the retrieval of the foreign body during the procedure.

Identification of the Trachea and of the Cricothyroid Membrane

Oxygenation via the anterior neck is the ultimate escape and last resort for oxygenation when all other methods have failed. In larger children, this should primarily be via the cricothyroid membrane, whereas in younger children access via the trachea is preferred.[5,6]

The trachea and the cricothyroid membrane should thus be identified in all patients with a suspected or known difficult airway before induction of anesthesia if time allows. In the majority of children, the identification can be done with inspection alone, or, if necessary, supplemented with palpation. However, in some patients, especially the obese or patients with airway malformations, it may be impossible to reliably identify the cricothyroid membrane and the trachea with inspection and palpation alone.[7]

In these cases, ultrasonographic identification should be performed. We describe two approaches that have each been shown to achieve a 90% success rate in the morbidly obese after a short training of the operator. The cricothyroid membrane was identified in all cases with at least one of the techniques, suggesting that the clinician should be proficient in both approaches.[8]

The transverse technique (the "TACA" technique: thyroid cartilage, airline, cricoid cartilage, airline):[8]

1. Place the transducer transversely on the anterior neck at the estimated level of the thyroid cartilage and move the transducer until the thyroid cartilage is identified as a hyperechoic triangular structure (Figure 14.12).
2. Move the transducer caudally until the cricothyroid membrane is identified: this is recognizable as a hyperechoic white line resulting from the echo of the air/tissue border of the mucosal lining on the inside of the cricothyroid membrane, often with parallel white lines (reverberation artifacts) below.
3. Move the transducer further caudally until the cricoid cartilage is identified (a black lying "C" with a white lining).
4. Finally move the transducer slightly back cephalic until the center of the cricothyroid membrane is identified.
5. The location of the cricothyroid membrane can be marked both transversely and sagittal on the skin with a pen. By identifying both the highly characteristic shapes of the thyroid and the cricoid cartilages, both the cephalic and caudal borders of the cricothyroid membrane have been identified.

The technique is demonstrated in an online video.[9]

The Longitudinal technique (the string-of-pearls technique):[8]

1. Palpate the sternal bone and place the ultrasound transducer transversely on the patient's anterior neck cephalic to the suprasternal notch to visualize the trachea (horseshoe-shaped dark structure with a posterior white line) (Figure 14.13).
2. Slide the transducer toward the patient's right side (toward the operator), so that the right border of the transducer is positioned midline of the trachea, and the ultrasound image of the tracheal ring is thus truncated into half on the screen.
3. Keep the right end of the transducer in the midline of the trachea, while the left end of the transducer is rotated 90 degrees into the sagittal plane, resulting in a longitudinal scan of the midline of the trachea. A number of dark (hypoechoic) rings will be seen anterior to the white hyperechoic line (air/tissue border), akin to a string of pearls. The dark hypoechoic "pearls" are the anterior part of the tracheal rings.
4. Maintain the transducer longitudinally in the midline and slide it cephalic until the cricoid cartilage comes into view (seen as a larger, more elongated, and anteriorly placed dark "pearl" compared to the other tracheal rings). Further cephalic, the distal part of the thyroid cartilage can be seen as well. The transducer now indicates the longitudinal course of the airway.

Chapter 14: Ultrasonography for Airway Management

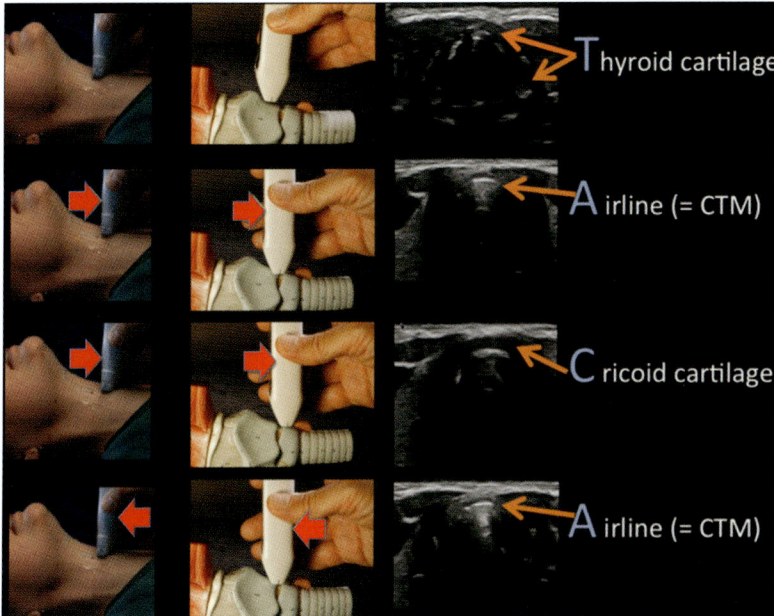

Figure 14.12 Transverse technique for identification of the cricothyroid membrane.
The transverse (thyroid-airline-cricoid-airline: TACA) method for identification of the cricothyroid membrane.
First row: the transducer is placed transversely on the neck where the thyroid cartilage is thought to be until the triangular shape of the thyroid cartilage (the "T") is identified.
Second row: the transducer is moved caudally until the "airline" (the "A") is seen: this is the hyperechoic (white) line from the tissue/air border on the luminal side of the cricothyroid membrane. The white line has similar echo lines deep to it: those are reverberation artifacts.
Third row: the transducer is moved further caudally until the cricoid cartilage (the "C") is seen as a black lying "C" with a posterior white lining. The white lining represents the tissue/air border on the luminal side of the anterior part of the cricoid cartilage.
Fourth row: subsequently, the transducer is moved a few millimeters back in cephalic direction and the approximate center of the "airline" (the "A"), the cricothyroid membrane, is thus identified and can be marked with a pen – by marking the midpoint of the footprint of the transducer.

5. Keep holding the ultrasound transducer with the right hand and use the left hand to slide a needle (as a marker that casts a shadow in the ultrasound image) between the transducer and the patient's skin until the needle's shadow is seen midway between the caudal border of the thyroid cartilage and the cephalic border of the cricoid cartilage.
6. Remove the transducer. Now the needle indicates the center of the cricothyroid membrane in the transverse plane and this can be marked on the skin with a pen.

The technique is demonstrated in an online video.[10]

Each of these two techniques has its own advantages. Some patients have limited space in the neck unable to accommodate the ultrasound transducer in a longitudinal midsagittal position (e.g., short necks, severe neck flexion deformity). Here, the transverse technique will be useful, and is the faster of the two techniques. The longitudinal technique, on the other hand, reveals additional information compared to the transverse technique; that is, the localization of the cricoid-tracheal interspace and of the tracheal interspaces. Apart from the ability to identify overlying blood vessels and direct the clinician to choose another tracheal interspace for elective tracheostomy or retrograde intubation, the longitudinal technique is useful in airway rescue situations where emergency access via the trachea would be needed instead of access via the cricothyroid membrane (e.g., smaller children, patients with tumors overlying the cricothyroid membrane, subglottic obstruction). We recommend that clinicians learn and become proficient in both techniques as either technique can overcome shortcomings of the other.

Prediction of the Optimal Diameter of the ETT

The internal diameter of the trachea can reliably be determined using ultrasound. Careful ultrasound scanning allows the identification of abnormal subglottic narrowing and selection of optimal size of

Section 2: Devices and Techniques to Manage the Abnormal Airway

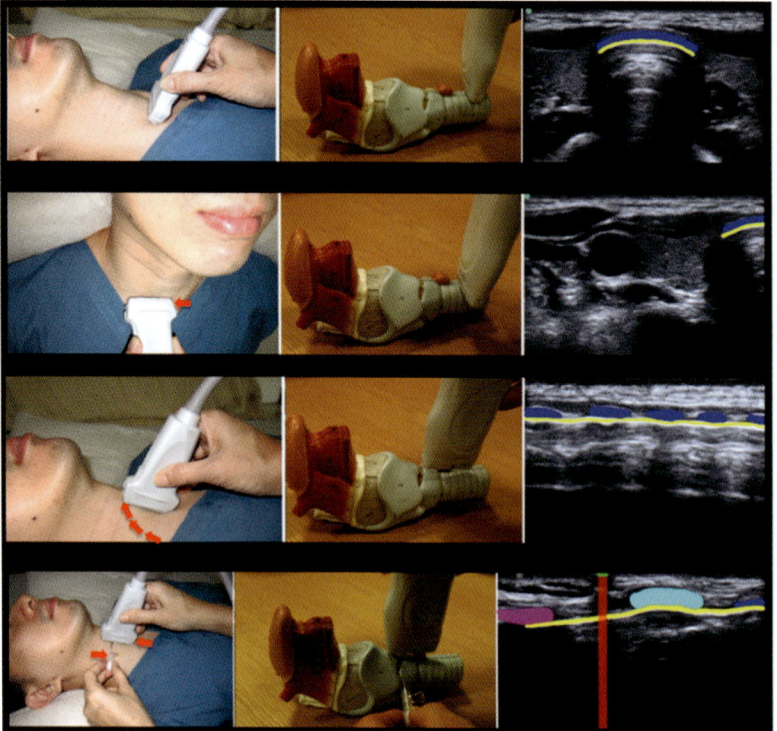

Figure 14.13 Longitudinal technique for identification of the cricothyroid membrane.

Upper row. Step one: the patient is lying supine and the operator stands on the patient's right side facing the patient. The sternal bone and the suprasternal notch are palpated, which can be done in even the morbidly obese patient. The linear high-frequency transducer is placed transversely over the neck just cranial to the suprasternal notch and the trachea is seen in the midline. The middle and the right photo show the ultrasound image and the relevant structures are highlighted on the photo to the right. Blue is the anterior part of a tracheal ring. Yellow indicates the tissue/air boundary inside the trachea. Everything below the tissue/air boundary is artifact.

Second row. Step two: the transducer is slid laterally toward the patient's right side, until the midline of the trachea is at the right border of the transducer, and the corresponding ultrasound image of the trachea (in the right photo) is truncated into half. Blue is the anterior part of a tracheal ring. Yellow indicates the tissue/air boundary inside the trachea.

Third row. Step three: staying midline with the right edge of the transducer, the left edge of the transducer is rotated into the sagittal plane to obtain a longitudinal image of the trachea. The anterior part of the tracheal rings appear as black hypoechoic round structures (like pearls) lying on a strong hyperechoic white line, which is the tissue/air boundary (and which looks like a string). Hence, the image is akin to a string of pearls. The blue markings represent the anterior parts of the tracheal rings. Yellow indicates the tissue/air boundary inside the trachea.

Fourth row. Step four: the transducer is slid cephalic and the anterior part of the cricoid cartilage (turquoise) is seen as a slightly elongated structure, which is significantly larger and more anterior than the tracheal rings (blue). Yellow indicates the tissue/air boundary inside the trachea. Immediately cephalic to the cricoid cartilage is the distal part of the cricothyroid membrane. The distal part of the thyroid cartilage (purple) is seen.

Step five: the cricothyroid membrane can be pointed out by sliding a needle (used only as a marker) underneath the ultrasonography transducer from the cranial end until it casts a shadow (red line) just cranial to the cricoid cartilage (turquoise). The green spot represents the reflection from the needle. Care is taken not to touch the patient with the sharp tip of the needle.

Step six: the transducer is removed, and the needle indicates the level of the distal part of the cricothyroid membrane. This spot can be marked with a pen so that it remains easily located should it be needed for subsequent difficult airway management.

tracheal tubes. Although technically feasible, routine use of this application appears useful only if uncuffed tubes are used and in long-term ventilated pediatric patients who may benefit from this noninvasive scan when upsizing or downsizing of tracheostomy tubes is required in the perioperative period.[1] A simple ultrasound-guided measurement of the minimal transverse diameter of the subglottic airway is a better guide for selection of the optimal tube diameter than age-related formulas in children below 5 years of age.[11] The method is based on the assumption that the minimal transverse diameter of the subglottic

Chapter 14: Ultrasonography for Airway Management

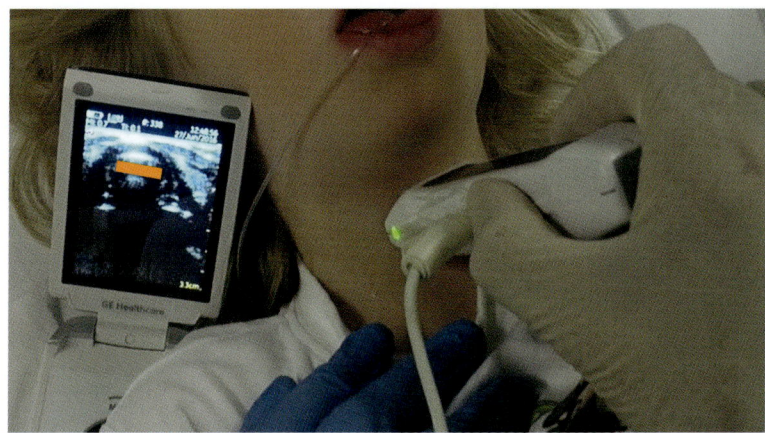

Figure 14.14 Measuring internal width of the trachea.
The linear transducer is placed at the level of the cricoid cartilage, thus measuring the internal diameter at the narrowest part of the upper airway (orange).

airway is equal to the outer diameter of a correctly fitting ETT. A high-frequency linear transducer is placed transversely over the cricoid cartilage and the diameter is measured during expiration (Figure 14.14).[11]

Correct Tracheal Tube Placement

Visualization of the tracheal tube passing the vocal cords and the detection of end-tidal carbon dioxide are considered the gold standards of verification of successful tracheal intubation. This may not always be achievable; for example, during difficult laryngoscopy or in patients with a low cardiac output. In addition, neither standard allows distinction between a tracheal and a bronchial intubation. Ultrasonography is able to provide an additional new way to confirm successful tracheal intubation and allows detection of inadvertent bronchial intubation. The tracheal tube position within the trachea can be verified using ultrasonography in two ways: direct (scans of the anterior neck during or immediately after intubation) or indirect (detecting ventilation at the pleura or diaphragm). Direct ultrasound scans of the anterior neck can be performed in three distinct areas: transversely (high on the neck at the level of the vocal cords where the dynamic, real-time tissue movement due to the tracheal tube can be detected), transversely (lower on the neck at the level of the suprasternal notch where both dynamic and static scanning are effective), and longitudinally (covering the visible length of trachea). The authors recommend placing a linear, high-frequency transducer transverse onto the neck immediately cranial to the suprasternal notch in the midline (Figure 14.7). The trachea is identified as a horseshoe-shaped dark structure with a strong white line tissue/air border artifact and a "comet-tail" artifact immediately posterior. The esophagus is most often seen posterolateral to the trachea on the patient's left side and has a "bullseye" appearance due to its concentric layers. Asking the patient to swallow will make the esophagus compress and expand, and will aid in its identification. Intubation should be performed following induction of anesthesia. If the tracheal tube enters trachea, a brief "snowstorm" artifact may be seen as the tracheal tube touches the anterior tracheal wall. No artifact may be seen if a layer of air separates the tracheal tube from the mucosa, precluding conduction of the ultrasound beam onto the tracheal tube. If the tube enters the esophagus, it will create a tissue/air border in the otherwise collapsed esophagus. This will appear as a strong white horizontal line, which may repeat itself several times (like a flutter) due to the "comet-tail"-like artifact. The esophagus will assume a shape similar to the trachea, and a "double-trachea" sign will appear (Figure 14.15). If the tracheal tube is seen passing into the esophagus, it should be removed without initiating positive-pressure ventilation. Successful intubation may or may not create an echo from within the trachea, so ventilation can be initiated provided the tube has not been identified in the esophagus.

Subsequently, the transducer is moved to the mid-axillary line on either side of the patient's chest. The pleural line is identified, posterior to the rib. During positive-pressure ventilation, a "lung-slide" sign should be visualized bilaterally (Figure 14.9).

Lung sliding appears as a to-and-fro movement synchronous with ventilation. The movement is

Section 2: Devices and Techniques to Manage the Abnormal Airway

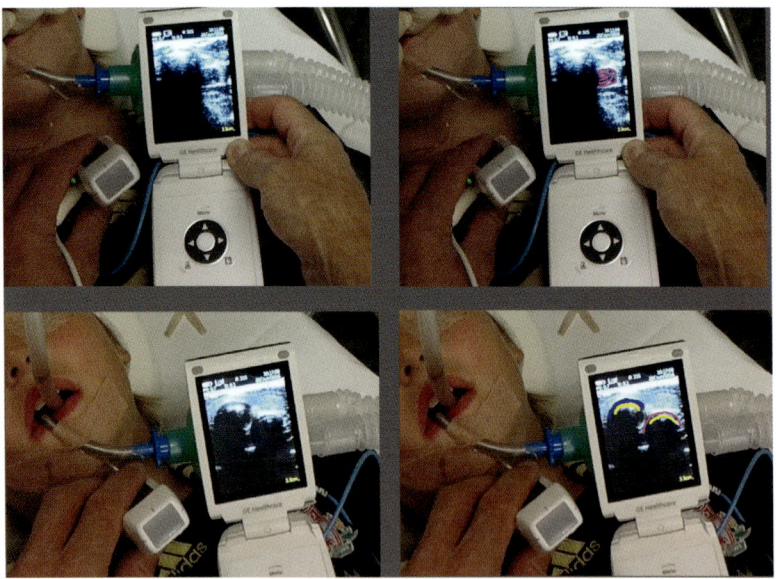

Figure 14.15 Detecting a tube in the esophagus.

Upper left: placing a linear probe transversely just cephalic to the suprasternal notch allows simultaneous observation of the trachea and the esophagus. Upper right (same image as upper left): the empty esophagus and its multilayered structure is marked with purple.

Lower left: when a tube (in this case a large-bore gastric tube) is in the esophagus, it appears as a second trachea, thus the "double trachea" sign. Lower right (same image as lower left): the anterior part of a tracheal ring (blue), the anterior wall of esophagus (purple). Yellow indicates the tissue/air border, which is now present in both the trachea and in the esophagus.

striking because the surrounding tissue is motionless. Applying M-mode scanning, which highlights a clear distinction between a wave-like pattern located above the pleural line and a sand-like pattern below, can enhance the detection of lung sliding. This is referred to as the "seashore" or the "sandy beach" sign. Detecting unilateral lung sliding confirms the intra-airway location of the tracheal tube, but does not rule out mainstem bronchus intubation. This requires subsequent examination of the other side of thorax. If lung sliding is also detected on the other side, this indicates that both lungs are being ventilated. If the lung is not ventilated, then there will be no lung sliding, but a lung pulse will typically be observed. The lung pulse arises from the beating heart pushing the lung and the pleura with each heartbeat (Figure 14.10). If there is one-sided lung sliding and a contralateral lung pulse, then a mainstem intubation is likely, and the tube should be withdrawn gradually until bilateral lung sliding is present.[12] If lung sliding cannot be detected on either side, but a bilateral lung pulse is present, an esophageal intubation (or non-tracheal tube position) is likely. If there is neither lung pulse nor lung sliding, then a pneumothorax should be suspected. The sensitivity for ultrasonographic distinction between tracheal and mainstem bronchus intubation is less precise than it is for distinction between esophageal and tracheal intubation.

In children above 9 months of age, the tracheal rapid ultrasound saline test (TRUST)[13] was recently reported to be accurate and rapid in a small study: the tube was deliberately inserted into the right mainstem bronchus and the tracheal cuff filled with saline. An ultrasound transducer was placed transversely at the level of the sternal notch and the tube then withdrawn until the sonographer noted the appearance of the saline-inflated cuff.[13] However, it is important to remember that using saline in a pediatric tracheal cuff is not licensed, and high and unmonitored tracheal cuff pressures may result in significant mucosal injury, swelling, and subsequent airway obstruction.

Indirect confirmation of intubation by visualization of bilateral diaphragmatic movements was shown to be useful for distinguishing between esophageal and endotracheal intubation in a pediatric population.[14] However, when the technique was used to distinguish between mainstem bronchus and endotracheal intubation, diaphragmatic ultrasound was not equivalent to chest radiography for determining ETT placement within the airway.[15]

Several studies in neonates have demonstrated that ultrasonographic localization of the tube tip is possible if ultrasound examinations are performed by specially trained investigators.[16] Comparable results are obtainable when using a direct observation of the tracheal tube tip with a longitudinal parasternal scanning approach,[17] using the distance between the tracheal tube tip and the apex of the aortic arch as reference. An 86% sensitivity to detect endobronchial-positioned tracheal tubes in babies weighing between 370 g and 3750 g is reported.

There are several advantages to using ultrasound over X-ray for tracheal tube detection in the neonatal population, including less patient handling, frequent assessment of tube position without X-ray exposure, and point-of-care confirmation in the delivery room (prior to prophylactic surfactant administration). Other advantages become apparent during complicated resuscitations, during neonatal transports, and in maintenance of a neutral thermal environment within the incubator.[17]

Confirmation or Exclusion of an Intraoperative Pneumothorax

Ultrasonography is as effective as chest radiography in detecting or excluding a pneumothorax.[18] It is even more sensitive in the ICU setting: ultrasonography was able to establish the diagnosis in the majority of patients in whom a pneumothorax was invisible on plain radiographs, but diagnosed by CT scan. In patients with multiple injuries, ultrasonography was faster and had a higher sensitivity and accuracy compared to chest radiography.[19]

The presence of lung sliding or lung pulse on ultrasonography indicates that two pleural layers are in close proximity to each other at that specific point under the transducer (i.e., there is no pneumothorax there). If there is free air (pneumothorax) in the part of the pleural cavity underlying the transducer, no lung sliding or lung pulse will be seen.[20] In the M-mode, the "stratosphere or barcode sign" will be seen: only parallel lines through all the depth of the image. If the transducer is placed right at the border of the pneumothorax, where the visceral pleura intermittently is in contact with the parietal pleura, the lung point will be seen. This is a sliding lung alternating with non-sliding, synchronous with ventilation. The lung point is highly suggestive of pneumothorax. If a pneumothorax is suspected, the rib interspaces of the thoracic cavity can be systematically "mapped" to confirm or rule out a pneumothorax. An online video is available to view the lung point.[21]

The detection of lung sliding has a negative predictive value of 100%, meaning that when lung sliding is seen, a pneumothorax of the part of the lung beneath the ultrasound probe is ruled out.[22] For diagnosis of occult pneumothorax, the abolition of lung sliding alone had a sensitivity of 100% and a specificity of 78%. The lung point had a sensitivity of 79% and a specificity of 100%.[20]

A systematic approach is recommended when examining the supine patient. The anterior chest wall can be divided into quadrants and the probe first placed at the most superior aspect of the thorax with respect to gravity (i.e., the caudal part of the anterior chest wall in supine patients). The probe is then positioned on each of the four quadrants of the anterior area, followed by the lateral chest wall between the anterior and posterior axillary lines and the rest of the accessible part of the thorax.[20]

Ultrasonography is the fastest way to confirm or exclude an intraoperative pneumothorax especially considering that an anterior pneumothorax is often undiagnosed in a supine patient subjected to plain anterior–posterior X-ray. Ultrasonography is an obvious first diagnostic choice if a pneumothorax is suspected during or after central venous cannulation or nerve blockade when the ultrasound machine is already in use for the procedure itself and immediately available.

References

1. Staface S, Engelhardt T, Teoh WH, Kristensen MS. Essential Ultrasound Techniques of the Pediatric Airway. *Paediatric Anaesthesia* 2016; **26**: 122–31.
2. Or DY, Karmakar MK, Lam GC, Hui JW, Li JW, Chen PP. Multiplanar 3D Ultrasound Imaging to Assess the Anatomy of the Upper Airway and Measure the Subglottic and Tracheal Diameters in Adults. *British Journal of Radiology* 2013; **86**: 20130253.
3. Kristensen MS, Teoh WH, Graumann O, Laursen CB. Ultrasonography for Clinical Decision-Making and Intervention in Airway Management: From the Mouth to the Lungs and Pleurae. *Insights Imaging* 2014; **5**: 253–79.
4. Walz PC, Schroeder JW, Jr. Prenatal Diagnosis of Obstructive Head and Neck Masses and Perinatal Airway Management: the Ex Utero Intrapartum Treatment Procedure. *Otolaryngology Clinics of North America* 2015; **48**: 191–207.
5. Holm-Knudsen RJ, Rasmussen LS, Charabi B, Bottger M, Kristensen MS. Emergency Airway Access in Children – Transtracheal Cannulas and Tracheotomy Assessed in a Porcine Model.

6. Johansen K, Holm-Knudsen RJ, Charabi B, Kristensen MS, Rasmussen LS. Cannot Ventilate–Cannot Intubate an Infant: Surgical Tracheotomy or Transtracheal Cannula? *Paediatric Anaesthesia* 2010; **20**: 987–93.

7. Teoh WH, Kristensen MS. Ultrasonographic Identification of the Cricothyroid Membrane. *Anaesthesia* 2014; **69**: 649–50.

8. Kristensen MS, Teoh WH, Rudolph SS, Hesselfeldt R, Borglum J, Tvede MF. A Randomised Cross-Over Comparison of the Transverse and Longitudinal Techniques for Ultrasound-Guided Identification of the Cricothyroid Membrane in Morbidly Obese Subjects. *Anaesthesia* 2016; **71**: 675–83.

9. AirwayManagement.dk. Identification of the Cricothyroid Membrane with Ultrasonography Transverse "TACA" Approach. Online Video Clip. http://airwaymanagement.dk/taca

10. AirwayManagement.dk Identification of the Cricothyroid Membrane with Ultrasonography Longitudinal "String of Pearls" Approach. Online Video Clip. http://airwaymanagement.dk/pearls

11. Schramm C, Knop J, Jensen K, Plaschke K. Role of Ultrasound Compared to Age-Related Formulas for Uncuffed Endotracheal Intubation in a Pediatric Population. *Paediatric Anaesthesia* 2012; **22**: 781–6.

12. Hiruma M, Watanabe T, Baba H. Using Lung Ultrasound in an Infant to Detect Bronchial Intubation Not Previously Identified by Auscultation. *Canadian Journal of Anesthesia/Journal canadien d'anesthésie* 2015; **62**: 1121–2.

13. Tessaro MO, Salant EP, Arroyo AC, Haines LE, Dickman E. Tracheal Rapid Ultrasound Saline Test (TRUST) for Confirming Correct Endotracheal Tube Depth in Children. *Resuscitation* 2015; **89**: 8–12.

14. Hsieh K-S, Lee C-L, Lin C-C, Huang T-C, Weng K-P, Lu W-H. Secondary Confirmation of Endotracheal Tube Position by Ultrasound Image. *Critical Care Medicine* 2004; **32**: S374–7.

15. Kerrey BT, Geis GL, Quinn AM, Hornung RW, Ruddy RM. A Prospective Comparison of Diaphragmatic Ultrasound and Chest Radiography to Determine Endotracheal Tube Position in a Pediatric Emergency Department. *Pediatrics* 2009; **123**: e1039–44.

16. Schmolzer GM, O'Reilly M, Davis PG, Cheung PY, Roehr CC. Confirmation of Correct Tracheal Tube Placement in Newborn Infants. *Resuscitation* 2013; **84**: 731–7.

17. Chowdhry R, Dangman B, Pinheiro JM. The Concordance of Ultrasound Technique versus X-Ray to Confirm Endotracheal Tube Position in Neonates. *Journal of Perinatology* 2015; **35**: 481–4.

18. Sartori S, Tombesi P. Emerging Roles for Transthoracic Ultrasonography in Pleuropulmonary Pathology. *World Journal of Radiology* 2010; **2**: 83–90.

19. Zhang M, Liu ZH, Yang JX, et al. Rapid Detection of Pneumothorax by Ultrasonography in Patients with Multiple Trauma. *Critical Care* 2006; **10**: R112.

20. Lichtenstein DA, Mezière G, Lascols N, et al. Ultrasound Diagnosis of Occult Pneumothorax. *Critical Care Medicine* 2005; **33**: 1231–8.

21. Airwaymanagement.dk Ultrasonography in Airway Management. Online Video Clip. http://airwaymanagement.dk/index.php?option=com_content&view=category&layout=blog&id=12&Itemid=115

22. Lichtenstein DA. A Bedside Ultrasound Sign Ruling Out Pneumothorax in the Critically Ill. *CHEST Journal* 1995; **108**: 1345.

Section 2 **Devices and Techniques to Manage the Abnormal Airway**

Chapter 15

Difficult Airway Cart

Alyson Walker and Britta S. von Ungern-Sternberg

Even though the CICO scenario is less common in children (< 0.5%) compared with adults (up to 10%), the difficult pediatric airway does exist and is associated with an increased morbidity and mortality, particularly in young infants.[1]

When dealing with a child with an anticipated or unanticipated difficult airway, an organized and regularly checked DAC tailored to a specific institution-based airway management plan is useful. The DAC not only contains all necessary equipment, but its structure and layout can also serve as an aide-mémoire in the stressful situation of a difficult airway. This chapter discusses considerations around designing a DAC, its contents, layout, and maintenance.

DAC Locations

A DAC should be immediately available in every clinical area where anesthesia and recovery may occur (e.g., operating theater areas, ED, theater recovery, ICU, radiology).[2,3] Institutions should standardize the contents and layout of their DAC in all sites as this consistency facilitates education of staff and facilitates patient care in disparate areas of the institution. The DAC should be close to patient care areas and easily located to ensure quick access in the event of an airway emergency. The DAC location must therefore be clearly signposted and easy for any staff member to find. The International Organization for Standardization (ISO) has developed standard signage to identify the location of airway equipment (Figure 15.1A and 15.1B).[4]

When the DAC is in use, a clear record of where it has been taken to should be displayed at the DAC location (e.g., on a wall-mounted whiteboard). This ensures the DAC is always easy to locate (Figure 15.2).

DAC Design and Layout

Regardless of the design and layout of the DAC, staff must be educated about the DAC system in place in

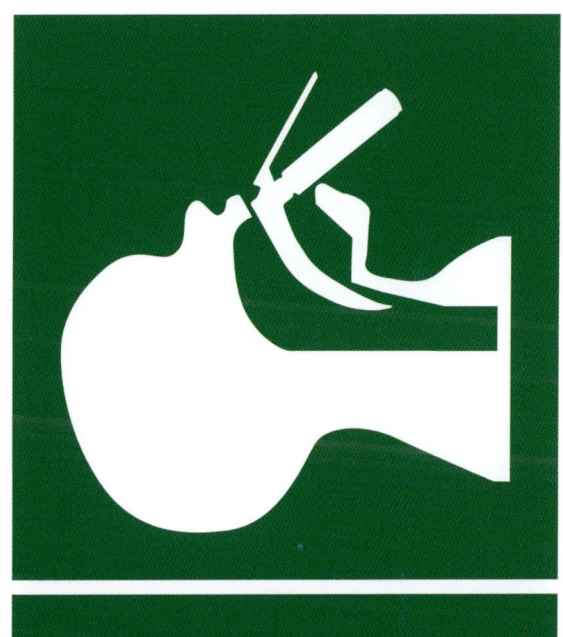

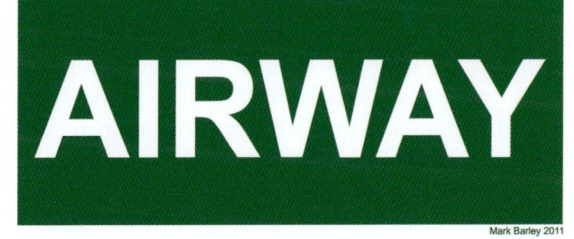

Figure 15.1A and 15.1B Examples of signposting for DAC.
(Images courtesy of Dr. Mark Barley.)

Section 2: Devices and Techniques to Manage the Abnormal Airway

Table 15.1 Contents of a DAC, Labeled According to Plans of Increasing Invasiveness

Drawer 1: label: "Failed oxygenation"
- LMA (without bars): sizes 1, 1.5, 2, 2.5, 3, 4, 5 (in duplicate)
- intubating LMA: sizes 3, 4, 5
- alternative SGA devices

Drawer 2: label: "Failed intubation Plan A"
- selection of "special" laryngoscopy blades (e.g., McCoy, Wisconsin, Miller)
- gum elastic bougie (5 fr, 10 fr)
- malleable stylet (2 fr, 5 fr)
- choice of visualization or intubation aid/video laryngoscope (according to local preference and availability)

Drawer 3: label: "Failed intubation Plan B"
- airway exchange catheters (7 fr, 8 fr, 11 fr, 14 fr, 19 fr)
- endoscopy masks (VBM sizes 1, 3, 5)

Drawer 4: label: "Rescue Plan C"
- cricothyroidotomy needle kit
- surgical cricothyroidotomy kit
- different-sized cannulas
- oxygenation device

Adapted from Weiss and Engelhart.[5] Figure 15.3

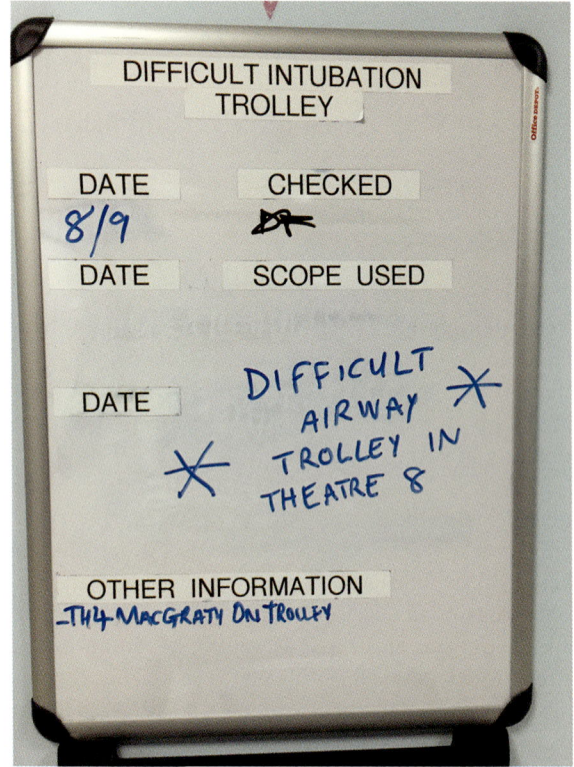

Figure 15.2 DAC communication board, located above the DAC. Theater complex staff members are able to clearly see where the DAC is located if it is in use.

their hospital, where the DAC is situated, and what the exact contents are. Each anesthetic/operating room should contain basic pediatric airway equipment. The DAC should only contain equipment necessary to manage the difficult airway. An exception to this caveat is institutions that provide occasional pediatric care; in which case, an all-encompassing pediatric airway trolley may be appropriate. Some institutions have one DAC for all difficult airways, while others advocate the use of two different DACs: one for the predicted difficult airway and another for the unpredicted difficult airway ("airway rescue trolley"). Depending on the hospital setting and the patient populations, it may be advantageous to have the pediatric DAC separate from the adult DAC. The cart should be a trolley, separate from any general anesthesia trolley, which is sturdy, mobile, and easy to clean. It is practical to have a working surface on top, which can be used to prepare the airway equipment.

Most DACs have 4–5 drawers, which are stocked with equipment for differing scenarios. The drawer layout should be logical, organized, and uncluttered with contents clearly labeled. In adult practice, it has been recommended that drawers be labeled using pictorial signs, which correlate with Plans A–D of difficult airway guidelines.[5] A similar approach is advocated in the pediatric setting by Weiss and Engelhardt, who have devised a difficult airway algorithm that correlates with the layout of their DAC (Table 15.1 and Figure 15.3).[5]

A DAC should be organized in a structured fashion to help clinical decision-making by guiding the operator along the difficult airway algorithm, particularly in the emergency situation. Even though there is no evidence that labeling the trolley in such a way increases the adherence to guidelines[2] or helps to guide management in a difficult airway, it may act as a visual prompt. There are different ways to categorize the drawers in a pediatric DAC; for example, by airway management strategy (Table 15.1 and Figure 15.3), by the purpose of the equipment

Table 15.2 Contents of a DAC, Organized According to Different Techniques (Figure 15.4)

Drawer 1: laryngoscopy
- video laryngoscope with different-sized blades/lighted stylet/lightwand

Drawer 2: face-mask fiberoptic intubation (fiberoptic scope stored next to DAC)
- laryngotracheal MAD
- nasal MAD
- Berman airway, Ovassapian airway
- bronchoscope airway (size 1, 3, 5)
- endoscopy mask (size 0, 2, 4)
- 18 G epidural catheter

Drawer 3: LMA-guided fiberoptic intubation
- bronchoscope swivel connector
- 180 cm J-tip 0.035″ wire
- 18 G epidural catheter
- Cook airway exchange catheter (8 fr, 11 fr, 14 fr) (may be stored on side of DAC)
- LMA or other SGA device, preferably without bars to ease insertion of bronchoscope

Drawer 4: CICO
- Melker size 3.5, 5.0
- safe oxygenation device (e.g., Enk OFM, Rapid O_2, Ventrain)
- scalpel bougie kit (size 10 blade, 5 fr portex, 8 fr frova, 11 fr CAE, ETTs 3, 4, 5)
- cannulas 18 G, 16 5 G, 14 G
- size 3.5 ETT connector

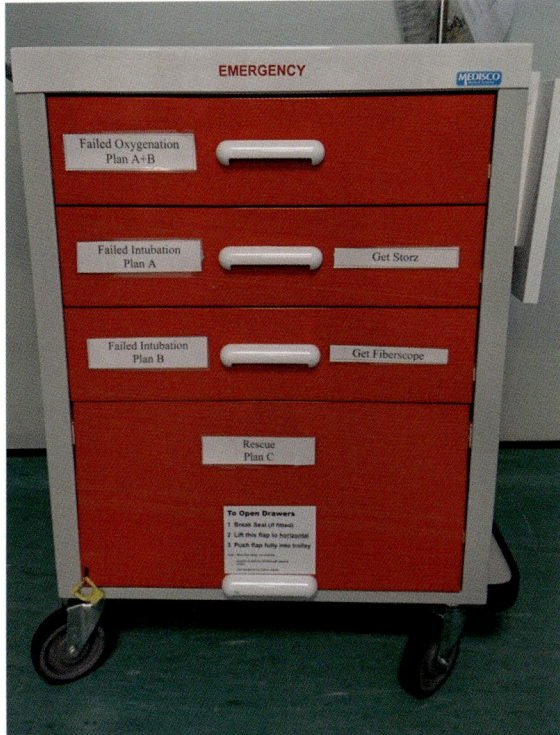

Figure 15.3 An example of a DAC organized according to plans of increasing invasiveness, designed to encourage a stepwise approach to the clinical situation. Note the seal on the "rescue" plan drawer, which must be broken before contents can be accessed. (Photograph courtesy of T Engelhardt.)

(Table 15.2 and Figure 15.4), or by the size of the child. It seems sensible for equipment that is likely to be used together to be stored in the same drawer. In the absence of clear evidence and varying practice, we recommend each institution/health authority tailor their DAC layout appropriate to their patient case mix, staff opinion/experience, and availability of equipment.

DAC Contents

The DAC is a means of keeping all equipment that the team may require to manage a difficult airway in one place. It is important to find a good balance between the availability of all necessary equipment and an excess of items. It is imperative that all staff are familiar with the DAC and regularly trained in its contents and use. Exact DAC contents vary locally, nationally, and internationally because of differing skill sets, experience, patient case mix, and equipment availability.[6] Content should regularly be reviewed as new equipment comes on the market, but care should be taken not to constantly change the DAC contents so as to maintain consistency. There is currently no internationally agreed-on list of pediatric DAC contents, but standardization is important to avoid confusion and improve familiarity with the equipment and its location in the DAC. Such standardization decreases latent human error, particularly when responding to emergencies in other clinical areas (e.g., during a medical emergency on a ward). The DAC contents should be selected with the least-experienced clinician in mind, and should contain devices that are highly successful with minimal

Section 2: Devices and Techniques to Manage the Abnormal Airway

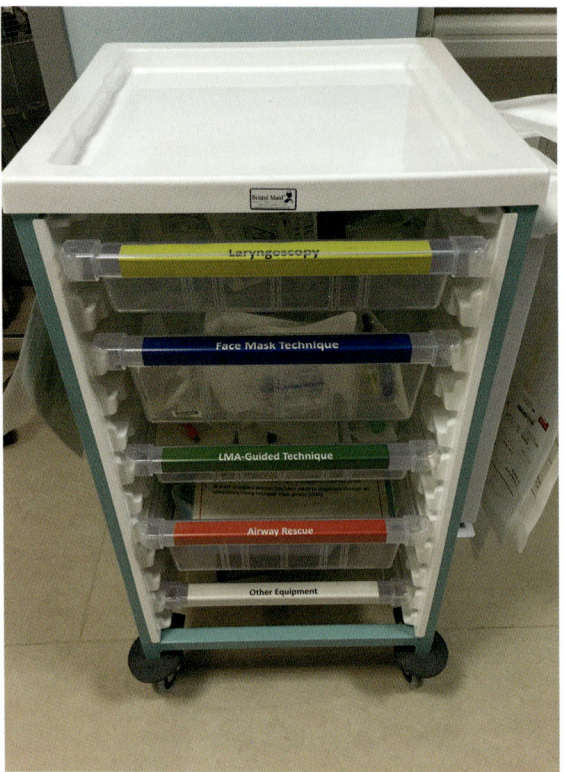

Figure 15.4 Example of a DAC organized according to task. This trolley correlates with the contents outlined in Table 15.2. A fiberoptic scope is stored next to this cart.

kinesthetic skill. Equipment for very experienced clinicians may also be stocked in the DAC, but should be used only by those with the requisite clinical skills.

Every piece of equipment on the DAC must be truly necessary and the whole team well trained in its use. Such a strategy will avoid clutter, particularly in the pediatric setting where several different sizes of each piece of equipment are necessary for different age groups. It is advisable to stock no more than two of each size of equipment to simplify restocking and limit clutter. Such streamlining will retain order and assist the user in finding what they need quickly, which is crucial in an emergency situation.

Often physically separate from the DAC due to size, fiberoptic scopes should be available, along with light sources and spare batteries. Bougies, Aintree intubation catheters (Cook Medical) and airway exchange catheters (Cook Medical) can be neatly stocked at the side of the DAC.

Some departments choose to stock relevant drugs on the DAC; for example, lidocaine, xylocaine, oxymetazoline, glycopyrrolate/atropine, and lubricant. These drugs must be regularly checked for stock levels and expiry dates.

Equipment for the CICO Scenario

The CICO situation is rare in pediatrics. It may be the case that oxygenation can be achieved using a simple solution (e.g., bimanual airway maneuvers, change of operator, SGA device, deepening of anesthesia).[5] FONA may be necessary in the scenario where *all* options to oxygenate have been attempted and failed, and there is no ENT surgeon on hand to perform surgical tracheostomy. In such a situation, it is useful for pediatric DACs to have a system in place, which prompts the clinician to stop and think: "is this the only option?" before proceeding to help avoid fixation error. A laminated copy of the institutional difficult airway algorithm should be attached to the DAC, which can be used as a checklist in an emergency (e.g., "Have I tried an LMA? Do I have time to wake the patient up?"), or a seal, which must be broken to access that drawer (Figure 15.3). An understanding of the influence of human factors in the CICO scenario is crucial.[7]

A useful technique in the CICO scenario is a surgical tracheostomy performed by a pediatric otolaryngology surgeon. When this is not possible, the anesthetist must decide between cannula and scalpel techniques. The evidence for which technique is most successful is scant, often derived from adult studies, based on small numbers, and/or animal models. It is important that the technique the anesthetist opts for is one that they are familiar with, have trained in, and that they perform with minimal delay.

The BD Insyte (Becton Dickinson and Company) cannula (14 G, 16 G or 18 G), a Ravussin needle (VBM Medizintechnik) or a Melker cricothyroidotomy/tracheotomy kit are often recommended for cannula cricothyroidotomy or tracheotomy. While a needle technique is not a definitive airway, it can be converted to a definitive airway using a Seldinger technique once the patient is oxygenated if necessary (e.g., using a Melker kit). The Melker kit was shown in a rabbit model to be a successful tool in the infant CICO scenario and superior to an Insyte technique.[8,9]

If a cannula technique is used, its position has to be checked (aspiration of air) and a safe oxygenation technique employed. Barotrauma can easily develop if too high pressures are used or if the cannula is displaced. The aim is primarily to oxygenate enough to avoid neurological damage or cardiac arrest; achievement of ventilation and control of carbon dioxide are secondary aims in this situation. The lowest effective oxygen pressure should be used via the oxygenation device. The oxygenation device should have an expiration port and should be a true "on–off" device. Devices that fit this description include the Enk OFM, Rapid O_2, and Ventrain. A 3.5 mm ETT connector and a 15 mm pediatric Ayres T-piece can be connected to a cannula/needle and used to oxygenate neonates/infants.[10,11]

If a cannula/Melker technique has been unsuccessful, it is reasonable to quickly move onto a scalpel technique. Some anesthetists may even wish to opt for a scalpel technique as their first choice. The "scalpel-bougie" technique using a size 10 scalpel blade, a bougie, and ETT is well described.[7,12] However, surgical cricothyroidotomy is generally contraindicated in very young infants. There are no designated tracheostomy kits available for young infants. As anesthetists, any cannula or Seldinger technique is close to our routine practice (particularly in comparison with surgical tracheostomy). However, it should be noted that the best technique available is still to be identified. Contents for a CICO kit have been described (see Table 15.3).[7]

Table 15.3 CICO Pack Contents, Royal Children's Hospital, Melbourne[7]

Equipment for cannula FONA
- BD Insyte cannula
- Rapid O_2 insufflator
- 5 ml syringe
- 10 ml saline ampoule

Equipment for scalpel FONA
- Portex 5 CH 50 cm tracheal tube guide (orange) (for size 3 ETT)
- Cook Frova intubating introducer 8 fr 35 cm (yellow, with stiffening cannula removed) (for size 4 ETT)
- Cook airway exchange catheter 11 fr 83 cm (yellow) (for size 5 ETT)
- Microcuff ETTs (3, 4, 5) (Halyard Health)
- lubricant

DAC Training

Familiarity with the DAC and its equipment is crucial to the success of difficult airway scenarios, and regular training is vital. All members of a department should receive training on the DAC location, contents, and use.[3] Training should be every 3–6 months.[6] Training in the use of the DAC increases the confidence of the clinician using it.[6] It is both the responsibility of each individual staff member and of the system in which they work to ensure that they remain up to date and familiar with the DAC. Training must be multidisciplinary, including all specialties involved in a difficult airway; for example, anesthesia, ENT, ICU. Regular use of the DAC when caring for elective patients may be beneficial so that the anesthetic team remains familiar with the DAC contents and skilled in their use.

Maintenance

Quality assurance measures should be in place to minimize DAC problems.[6] Checking and restocking the DAC needs to be well organized to ensure appropriate stock at all times. Some institutions seal the trolley to avoid stock being taken for convenience rather than urgent need, which may lead to lack of equipment in the emergency situation. It is highly recommended to check the DAC regularly, ideally daily, and to record this check.[2,13] Equipment must be replaced as soon as it is used and it must remain in date. Poor maintenance may lead to critical incidents due to missing or faulty equipment.[6] Expired equipment can be decommissioned and labeled in an airway training area for teaching purposes. It is important to have in place a system that prevents unwanted equipment removal or additions. A numbered breakable seal system is one such system and decreases possible problems, which may be encountered with a key system (namely the risk of mislaying the key at a crucial clinical moment).

Paperwork

It is useful to securely attach pertinent documentation to the cart, such as relevant airway guidelines, a contents checklist for restocking, and a logbook to record when the cart has been checked. The presence of an airway algorithm may guide decision-making in situations that can become emergent. It may be useful to stock difficult airway-alert system documentation and cards, along with data-collection forms for each time the DAC is used. Difficult airways should be clearly recorded in the patient notes (paper and electronic) and this information be easily available to other healthcare professionals who will be caring for them. Pictorial guides for fiberoptic intubation setup, including which ETT sizes correspond to which scopes and what size LMAs accommodate what ETTs, are useful, particularly if this is a technique the anesthetist does not use very regularly.

Institutional Infrastructure

Over and above having a well-organized DAC and appropriately trained staff, it has been suggested that an overarching team responsible for difficult airways may be worthwhile. Nykiel-Bailey and colleagues[13] describe the implementation of a pediatric difficult airway consultation service following three critical incidents where morbidity occurred after failed difficult airway management. This interdisciplinary service identifies patients with suspected or known difficult airways, develops detailed management plans, and facilitates communication between relevant services. They manage children in settings where airway management may be required as part of the patient's medical care (e.g., oncology ward). Since the majority of difficult pediatric airways are predictable, care of the child with a difficult airway should start early where possible to avert potential airway crises. A management plan that allows care to be planned, equipment to be gathered, and staff to be trained is the gold standard. A multidisciplinary approach is often key to the success of difficult airway situations (e.g., anesthesiology, otolaryngology, pediatric intensive care unit). Examples of situations where a difficult airway consultation service may be useful include EXIT procedures, elective tracheostomy, and extubation of patients with difficult airways.

References

1. von Ungern-Sternberg BS. Rare Events can be Fatal and Must Not be Ignored – How Much Needs to Happen before We Act? *Pediatric Anesthesia* 2015; **25**: 332–3.

2. The Royal College of Anaesthesia and The Difficult Airway Society. Children. In Fourth National Audit Project (NAP4): Major Complications of Airway Management in the United Kingdom. March 2011. Website. http://www.rcoa.ac.uk/system/files/CSQ-NAP4-Section2.pdf

3. Difficult Airway Society (July 2005). Recommended Equipment for Management of Unanticipated Difficult Intubation. Website. https://www.das.uk.com/content/equipmentlistjuly2005.htm

4. Barley M. Anaesthetic Emergency Signage. Website. http://www.das.uk.com/content/anaesthetic-emergency-signage

5. Weiss M, Engelhardt T. Proposal for the Management of the Unexpected Difficult Pediatric Airway. *Pediatric Anesthesia* 2010; **20**: 454–64.

6. Calder A, Hegarty M, Davies K, et al. The DAT in Pediatric Anaesthesia: an International Survey of Experience and Training. *Pediatric Anesthesia* 2012; **22**: 1150–4.

7. Sabato SC, Lon E. An Institutional Approach to the Management of the "Can't Intubate, Can't Oxygenate" Emergency in Children. *Pediatric Anesthesia* 2016; **26**: 784–93.

8. Stacey J, Heard AMB, Chapman G, et al. The "Can't Intubate Can't Oxygenate" Scenario in Pediatric Anaesthesia: a Comparison of Different Devices for Needle Cricothyroidotomy. *Pediatric Anesthesia* 2012; **22**: 1155–8.

9. Prunty SL, Aranda-Palacios A, Heard AMB, et al. The "Can't Intubate Can't Oxygenate" Scenario in Pediatric Anesthesia: a Comparison of the Melker Cricothyroidotomy Kit with a Scalpel Bougie Technique. *Pediatric Anesthesia* 2015; **25**: 400–4.

10. Bolton P. Emergency Jet Ventilation in Children. *Pediatric Anesthesia* 2009; **19**: 425–7.

11. Sims C, von Ungern-Sternberg BS. The Normal and the Challenging Pediatric Airway. *Pediatric Anaesthesia* 2012; **22**: 521–6.

12. Heard AMB, Green RJ, Eakins P. The Formulation and Introduction of a "Can't Intubate, Can't Ventilate" Algorithm into Clinical Practice. *Anaesthesia* 2009: **64**; 601–08.

13. Nykiel-Bailey SM, McAllister JD, Schrock CR, et al. Difficult Airway Consultation Service for Children: Steps to Implement and Preliminary Results. *Pediatric Anesthesia* 2015; **25**: 363–71.

Section 3 Special Topics

Chapter 16: Extubation in Children with Difficult Airways

Luis Sequera-Ramos, Alec Zhu, Benjamin Kiesel, and Narasimhan Jagannathan

General Principles in Pediatric Airways

There are some unique considerations when caring for the airway in infants and small children. They have relatively larger oropharyngeal structures (tongue, tonsils, and adenoids), and a large and floppy epiglottis, which can predispose to upper airway obstruction. A larger occiput may increase the neck flexion observed while in supine position as compared with adults, which can also lead to airway obstruction. The shorter and narrower trachea may increase the risk for tracheal tube malposition after intubation, and has a greater risk for secretions, edema, or foreign body to produce disproportionate negative effects in airflow resistance.[1] Children run the highest risk of problems from stridor and glottic edema because of their smaller diameter airways. Post-extubation stridor incidence ranges from 2% in children having elective surgical procedures to 40% in pediatric trauma and burn victims.[2-4] Additionally, infants have less physical space in the oropharynx and within the tracheal tube for an advanced bridging technique such as SGA devices and/or airway exchange catheter.

Physiological differences in children that can have a direct impact on airway management during tracheal extubation when compared to adults include a greater metabolic rate with increased consumption of oxygen per unit of time (~6 ml/(kg min))[5] and decreased physiologic reserve (reduced FRC). These two factors mainly account for a decreased time to hypoxia during hypoventilation and/or apneic periods.[6,7] Children, particularly infants, tend to desaturate more rapidly, even when no other cardiorespiratory conditions exist. A more cartilaginous, compliant chest wall means children rely more on muscle tone to maintain sufficient breathing.[8] This leads to a higher incidence of fatigue, atelectasis, and oxygen desaturations. Additionally, the tidal volumes of infants and young children relative to their body sizes are less than that of adults, making children more susceptible to iatrogenic barotrauma from high positive-pressure ventilation and decreasing the effect of deeper breathing to increase minute ventilation sufficiently to sustain adequate oxygenation/ventilation.

Extubation in the Pediatric Difficult Airway

Extubation is an elective process. The goals when planning for extubation should include maintaining adequate ventilation and oxygenation, while minimizing delay if reintubation is needed.[9] As mentioned before, in children, oxygen desaturation tends to develop faster, emphasizing the importance of having a clear plan (e.g., equipment, personal) to recover the airway if extubation were to fail. Frequently, failures occur due to upper airway obstruction and hypoventilation syndromes.[10] In patients with a difficult airway, the chance of upper airway obstruction is greater and the management may be more complicated at the end of the surgery, especially when the access to the airway is limited. Additionally, co-existing comorbidities, such as congenital cardiac disease may also increase the complexity of their care. Furthermore, the incidence of airway-related perioperative complications, such as laryngospasm, is higher in children.[11] Particular patient features and odds to successfully maintain spontaneous ventilation should guide the timing and initial approach to safely remove the tracheal tube. The entire care team participating in the process of tracheal extubation should be aware of the plan of action if extubation fails.

Most anesthesia providers agree that children with a difficult airway and those with increased risk for aspiration should be extubated awake, once spontaneous ventilation is appropriate and protective airway reflexes return.[12]

Basic Considerations

Potential problems arising during extubation are shown in Table 16.1. Patients with difficult airway are considered "at risk" for extubation failure. Preexisting airway difficulties can become more pronounced during surgery with significant airway deterioration secondary to distorted anatomy, secretions, blood, and edema.[9] Additionally, surgical implants, cervical spine fixation, and mandibular retractors can restrict the access to the airway. The cuff-leak test can be performed at the end of the case when significant airway edema is suspected, but is not specific to predict if extubation will be successful.[13]

In preparation for extubation, other risk factors for extubation failure must be optimized to increase the likelihood of success. These include positioning, neuromuscular blockade reversal, appropriate analgesia and temperature, as well as cardiovascular, neurological, and metabolic status: these may complicate or even preclude extubation. Positioning the patient head-up may be beneficial in obese patients, and the left lateral position is advocated for the non-fasted patient. Oropharyngeal (under direct visualization) and ETT suctioning may be needed as well.

Alveolar recruitment maneuvers and preoxygenation may be preferred at the end of the surgery, and an expired fraction of oxygen < 0.9 or as close to the FiO_2 as possible: optimal oxygenation may require longer time to be achieved as age increases.[14] Continuous oxygenation is especially important in infants and can be provided with the use of a nasal cannula or high-flow nasal cannula[15,16] through the entire process, but SGA devices[17] and/or anesthesia face masks can also be utilized. High-flow oxygen via a nasal cannula can increase the apneic time in small children[18] and new devices seem to be promising to monitor ventilation in the recovery unit.[19] Gastric distention can restrict diaphragmatic incursion and limit ventilation, possibly leading to hypoventilation, especially in infants; gastric decompression may be beneficial in these patients, but does not necessarily decrease the risk of vomiting,[20] and aspiration can may still occur during emergence.[21]

Table 16.2 describes potential complications after extubation. A failed extubation is described as the inability to maintain adequate oxygenation and ventilation after tracheal tube removal, requiring reintubation.[22,23]

Additional forethought is needed when surgical factors require emergence from anesthesia to be smooth, avoiding increase in intracranial pressure, coughing, bucking, or straining, as they can cause suture disruption or hematoma formation and compromise surgical outcome. Cardiovascular changes associated to emergence with the tracheal tube in place may also be deleterious in patients with congenital cardiac conditions.

To allow for continuous oxygenation and ventilation after extubation, there are different devices and approaches that have been described in patients with a difficult airway. In children, additional considerations include less size-appropriate equipment availability when compared to adults.

Table 16.1 Problems Encountered During Extubation

Problems at extubation

• related to airway reflexes:
     ○ exaggerated laryngeal reflexes: coughing, breath-holding, bucking, increase in heart rate and blood pressure, laryngospasm
     ○ reduced airway reflexes: decreased muscular tone, impaired upper airway patency, obstructive sleep apnea, obesity, airway edema
     ○ dysfunctional laryngeal reflexes: paradoxical vocal cords motion
 • depletion of oxygen stores at extubation
 • airway injury
 • physiological deterioration in other systems
 • human factors: equipment, inadequate assistance, fatigue, poor communication

Adapted from the Difficult Airway Society Guidelines 2012[9]

Table 16.2 Complications During Extubation of Pediatric Patients with Difficult Airways

Acute/ immediate	Subacute	Severe complication
Laryngospasm	Sore throat	Pneumothorax
Bronchospasm	Hoarseness	Cardiac arrest
Laryngeal edema	Aspiration	Severe airway trauma
Epistaxis	Laryngeal edema	Death
Emesis	Hypoxemia	Aspiration
Airway trauma	Arrhythmias	Positive-pressure pulmonary edema
Aspiration	Atelectasis/ lung collapse	

Modified from Fiadjoe et al. and Jagannathan et al. 2016[23,24]

Extubation Strategies

All patients should be assessed for readiness to extubate the trachea. Some valuable criteria to consider include the capacity to maintain adequate arterial oxygenation (in patients where an arterial line allows to monitor) with low positive airway pressure, as well as to maintain adequate ventilation, return of full strength (evidenced by sustained hip flexion in infants), if neuromuscular blockade was used, return of airway protective reflexes, easily managed secretions, appropriate hemodynamic function, regular respiratory effort and negative inspiratory pressure > −20 cmH$_2$O. Additionally, medications that could provide some benefit to facilitate extubation should be considered (e.g., lidocaine, dexamethasone, dexmedetomidine, caffeine citrate, methylxanthines).

The surgical procedure may have a direct effect on the airway at the time of extubation (e.g., airway edema, blood, and airway secretions), and this may be more robust after surgery of the head and neck. It is also important to consider the risk of aspiration as these patients should be extubated awake with airway reflexes present while spontaneously breathing. In patients with a "high risk" for reintubation, postponing extubation and/or placing a tracheostomy tube should be considered. Advanced techniques for extubation should be performed by an experienced provider with training in rescue techniques, and a clear plan for post-extubation care should be established before extubation is attempted, and whether the patient will be transported to the postanesthesia recovery unit or to the ICU.

Advanced Airway Techniques for Extubation in Children

Basic Adjuncts

A suction source should be readily available before attempting extubation. Soft tissues of the oropharynx are at risk of trauma if suction is not applied under direct vision, especially if there is increased risk of secretions, blood, or surgical debris.[25,26] Adequate sizes of face masks and oral airway and/or nasal airways also should be available. Appropriately sized SGA device of choice and ETT with a stylet should be at reach as well.

Awake extubation and transition onto face mask with possible use of a nasal or oropharyngeal airway can be used in patients with a low risk for reintubation, in which mild-to-moderate upper airway obstruction could be easily overcome by the oral airway.

Difficult airway guidelines for extubation describe three advanced methods to bridge extubation: airway exchange catheter, an SGA device, and a remifentanil technique.[9,27]

Airway Exchange Catheter and Reintubation Guides

Devices used to bridge extubation and allow reintubation in pediatric patients include the Cook airway exchange catheter, Sheridan tracheal tube exchanger (Teleflex) and the CardioMed endotracheal ventilation catheter (ETVC) (CardioMed Supplies Inc) (Table 16.3 and Figure 16.1). They all are radiopaque or have radiopaque stripes. Cook airway exchange catheters are long, hollow tubes made out of polyurethane, with a distal hole and two distal side holes, and markings between 5 cm and 35 cm from the distal end, it comes along with a Rapi-Fit adapter, which allows to connect to either a 15 mm connector or a Luer lock jet ventilation. The Sheridan tube exchange catheter is made of a thermolabile material, has depth markings on both sides, and has no side

Table 16.3 Airway Exchange Devices Used in Pediatric Patients

Catheter OD	Catheter length (cm)	Catheter ID (mm)	ETT that can fit the catheter (ID in mm)
Cook airway exchange catheter			
8 fr	45	1.6	≥ 3.0
11 fr	83	2.3	≥ 4.0
14 fr	83	3.0	≥ 5.0
Sheridan tracheal tube exchanger			
2.0 mm	56		2.5 to 4.0
3.3 mm	81		4.0 to 6.0
CardioMed endotracheal ventilation catheter			
4.0 mm	85		> 6.0

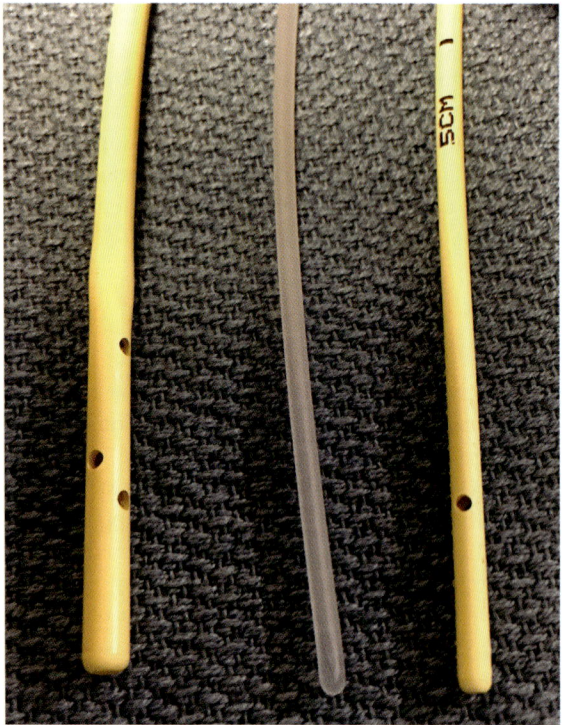

Figure 16.1 CardioMed catheter (left), Sheridan catheter (middle) and Cook airway exchange catheter (right).

holes. The ETVC has eight helically arranged side holes (to facilitate jet ventilation) and a distal end hole.

Cook airway exchange catheters have been described as useful tools for trial of extubation in ICU patients with a difficult airway.[28] In a prospective study with 20 pediatric patients with known difficult airways, Cook airway exchange catheters were used to bridge extubation and provide passive oxygenation, and allowing to successfully reintubate five patients who failed the extubation trial.[29]

Airway exchange catheters have been used as a bridge to allow reintubation, if needed after extubation. In infants and small children, the reduced diameter of the pediatric airway can limit the utility of these catheters and may have a bigger impact on airway flow and resistance than in adults. The smallest available Cook airway exchange catheter is 2.7 mm (8 fr) in diameter,[30] which can be accommodated by a size 3.0 mm ID ETT. An extraluminal approach to place an airway exchange catheter may be considered to minimize occupying the diameter of a tracheal tube by the airway exchange catheter.

Passive oxygenation and jet ventilation via airway exchange catheter have been described, but the risk of severe complications and barotrauma, especially with jet ventilation, may be significant. We do not recommend the use of jet ventilation in children unless a life-or-death situation is encountered. Airway exchange catheters are designed to maintain a guide to reintubate the patient if promptly needed and oxygenation through standard delivery methods can be applied (e.g., nasal cannula, face), while the catheter is in place. Additionally, oxygenation via the airway exchange catheter has not been proven to be better than other methods. Poor patient compliance, inadequate fixation of the airway exchange catheter, and airway manipulation can lead to dislodgement. Other complications include direct tracheal mucosa perforation and interstitial pulmonary emphysema.[31]

Especial attention should be taken when using these devices to avoid keeping the distal end of the catheter below or at the level of the carina as it can stimulate the airway. Although most authors describe that patients can tolerate these devices without major issues and could phonate and tolerate the catheter for up to 72 hours,[32] topical lidocaine has been suggested as a possible additive if they are not well tolerated, although this can also decrease protective airway reflexes. Described techniques using an airway exchange catheter include inserting the airway exchange catheter before extubation or during respiratory deterioration (to maintain oxygenation), reintubation using an airway exchange catheter, and high-pressure source (jet) ventilation during airway exchange catheter airway rescue.

SGA Devices as a Bridge for Extubation

SGA device-bridged extubation has been described mainly in adults,[9] but these techniques may be useful in children. In infants and small children, the limited physical space in the oropharynx can be a limitation for these methods.

Bridging an extubation using an SGA device can be considered in patients who require smooth emergence[33] with minimal airway and cardiovascular responses to avoid surgical disruption, such as smokers, asthmatics, and patients with reactive airways.[9,34,35] An SGA device can allow for fiberoptic inspection of the periglottic area, the vocal cords, and the trachea in patients undergoing airway or neck surgery[36] when mask ventilation can be difficult. It

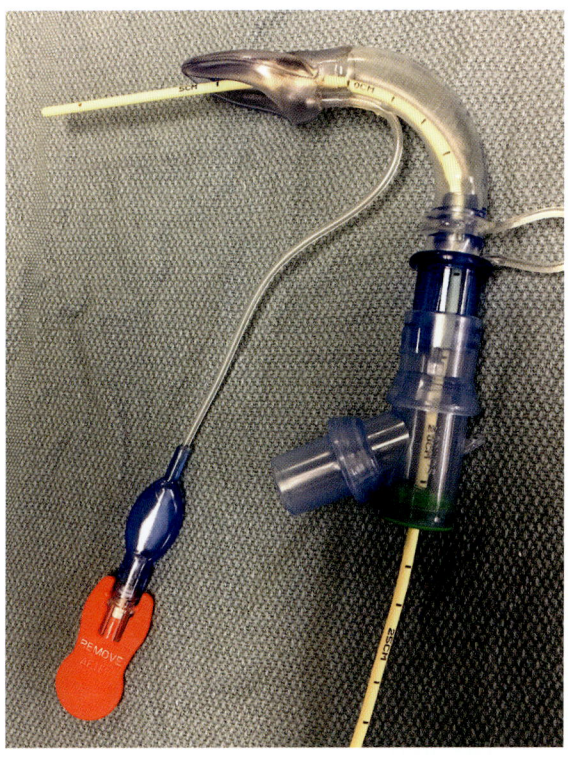

Figure 16.2 Left to right: An airway exchange catheter passed through an air-Q; the elbow connector allows connecting the breathing circuit and provides continuous ventilation/oxygenation.

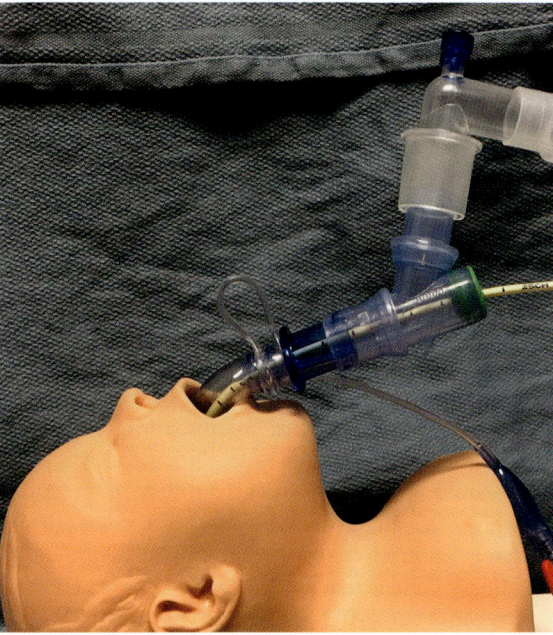

Figure 16.3 Demonstration of an airway exchange catheter placed through an elbow adapter to allow for continuous oxygenation via an air-Q (infant manikin model).

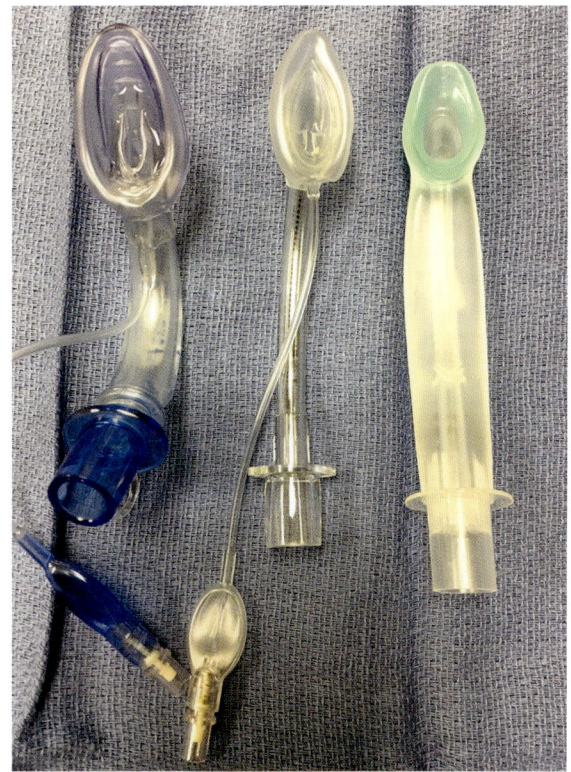

Figure 16.4 SGA devices. From left to right: air-Q, LMA Classic, and i-gel. All the devices shown are size 1.

can also function as a conduit for immediate reintubation[37,38] or as a conduit for an airway exchange catheter placement[39,40] to allow reintubation should extubation trial fail.

The Bailey's maneuver consists of blindly advancing the SGA behind the tracheal tube, and posterior removal of the tube, allowing ventilation via the SGA device.[41] This technique may be inappropriate in patients in whom reintubation can be difficult or are at risk of regurgitation. Other techniques include retrofitting the SGA device through the ETT, and placing an airway exchange catheter through the ETT, removing the tube and railroading the SGA device into position over the existing airway exchange catheter. Using a fiberoptic scope elbow adaptor between the SGA device and the breathing circuit can keep the AEC in place while confirming appropriate ventilation via the SGA device (Figures 16.2 and 16.3). SGA devices that are designed to serve as a conduit to intubation are likely to be better fit for bridging extubation: these include the air-Q and the i-gel, although the LMA Classic has also been described (Figure 16.4).

Exchange of the ETT for the SGA device or the airway exchange catheter should be done under a deep plane of anesthesia, and topical local anesthetic could be considered. Suction should be performed before to remove secretions and assess proper anesthesia level. These techniques should be avoided in patients at increased risk for aspiration; in which, use of an SGA device is contraindicated. Neuromuscular blockade reversal for these techniques should be given after suction and correct deepening has been confirmed.

J-tipped wire catheters, ureteral stents, and guide-wire sheaths have also been used as bridges for extubation[30] and as potential reintubation guides in infants and small children with difficult airways.[42,43] They could be especially useful in those populations in which the airway flow around a regular airway exchange catheter can be limited during spontaneous breathing. Guidewires can be Teflon-coated and their floppy and curve-tip design can minimize trauma during placement. They can be placed intraluminally (through the ETT) or extraluminally (parallel). Risks of this approach include dislodgement of the guide, direct and indirect airway trauma by coughing, and laryngospasm.[30]

Finally, reintubation using any of these adjuncts can be unsuccessful and/or traumatic. Further research is needed to assess the rate of success, benefits, and risk of these techniques in the pediatric population.

Continuous remifentanil infusion throughout extubation has been recommended in patients prone to develop coughing, agitation, or hemodynamic disturbances during emergence from anesthesia (e.g., neurosurgical, maxillofacial, plastics or patients with significant cardiovascular or cerebrovascular disease).[9]

Positive-Pressure Ventilation

In preterm infants, the use of nasal CPAP and nasal noninvasive intermittent positive ventilation have been shown to reduce the risk for reintubation.[44] Noninvasive ventilation has been largely studied in cardiac surgery and is generally considered useful and safe to use to decrease extubation failure.[45] It has also been described in children with mediastinal masses[46] and in children with muscular weakness and who are difficult to wean off mechanical ventilation.[47]

Heliox

In pediatric patients, it is thought that helium improves the work of breathing by reducing turbulent flow when mixed with oxygen (heliox) at a 70/30 or 80/20 proportion.[48,49] It is administered via a non-rebreathing mask, especially when avoiding intubation.[50] Heliox has been studied experimentally for its theoretical capacity to decreased airflow resistance, particularly during expiration.[51] It has been described as a temporizing measure in upper airway obstruction, especially for glottis and subglottic airway stenosis, and for asthma.[52,53]

References

1. Litman RS, Fiadjoe JE, Stricker PA, et al. The Pediatric Airway. In Cote CJ, Lerman J, Anderson JB, eds. *A Practice of Anesthesia for Infants and Children*. 5th ed. Philadelphia: Elsevier; 2013: 269–70.

2. Koka BV, Jeon IS, Andre JM, et al. Postintubation Croup in Children. *Anesthesia & Analgesia* 1977; **56**: 501–5.

3. Principi T, Fraser DD, Morrison GC, et al. Complications of Mechanical Ventilation in the Pediatric Population. *Pediatric Pulmonology* 2011; **46**: 452–7.

4. Nascimento MS, Prado C, Troster EJ, et al. Risk Factors for Post-Extubation Stridor in Children: the Role of Orotracheal Cannula. *Einstein (São Paulo)* 2015; **13**: 226–31.

5. Keens TG, Bryan AC, Levison H, et al. Developmental Pattern of Muscle Fiber Types in Human Ventilatory Muscles. *Journal of Applied Physiology: Respiratory, Environmental and Exercise Physiology* 1978; **44**: 909–13.

6. Patel R, Lenczyk M, Hannallah RS, et al. Age and the Onset of Desaturation in Apnoeic Children. *Canadian Journal of Anesthesia/Journal canadien d'anesthésie* 1994; **41**: 771–4.

7. Rinderknecht AS, Mittiga MR, Meinzen-Derr J, et al. Factors Associated with Oxyhemoglobin Desaturation during Rapid Sequence Intubation in a Pediatric Emergency Department: Findings from Multivariable Analyses of Video Review Data. *Academic Emergency Medicine* 2015; **22**: 431–40.

8. Papastamelos C, Panitch HB, England SE, et al. Developmental Changes in Chest Wall Compliance in Infancy and Early Childhood. *Journal of Applied Physiology* 1995; **78**: 179–84.

9. Popat M, Mitchell V, Dravid R, et al. Difficult Airway Society Guidelines for the Management of Tracheal Extubation. *Anaesthesia* 2012; **67**: 318–40.

10. Cooper RM. Strengths and Limitations of Airway Techniques. *Anesthesiology Clinics* 2015; **33**: 241–55.

11. Orliaguet GA, Gall O, Savoldelli GL, et al. Case Scenario: Perianesthetic Management of Laryngospasm in Children. *Anesthesiology* 2012; **116**: 458–71.

12. Klucka J, Stourac P, Stoudek R, et al. Controversies in Pediatric Perioperative Airways. *BioMed Research International* 2015; **2015**: 368761.

13. Infosino A. Pediatric Upper Airway and Congenital Anomalies. *Anesthesiology Clinics of North America* 2002; **20**: 747–66.

14. Oshan V, Plant N, Gopal P, et al. The Effect of Age and Increasing Head-Up Tilt on Pre-Oxygenation Times in Children: a Randomised Exploratory Study. *Anaesthesia* 2016; **71**: 429–36.

15. Kotecha SJ, Adappa R, Gupta N, et al. Safety and Efficacy of High-Flow Nasal Cannula Therapy in Preterm Infants: A Meta-Analysis. *Pediatrics* 2015; **136**: 542–53.

16. Al-Mandari H, Shalish W, Dempsey E, et al. International Survey on Periextubation Practices in Extremely Preterm Infants. *Archives of Disease in Childhood. Fetal and Neonatal Edition.* 2015; **100**: F428–31.

17. Sohn L, Sawardekar A, Jagannathan N. Airway Management Options in a Prone Achondroplastic Dwarf with a Difficult Airway after Unintentional Tracheal Extubation during a Wake-Up Test for Spinal Fusion: to Flip or Not to Flip? *Canadian Journal of Anesthesia/Journal canadien d'anesthésie* 2014; **61**: 741–4.

18. Riva T, Seiler S, Stucki F, et al. High-Flow Nasal Cannula Therapy and Apnea Time in Laryngeal Surgery. *Paediatric Anaesthesia* 2016; **26**: 1206–8.

19. Nagoshi M, Morzov R, Hotz J, et al. Mainstream Capnography System for Nonintubated Children in the Postanesthesia Care Unit: Performance with Changing Flow Rates, and a Comparison to Side Stream Capnography. *Paediatric Anaesthesia* 2016; **26**: 1179–87.

20. Jones JE, Tabaee A, Glasgold R, et al. Efficacy of Gastric Aspiration in Reducing Posttonsillectomy Vomiting. *Archives of Otolaryngology – Head and Neck Surgery* 2001; **127**: 980–4.

21. Tan Z, Lee SY. Pulmonary Aspiration under GA: a 13-Year Audit in a Tertiary Pediatric Unit. *Paediatric Anaesthesia* 2016; **26**: 547–52.

22. Epstein SK. Decision to Extubate. *Intensive Care Medicine* 2002; **28**: 535–46.

23. Jagannathan N, Shivazad A, Kolan M. Tracheal Extubation in Children with Difficult Airways: a Descriptive Cohort Analysis. *Paediatric Anaesthesia* 2016; **26**: 372–7.

24. Fiadjoe JE, Nishisaki A, Jagannathan N, et al. Airway Management Complications in Children with Difficult Tracheal Intubation from the Pediatric Difficult Intubation (PeDI) Registry: a Prospective Cohort Analysis. *The Lancet Respiratory Medicine* 2016; **4**: 37–48.

25. Bogetz MS, Lockhart SH. Suction at the Ready. *Canadian Journal of Anesthesia/Journal canadien d'anesthésie* 1991; **38**: 686.

26. Bogetz MS, Tupper BJ, Vigil AC. Too Much of a Good Thing: Uvular Trauma Caused by Overzealous Suctioning. *Anesthesia & Analgesia* 1991; **72**: 125–6.

27. Apfelbaum JL, Hagberg CA, Caplan RA, et al. Practice Guidelines for Management of the Difficult Airway: an Updated Report by the American Society of Anesthesiologists Task Force on Management of the Difficult Airway. *Anesthesiology* 2013; **118**: 251–70.

28. Lin TC, Soo LY, Chen TI, et al. Perioperative Airway Management in a Child with Treacher Collins Syndrome. *Acta Anaesthesiologica Taiwanica: Official Journal of the Taiwan Society of Anesthesiologists* 2009; **47**: 44–7.

29. Wise-Faberowski L, Nargozian C. Utility of Airway Exchange Catheters in Pediatric Patients with a Known Difficult Airway. *Pediatric Critical Care Medicine* 2005; **6**: 454–6.

30. Hammer GB, Funck N, Rosenthal DN, et al. A Technique for Maintenance of Airway Access in Infants with a Difficult Airway Following Tracheal Extubation. *Paediatric Anaesthesia* 2001; **11**: 622–5.

31. Duggan LV, Law JA, Murphy MF. Brief Review: Supplementing Oxygen through an Airway Exchange Catheter: Efficacy, Complications, and Recommendations. *Canadian Journal of Anesthesia/Journal canadien d'anesthésie* 2011; **58**: 560–8.

32. Mort TC. Continuous Airway Access for the Difficult Extubation: the Efficacy of the Airway Exchange Catheter. *Anesthesia & Analgesia* 2007; **105**: 1357–62.

33. El-Orbany M. The Use of a Supraglottic Airway Device as an Extubation Bridge for the Difficult Airway. *Canadian Journal of Anesthesia/Journal canadien d'anesthésie* 2014; **61**: 387–8.

34. Koga K, Asai T, Vaughan RS, et al. Respiratory Complications Associated with Tracheal

Extubation. Timing of Tracheal Extubation and Use of the Laryngeal Mask during Emergence from Anaesthesia. *Anaesthesia* 1998; **53**: 540–4.

35. Fujii Y, Saitoh Y, Tanaka H, et al. Cardiovascular Responses to Tracheal Extubation or LMA Removal in Children. *Canadian Journal of Anesthesia/Journal canadien d'anesthésie* 1998; **45**: 178–81.

36. Ellard L, Brown DH, Wong DT. Extubation of a Difficult Airway after Thyroidectomy: Use of a Flexible Bronchoscope via the LMA-Classic. *Canadian Journal of Anesthesia/Journal canadien d'anesthésie* 2012; **59**: 53–7.

37. Jagannathan N, Sohn L, Ramsey M, et al. A Randomized Comparison between the i-gel and the air-Q Supraglottic Airways when Used by Anesthesiology Trainees as Conduits for Tracheal Intubation in Children. *Canadian Journal of Anesthesia/Journal canadien d'anesthésie* 2015; **62**: 587–4.

38. Jagannathan N, Sohn LE, Sawardekar A, et al. A Randomized Trial Comparing the Ambu Aura-i with the air-Q Intubating Laryngeal Airway as Conduits for Tracheal Intubation in Children. *Paediatric Anaesthesia* 2012; **22**: 1197–204.

39. Raveendran R, Sastry SG, Wong DT. Tracheal Extubation with a Laryngeal Mask Airway and Exchange Catheter in a Patient with a Difficult Airway. *Canadian Journal of Anesthesia/Journal canadien d'anesthésie* 2013; **60**: 1278–9.

40. Komasawa N, Ueki R, Iwasaki Y, et al. Use of the air-Q Laryngeal Airway and Tube Exchanger in a Case of Difficult Tracheal Extubation after Maxillectomy. *Masui* 2012; **61**: 1125–7.

41. Nair I, Bailey PM. Use of the Laryngeal Mask for Airway Maintenance Following Tracheal Extubation. *Anaesthesia* 1995; **50**: 174–5.

42. Xue FS, Zhang YM, Liao X, et al. Extubation and Endotracheal Tube Exchange Using a Guidewire Sheath in Management of Difficult Pediatric Airways. *Paediatric Anaesthesia* 2009; **19**: 646–8.

43. Sharma R, Panda A, Kumar A. Sheath of Guidewire of Ureteric Stent as an Aid to Extubation in Difficult Pediatric Airway. *Paediatric Anaesthesia* 2008; **18**: 1252–3.

44. Davis PG, Henderson-Smart DJ. Nasal Continuous Positive Airways Pressure Immediately after Extubation for Preventing Morbidity in Preterm Infants. *The Cochrane Database of Systematic Reviews* 2003: Cd000143.

45. Gupta P, Kuperstock JE, Hashmi S, et al. Efficacy and Predictors of Success of Noninvasive Ventilation for Prevention of Extubation Failure in Critically Ill Children with Heart Disease. *Pediatric Cardiology* 2013; **34**: 964–77.

46. Bassanezi BS, Oliveira-Filho AG, Miranda ML, et al. Use of BiPAP for Safe Anesthesia in a Child with a Large Anterior Mediastinal Mass. *Paediatric Anaesthesia* 2011; **21**: 985–7.

47. Reddy VG, Nair MP, Bataclan F. Role of Non-Invasive Ventilation in Difficult-to-Wean Children with Acute Neuromuscular Disease. *Singapore Medical Journal* 2004; **45**: 232–4.

48. Ho AM, Dion PW, Karmakar MK, et al. Use of Heliox in Critical Upper Airway Obstruction. Physical and Physiologic Considerations in Choosing the Optimal Helium:Oxygen Mix. *Resuscitation* 2002; **52**: 297–300.

49. Ho AM, Lee A, Karmakar MK, et al. Heliox vs Air-Oxygen Mixtures for the Treatment of Patients with Acute Asthma: a Systematic Overview. *Chest* 2003; **123**: 882–90.

50. Polaner DM. The Use of Heliox and the Laryngeal Mask Airway in a Child with an Anterior Mediastinal Mass. *Anesthesia & Analgesia* 1996; **82**: 208–10.

51. Martin AR, Katz IM, Terzibachi K, et al. Bench and Mathematical Modeling of the Effects of Breathing a Helium/Oxygen Mixture on Expiratory Time Constants in the Presence of Heterogeneous Airway Obstructions. *Biomedical Engineering Online* 2012; **11**: 27.

52. Green J, Walters HL, 3rd, Delius RE, et al. Prevalence and Risk Factors for Upper Airway Obstruction after Pediatric Cardiac Surgery. *The Journal of Pediatrics* 2015; **166**: 332–7.

53. Tobias JD. Heliox in Children with Airway Obstruction. *Pediatric Emergency Care* 1997; **13**: 29–32.

Section 3 Special Topics

Chapter 17: Airway Management in the Child with an Airway Injury

Somaletha T. Bhattacharya

A traumatized airway can be challenging and requires timely intervention. Improper management can result in high mortality and morbidity, especially in the younger age group. Airway injuries in children occur as a result of direct injury to the airway, or indirect, as in anaphylaxis. Direct injury to the airway can be the result of penetrating or blunt trauma to the upper torso (head, neck, and chest).

Injuries to the facial structures are sustained as a result of high-velocity impact or a fall onto the face. In children, due to the large cranium-to-body ratio, the skull and brain is usually injured in pediatric facial fractures.[1,2] The mandible is reported to be the commonest fractured facial bone in children, with the condyle being the most common site.[3,4] Mid-facial injuries are uncommon in children below 5 years of age.[3] Maxillary alveolar ridge fracture is the commonest fracture seen in children below 6 years of age.[5] Mid-facial injuries are classified by the Le Fort classification. Le Fort I is a horizontal fracture extending from the floor of the nose, involving the lateral and medial wall of the maxillary sinus, up to the pterygoid plate. It separates the alveolus and palate from the rest of the maxilla. Le Fort II is a pyramidal fracture, which extends from the nasal bridge, to the medial wall of maxilla – involving the inferior orbital rim, infraorbital foramen, and below the zygoma – to the pterygoid plate. It separates the midface from the cranium. Le Fort III is a transverse fracture, which extends from the nasofrontal bridge to the medial and lateral orbital walls, including the nasolacrimal bone, infraorbital fissure, the zygomatic arch, and ultimately the pterygoid plate. A Le Fort III fracture separates the face from the rest of the skull (Figure 17.1). Injuries to the neck area by blunt or penetrating causes can result in airway compromise. The neck includes structures containing air (pharynx, hypopharynx, trachea, esophagus), blood (veins, arteries), muscles and bones (cervical spine, thyroid, cricoid and hyoid cartilages, bones). Injuries to the neck area can lead to airway compromise by direct injury to the airway (tracheal transection), airway compression by hematoma, and subcutaneous emphysema and airway obstruction by secretions, blood, or foreign bodies.

Cervical spine injury is uncommon in children, but when present, can lead to increase in mortality and morbidity. Children less than 8 years of age are prone to ligamentous and spinal cord injury without radiographic abnormality (SCIWORA).[6] Children less than 8 years of age are prone to axial injuries such as atlantoaxial dislocation and atlanto-occipital dislocation, which can be fatal.[7] The most common injury seen in this age group is atlantoaxial rotatory subluxation, which is characterized by chin rotation to the contralateral side and flexion of the neck ("cock robin" torticollis).[8] Spinal cord injury should be suspected in patients who are unconscious, children less than 3 years of age with a Glasgow Coma Scale of less than 14, patients with focal or abnormal neurological findings, neck hematomas, neck tenderness (especially posterior midline), limited neck mobility (even with SCIWORA), and in patients with predisposing factors such as motor vehicle and diving injuries.[9] Computed tomography (CT) scans are highly sensitive in detecting cervical spine injury in high-risk patients and MRI has become the standard method in ruling out ligamentous injury.[10] Cervical immobilization is recommended for trauma patients, especially those with high risk for spinal injury.

Thoracic traumas in children are usually a result of blunt injury to the chest. According to the National Pediatric Trauma Registry, most injuries are due to motor vehicle accidents. Penetrating injuries account for less than 20% of thoracic traumas and are usually due to gunshots or injury with a sharp object. Unlike an adult chest, the pediatric chest is more cartilaginous and is more compliant.[11] Hence, a blunt injury to the chest rarely results in rib fractures, but causes

Section 3: Special Topics

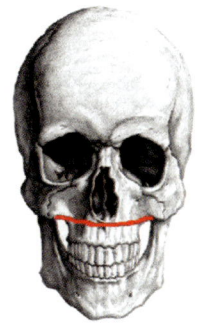
Le Fort I fracture

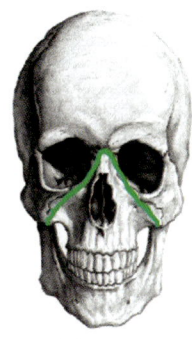
Le Fort II fracture

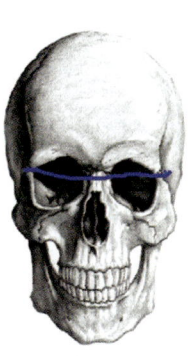
Le Fort III fracture

Figure 17.1 Le Fort fractures.

more injury to the internal organs in the chest by the absorbed kinetic energy of the force. Children are more prone to lung contusions, resulting in ventilation perfusion mismatch, pneumothorax, hemothorax, and cardiac contusion, and injuries to the trachea, esophagus, and diaphragm.

Laryngotracheal injuries are rare in children, but a high degree of suspicion of laryngotracheal injury is necessary in patients with injury to the neck and/or upper torso. These patients may present with symptoms and signs of respiratory distress, hoarseness or aphonia, difficulty and/or pain in swallowing, cough, hemoptysis, or subcutaneous emphysema with or without any visible injury to the skin. A change in voice and dyspnea are red flags for airway injury. Subcutaneous emphysema confined only to neck is also pathognomonic of injury to aerodigestive structures. All patients suspected of having laryngotracheal injuries should undergo a neck X-ray and CT three-dimensional imaging of trachea.[12] Ultrasonography is useful for visualizing the mobility of the vocal cords and arytenoid cartilages, asymmetric positioning of the arytenoid cartilages, and for looking for any thickening of the vocal cords, fractures of thyroid cartilage, and hematoma.[13] Flexible fiberoptic endoscopy of the airway is a good tool for assessment of laryngeal trauma and should be done prior to intubations in these patients.

Thermal injuries in the pediatric age group occur as a result of burns, scald injury, and chemical injury. These can affect both the upper airways and lower airways. Inhalational injury in burns leads to increased mortality and morbidity. Airway injury in burns can be the result of (a) airway edema due to direct injury to the head and neck, and indirectly during fluid resuscitation, (b) airway obstruction from the presence of foreign materials like carbonaceous secretions and fibrin casts or compression by eschar around the neck, (c) chemical injury due to inhalational of toxic chemical substances such as aldehydes and oxides of sulfur and nitrogen, and hydrochloric acid in smoke, and (d) hypoxia due to diminished oxygen-carrying capacity due to carbon monoxide and cyanide.[14] Inhalational injury should be suspected in patients with singed eyebrows or nasal hairs, the presence of soot or carbonaceous material in the oropharynx or nasopharynx, and in patients found in an enclosed area in the event of a fire. Chest compliance can be severely affected by circumferential eschar involving the chest area. Lung compliance is also decreased by interstitial edema and mucosal edema. Symptoms and signs of airway involvement are stridor, hoarseness, tachypnea, dyspnea, and respiratory distress. Scald injury affecting the airways occurs when the head-and-neck area are involved. This usually occurs as a result of hot liquid spilling from a height onto the patient, usually in the toddler age group. Caustic ingestion generally causes injury to the aerodigestive system. Caustic substances cause injury due to chemicals resulting in necrosis of the tissue when in contact, and thermal injury as a result of an exothermic reaction. Iatrogenic thermal injuries to the airways can occur in the operating room during laser therapy, and from the use of cautery in the head-and-neck area in the presence of high oxygen concentration. Chest X-ray is not a good indicator of lung involvement in the acute early stage. Flexible fiberoptic endoscopy of the airway is the most efficient way of diagnosing inhalational injury. Thermal injuries can affect the airway in the later stages due to contractures, fibrosis, and distortion of the normal anatomy.

Iatrogenic injuries to the airway usually result during airway intervention. A difficult airway can result in multiple attempts to secure the airway by multiple providers with different devices. This can cause airway edema, bleeding, injury to the glottic structures, and injury to the trachea, carina, and bronchus with bougies and airway exchange catheters. Intubation with a tight ETT or overinflated cuff can result in croup and subglottic stenosis, especially in newborns and infants. Domino and colleagues analyzed the claims for airway injury during anesthesia in the ASA Closed Claims Project database and reported this at 6% of 4460 claims, with the larynx (33%) as the major site of injury.[14]

In all trauma patients, if possible, a good history regarding mechanism of injury, any significant medical and surgical history, and allergies can be helpful in management. A quick assessment of the nervous system (level of consciousness and Glasgow Coma Scale), respiratory system (airway patency, signs of respiratory distress), cardiovascular system (hemodynamic stability), and musculoskeletal system (cervical spine, bony injuries) is useful for management. A quick primary survey should be conducted in accordance with the Advanced Trauma Life Support guidelines.

Airway Management

The circulation, airway, and breathing (CAB) of resuscitation is applicable here. Pulse oximetry provides information regarding oxygen saturation, but not of oxygen content, delivery, or impending respiratory failure until it is often too late. A cervical collar should be applied until injury to the cervical spine is ruled out. It is important to have a parent or caretaker present to calm the already-traumatized child.[15]

Look for any signs of upper airway obstruction (inspiratory stridor, snoring, noisy respiration). Clear the airway of secretions, blood, tissue, and foreign bodies (teeth, dentures, food particles). If using suction, be gentle and, if possible, suction the posterior part of oropharynx under direct vision. Blind suctioning of the back of pharynx may stimulate the gag reflex and vomiting. Assess airway patency. Auscultation of the neck provides information of airway patency. If obstructed, maintain airway patency by positioning the patient laterally (if there is no spinal injury), use jaw thrust and chin lift, and use airway adjuncts such as an appropriately sized oropharyngeal airway, nasopharyngeal airway (avoid in base-of-skull fracture and nasal fractures), or even an SGA. All patients should be provided with oxygen at high flows via a mask.

Assessment of the airway may not be easy in a child, especially in trauma. The mnemonic "LEMON" used in trauma situations may be helpful in older children:[16] Look (L) at the external appearance. Observe the lateral profile and imagine a line drawn straight down from the upper lip. If the chin is behind the line, this indicates micrognathia or retrognathia; if the chin is in front of the line, this indicates prognathia. This is useful to do in all patients. Low-set ears may indicate an abnormal or difficult airway. Evaluate (E) the 3–3–2 rule: Determine whether the patient can open his or her mouth to accommodate three fingers, which will inform on temporomandibular joint mobility. The distance from the mentum to hyoid bone equals three of the patient's fingers and two fingers from the hyoid to thyroid. Mallampati score (M) is assessed by the patient opening his or her mouth to say "Ah." Obstruction (O) is assessed by looking for obstructers such as tissue edema, blood, secretions, and foreign bodies. Neck (N) immobility can be caused by injury, disease, or surgery.

The ability of a patient to phonate, cry, swallow, and cough indicates the capability to maintain and clear the airway. Airway or respiratory problems should be suspected in patients with signs of obstruction such as inspiratory stridor (upper airway), expiratory stridor (lower airway), snoring, noisy respiration, brassy inadequate cough, and hemoptysis. Difficulty phonating (aphonia, hoarseness, low voice) may be due to glottic edema, vocal cord injuries, or impending respiratory failure. Difficulty in swallowing may be due to airway edema or obstruction or injury to the aerodigestive system. Impending respiratory failure may be preceded by increased respiratory rate, nasal flaring, sternal and/or subcostal retractions, a see-saw pattern of breathing, and grunting. The silent toddler can also be a sign of respiratory failure.

Examination of the airway should include the ability to open the mouth, cough, and protrude the tongue. Look for injury to dentition, pain (especially in the posterior midline of neck), surgical emphysema (injury to laryngotracheal structure, esophageal injury), swelling or open wounds on the neck, and bruises or open wounds in the chest area. Hyperresonance or dullness on percussion of the chest indicates pneumothorax or hemothorax respectively. Look for any chest wall deformity (fractured ribs) or instability (flail chest). Auscultation will provide information on air entry and any adventitious sounds.

Injury to the mandibular condyle can limit mouth opening, and bilateral factures of mandible can displace the tongue posteriorly. In this case, the tongue can be pulled forward with forceps or a tongue stitch.

CT scan during primary survey is the diagnostic tool used for most injuries due to the speed in which results can be obtained. In children, the risk of radiation must be weighed up against the benefits of imaging. The "focused assessment with computed tomography in trauma" (FACTT), an imaging modality introduced by Kanz and colleagues, has been shown to shorten the time taken to make a definitive diagnosis.[17] Ultrasonography has been suggested to be helpful in assessment of vocal cord mobility and fractures of the laryngeal cartilage.[13] Experience is required to make the correct diagnosis with ultrasonography. Flexible fiberoptic endoscopy of the airway is the best tool for assessing airway integrity and trauma to the airway.

All patients with significant trauma should be presumed to have cervical spine injury. The cervical spine should be stabilized in an appropriate cervical collar until the spine is cleared of injury. It is advisable to remove the front of the collar and maintain in-line stabilization to facilitate intubation. In patients with cervical spine injury, manual in-line immobilization during airway management is of utmost importance. Brown and Raja[18] recommend two methods of spine immobilization. The first method consists of the assistant approaching the head from the upper torso, resting his or her forearms on the upper chest and clavicles, with the wrists and hands alongside the neck bilaterally, so that the hands with spread fingers can grip and immobilize the occipital–parietal area. In the second method, the assistant crouches below the table or stretcher to the left of the individual managing the airway. The assistant reaches over the head and immobilizes the base of the occiput with the heels of both hands. The fingers are extended along the neck to the top of the patient's shoulders. The assistant should provide instant feedback regarding any movement of the spine during airway manipulation.

Bag-mask ventilation should be initiated in patients who are apneic or who have inadequate respiratory effort. It should be done with caution or avoided in patients with subcutaneous surgical emphysema. In case of problems with bag-mask ventilation, an SGA device should be used.

As a means of providing a protective definite airway, intubation is an easy decision in some cases, such as the unconscious patient, the hemodynamically unstable patient, the hypoxic patient, and the patient with impending respiratory failure. However, based on the clinical picture, the decision is not whether to intubate, but when the right time to intubate is. This decision should be a team effort. When time permits, the intubation should be done in a controlled fashion and in a controlled environment (i.e., the operating room). Intubation in particularly difficult situations should be done by the most experienced person, especially with young pediatric patients. The chosen techniques must be ones that the airway expert is familiar with.

When the decision to intubate a patient is taken, it is important to have not just one definite plan, but multiple backup plans in case the first is unsuccessful. Requirements for intubation are a cohesive team (T), a variety of airway (A) equipment, the required pharmacological (P) agents, and a working suction (S) (TAPS). Direct laryngoscopy (previously the first choice for intubation) is slowly being replaced by the various video laryngoscopes in most trauma cases. In suspected airway injury (laryngotracheal injuries), flexible fiberoptic bronchoscopy may be a suitable method to assess the extent of injury. In the teenage age group, this can be done with minimal sedation and topical anesthesia. In younger age groups, the procedure can be done through an LMA under anesthesia maintaining spontaneous respiration. Flexible fiberoptic bronchoscopy is used for intubation in cases where laryngoscopy (direct/video assisted) is impossible or has failed. Flexible fiberoptic bronchoscopy can be difficult in the presence of secretions and blood. If intubation is difficult or impossible, and ventilation cannot be achieved, the next urgent step is a surgical airway (cricothyroidotomy or tracheotomy). An experienced surgeon should ideally perform the procedure. Cricothyroidotomy is not an easy procedure in the very young, even for the experienced.

In most cases of trauma, rapid-sequence intubation is the method used. All patients should be preoxygenated prior to rapid-sequence intubation. There is a lot of debate regarding the use of cricoid pressure (Sellick maneuver). Cricoid pressure, when applied properly, should prevent aspiration, but improper technique tends to cause more harm than good. It can distort the anatomy of the airway and convert it to a difficult airway for intubation; applied too early can cause retching and incomplete compression of esophagus, and lead to aspiration. In younger age groups, it is possible not only to compress the esophagus, but also the trachea, making insertion of an ETT impossible.

The choice of drugs and dosages for rapid-sequence intubation in a traumatized airway will depend on the hemodynamic status of the patients. The available induction drugs are propofol, ketamine, etomidate, methohexitone, midazolam, and sevoflurane, in combination with short-acting narcotics (remifentanil, alfentanil, fentanyl).

Management of Airway in Thermal Injuries

In acute thermal injuries, when and whether to intubate is an important decision. Delays in intubating a patient can result in an easy airway becoming a difficult airway due to swelling of facial structures and airway edema. However, intubating the trachea when it is not warranted has its own consequences. Children with intraoral scald burns may not appear to be in any distress initially, but with time, edema will most likely set in and may result in airway obstruction and distress.

Not all inhalational injuries require prophylactic tracheal intubation. The classical teaching has been to intubate any inhalation injuries: singed nasal hairs, presence of carbonaceous sputum, facial burns, and hoarseness of voice may indicate airway involvement. These may be unreliable, however, and not predictive of airway involvement.[19,20] According to the recent American Burns Association practice guidelines (2001), intubation is indicated if the upper airway patency is threatened, gas exchange or compliance mandates ventilatory assistance, or if mental status is inadequate to maintain the airway. Prophylactic steroids and antibiotics are not recommended in the initial management of inhalational injury, according to the practice guidelines. All patients who are not intubated should be continuously evaluated for any airway compromise, as evidenced by progressive hoarseness of voice, stridor, and retractions. Edema formation can be reduced to some extent by upright positioning of the head and avoidance of excess fluid therapy.[21] Laryngeal examination with serial fiberoptic nasendoscopy has been recommended as a simple and less invasive method for assessing supraglottic edema and the need for airway intervention,

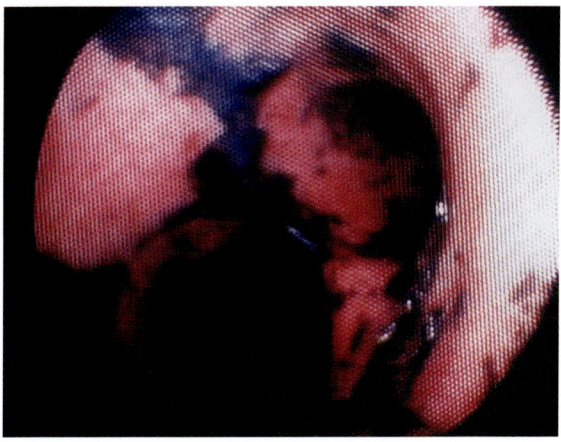

Figure 17.2 Bronchoscopy of airway: carbonaceous material.

especially in the early phases of resuscitation.[19,20] Bronchoscopy is indicated for assessing subglottic airway and the presence of carbonaceous material (Figure 17.2). Bronchoscopy requires sedation/anesthesia and is more invasive than nasendoscopy. Presence of carboxyhemoglobin in carbon monoxide poisoning can be detected only by measuring the level of carboxyhemoglobin in arterial blood or the oxygen-carrying capacity of hemoglobin by a co-oximeter. Certain pulse oximeters can read both oxyhemoglobin and carboxyhemoglobin. The timing of measurement is important as the level of carboxyhemoglobin falls by 50% from injury level in 4 hours if the patient is breathing room air, and in 1 hour if patient is on 100% oxygen.[15]

In chemical burns involving the airway, the chemical agent should be removed if possible. In most cases, immediate airway intervention and protection is required (intubation/tracheostomy). Airway mucosa may be ulcerated and edematous, and the structure distorted. Airway protection is required prior to dilution of the chemical, especially in cases where the oral airway is involved. Figure 17.3 shows the laryngoscopic view of a child who had a caustic injury in the past. The posterior part of the tongue was fused to the palate. It was impossible to insert an oral or nasopharyngeal airway, and required a tracheostomy under spontaneous respiration with a mask.

When intubation is required in acute thermal burns, it should be performed by the most experienced provider and, if possible, in an area with essential equipment, personnel, and pharmacology. Preoxygenation should be provided. Mask

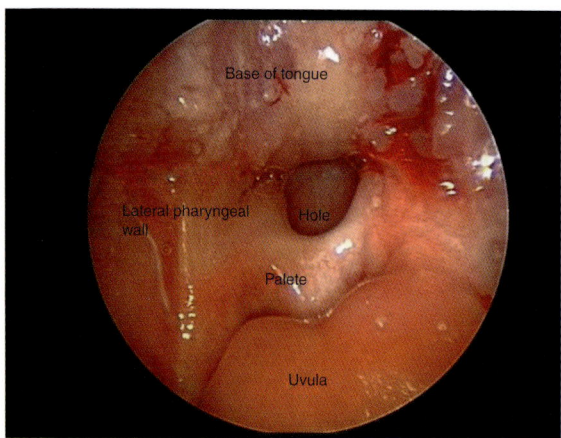

Figure 17.3 Laryngoscopic view: caustic airway injury.

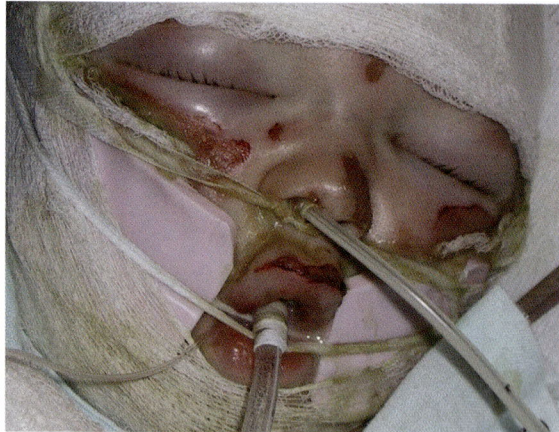

Figure 17.4 Otoform elastomer: used in securing tube with ties in burns.

ventilation may be difficult due to facial burns and swelling and an SGA device may be useful. Aspiration may be a risk factor in most cases. Induction agents should be based on hemodynamic stability and the need for maintaining spontaneous respiration. Muscle relaxants are indicated if ventilation is possible. The current recommendation is to avoid succinylcholine in patients 48 hours after burn injury due to the increase in extrajunctional acetylcholine receptors resulting in hyperkalemia with the use of succinylcholine.[22] Direct laryngoscopy may be difficult due to facial swelling, airway edema, and presence of soot. Video laryngoscopy, fiberoptic intubation, or intubation through an SGA may be indicated in difficult airways. A cuffed tube is recommended due to the change in airway compliance. In the presence of edema, a smaller-sized tracheal tube may be required. Ideally, the cuff pressure should be measured and kept between 20 cm and 30 cm of water. Securing the tracheal tube may be difficult in facial burns. The tube must be secured well to prevent extubation. The tube is secured either with ties or tapes encircling the patient's head, or with wires to a tooth.[22] Figure 17.4 shows the method used at Shriners Hospital for Burns in Boston: the tube is secured with tape using otoform elastomer to prevent injuries to the tissue from the tape. Eschars encircling the neck area may obstruct the airway and those around the chest and abdomen may interfere with ventilation. In these cases, escharotomies are indicated.

In the case of iatrogenic airway fires in operating rooms, extinguish and remove the source of ignition and switch off all gas flows. If the endotracheal tube is on fire, extinguish it with saline and remove the tube. Reestablish the airway and mask-ventilate with air. Assess the airway for extent of injury and fragments of tube with bronchoscopy.

Airway management of patients with burn contractures of the neck and caustic injury to the airway can be challenging and requires skill and competency. The safest method normally recommended for a difficult airway is an awake intubation. Unfortunately, this is not easy in young children or uncooperative older patients. Patients with burns contracture of the neck can have a small mouth opening due to fibrosis of tissues around the mouth, restricted neck extension with fixed flexion of the neck, constricted nasal passages, minimal-to-no submandibular space, and altered and distorted airways (Figures 17.5 and 17.6). Contractures of the neck make the airway more difficult as time progresses. X-ray of the airway (head and neck) in lateral and anterior–posterior view and CT scan of the airway are useful in assessing the oropharyngeal space and distortion and narrowing of the airway. A good history of snoring (obstructed airway), sleeping position (best position for airway patency when unconscious), and evaluation of the airway helps in planning. If awake fiberoptic bronchoscopy is the path chosen, the patient may be minimally sedated with use of midazolam, fentanyl, or dexmedetomidine, while still maintaining spontaneous respiration and cooperation. Antisialagogue and topicalization of the airway with nebulized lidocaine, gargling viscous lidocaine, or spraying with lidocaine are combined to assist in the fiberoptic intubation. In children, often anesthesia must be induced prior to

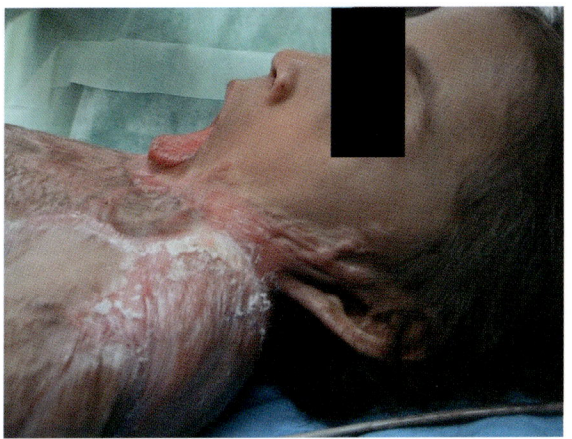

Figure 17.5 Burns contracture of the neck.

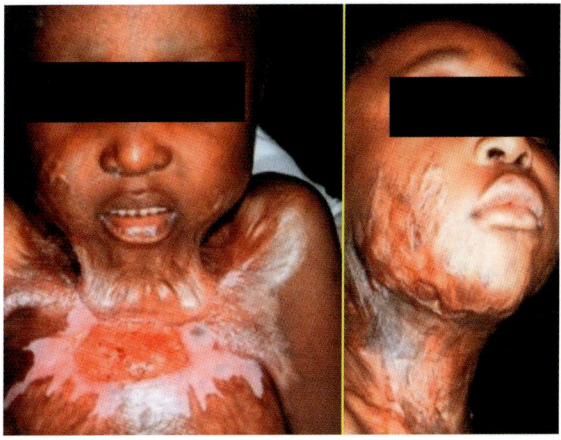

Figure 17.6 Burns contracture of neck before and after release.

securing the airway. Inhalational induction helps maintain spontaneous respiration, and patency of airway can be maintained by nasopharyngeal or oropharyngeal airways, or supraglottic devices, depending on the interincisor distance and nare patency. In cases where this is impossible, a quick excision of the neck contracture or circumoral contracture under local anesthesia by the surgeon under ketamine anesthetic can help further increase the degree of extension of the neck and opening the mouth. In each individual case, the method used for airway management will depend on the patient, the anatomy of the airway, the availability of various airway equipment, and the skill, competency, and preferences of the provider. Unlike other cases of difficult airway, where surgical airway may be the final choice, surgical airway in patients with neck contractures is difficult, even for the most experienced surgeon due to the distorted anatomy. Muscle relaxants should be used only if ventilation is possible. Mask ventilation may be difficult due to difficulty in using adjuncts like chin lift and jaw thrust. Supraglottic devices are useful for ventilation and for assisting fiberoptic intubation. Due to the fixed flexion deformity, fiberoptic intubation is also not easy. To help advance the ETT over the fiberscope into the trachea, Asai and colleagues[23] recommend reducing the gap between the scope and trachea, use of a flexible or armored tube, and 90-degree anticlockwise rotation of the tracheal tube. Introduction of video laryngoscopes with monitors have helped in the intubating of these patients, provided there was space to insert not only the laryngoscope blade, but also the ETT. Figure 17.7 depicts three individuals inserting

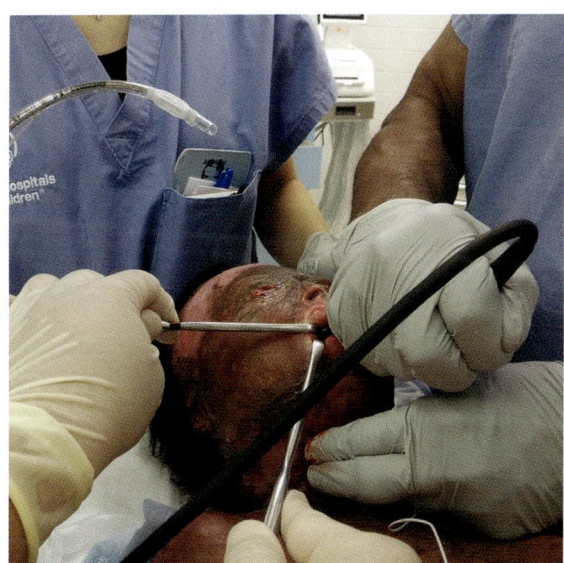

Figure 17.7 GVL and retractors to assist intubation.

the ETT with a GVL: one holding the GVL and applying pressure on the laryngeal area to obtain a Cormack–Lehane grade I–II view, while the second is using surgical retractors to provide space for the third person to insert the ETT and ultimately intubate the patient. Once intubated, care must be taken to make sure the patient is not accidentally extubated when the neck is finally extended.[24] In their review, Prakash and colleagues[24] recommend meticulous planning, preparation of the patient, skilled assistance, expertise in dealing with difficult airway and multiple airway strategies during induction, and maintenance and emergence of anesthesia. In all cases, it is also important to know when to stop and not persist when multiple attempts have failed.

In conclusion, dealing with an injured airway in a child requires skill and expertise in airway evaluation and management, a cohesive team, multiple plans in cases of failure of one, proper preparation, and timely intervention.

The author wishes to thank Dr. Robert L Sheridan MD (Burns Unit – Shriners Hospitals for children in Boston) for Figures 17.2, 17.4, 17. 5, and 17.6.

References

1. Ferreira PC, Amarante JM, Silva PN, et al. Retrospective Study of 1251 Maxillofacial Fractures in Children and Adolescents. *Plastic and Reconstructive Surgery* 2005; **115**: 1500–8.

2. Chao MT, Losee JE. Complications in Pediatric Facial Fractures. *Craniomaxillofacial Trauma and Reconstruction* 2009; **2**: 103–12.

3. Zimmermann CE, Troulis MJ, Kaban LB. Pediatric Facial Fractures: Recent Advances in Prevention, Diagnosis and Management. *International Journal of Oral and Maxillofacial Surgery* 2006; **35**: 2–13.

4. Oji C. Fractures of the Facial Skeleton in Children: a Survey of Patients Under the Age of 11 Years. *Journal of Cranio-Maxillofacial Surgery* 1998; **26**: 322–5.

5. Iida S, Matsuya T. Paediatric Maxillofacial Fractures: their Aetiological Characters and Fracture Patterns. *Journal of Cranio-Maxillofacial Surgery* 2002; **30**: 237–41.

6. Pang D. Spinal Cord Injury Without Radiographic Abnormality in Children, 2 Decades Later. *Neurosurgery* 2004; **55**: 1325–42.

7. Patel JC, Tepas DL III, Molitt DC, et al. Pediatric Cervical Spine Injuries – Defining the Disease. *Journal of Pediatric Surgery* 2001; **36**(2): 373–6.

8. Leonard JC. Cervical Spine Injury. *Pediatric Clinics of North America* 2013; **60**: 1123–37.

9. Leonard JC, Kuppermann N, Olsen C, et al. Factors Associated with Cervical Spine Injury in Children after Blunt Trauma. *Annals of Emergency Medicine* 2011; **58**: 145–55.

10. Tilt L, Babineau J, Fenster D, Ahmad F, Roskind CG. Blunt Cervical Spine Injury in Children. *Current Opinion in Pediatrics* 2012; **24**: 301–6.

11. Smyth BT. Chest Trauma in Children. *Journal of Pediatric Surgery* 1978; **14**: 41–7.

12. Poli-Merol ML, Belouadah M, Parvy F, Chauvet P, Egreteau L, Daoud S. Tracheobronchial Injury by Blunt Trauma in Children: is Emergency Tracheobronchoscopy Always Necessary? *European Journal of Pediatric Surgery* 2003; **13**: 393–402.

13. Jakubowska A, Zawadzka-Glos, Brzewski M. Usefulness of Ultrasound Examination in Larynx Traumas in Children. *Polish Journal of Radiology* 2011; **76**: 7–12.

14. Domino KB, Posner KL, Caplan RA, Cheney FW. Airway Injury during Anesthesia. *Anesthesiology* 1999; **91**: 1703.

15. Mlcak RP, Suman OE, Herndon DN. Respiratory Management of Inhalational Injury. *Burns* 2007; **33**: 2–13.

16. Murphy MF, Walls RM. Identification of the Difficult and Failed Airway. In Walls RM, Luten RC, eds. *Manual of Emergency Airway Management*. 3rd ed. Philadelphia: Lippincott Williams & Wilkins; 2008: 81–93.

17. Kans KG, Paul AO, Lefering R, et al. Trauma Registry of the German Trauma Society. Trauma Management Incorporating Focused Assessment with Computed Tomography in Trauma (FACTT) – Potential Effect on Survival. *Journal of Trauma Management and Outcomes* 2010; **4**: 4.

18. Brown CA, Raja AS. The Traumatized Airway. In Haberg CA, ed. *Benumof and Hagberg's Airway Management*. 3rd ed. Elsevier Health Sciences; 2012: 859–75.

19. Ikonomidis C, Lang F, Radu A, Berger MM. Standardizing the Diagnosis of Inhalational Injury Using Descriptive Score Based on Mucosal Injury Criteria. *Burns* 2012; **38**: 513–19.

20. Madnani DD, Steele NP, de Vries E. Factors that Predict the Need for Intubation in Patients with Smoke Inhalation Injury. *Ear Nose and Throat Journal* 2006; **85**: 278–80.

21. Oscier C, Emerson B, Handy JM. New Perspectives on Airway Management in Acutely Burned Patients. *Anaesthesia* 2014; **69**: 105–10.

22. Bittner EA, Shank E, Woodson L, Martyn JAJ. Acute and Perioperative Care of the Burn-Injured Patient. *Anesthesiology* 2015; **122**: 448–64.

23. Asai T, Shingu K. Difficulty in Advancing a Tracheal Tube over a Fiberoptic Bronchoscope: Incidence, Causes and Solutions. *British Journal of Anaesthesia* 2004; **92**: 870–81.

24. Prakash S, Mullick P. Airway Management in Patients with Burn Contractures of the Neck. *Burns* 2015; **41**: 1627–35.

Section 3 Special Topics

Chapter 18

Airway Management Outside of the Operating Room: the Emergency Department

Aaron Donoghue

Introduction

For pediatric patients, tracheal intubation in the ED is a fundamental lifesaving procedure, but one that occurs with a much lower frequency than other care areas in the hospital. The challenges associated with intubation of a pediatric patient in the ED relate to a variety of aspects of the procedure, including the underlying epidemiology, the uniformly higher level of acuity than other settings, and actual or potential underlying pathophysiology that directly impacts decision-making with regard to airway management. This chapter will review these phenomena, with particular attention to choice and application of medications for facilitating intubation, as well as several typical pathophysiologic states that lead to the need for ED airway management in children.

General Epidemiology

Indications for intubation in the ED for pediatric patients vary from other acute care settings. Studies done at both pediatric and non-pediatric hospitals have demonstrated that traumatic injury is the leading indication for ED intubation in children, with known or suspected traumatic brain injury representing the leading diagnosis.[1,2] Seizures and seizure-related complications, poisonings and intoxications, and out-of-hospital cardiac arrest account for a significant proportion of children undergoing intubation in the ED. This epidemiology mirrors that of adult patients requiring airway management in the ED.

One of the important implications of the epidemiology of ED airway management for children is that most children requiring intubation in this setting have existing or impending respiratory failure based on underlying neurological disease. This is different than children undergoing intubation in the ICU, where primary failure of oxygenation or ventilation based on lung or cardiovascular disease is more prevalent.[3] In theory, this should mean that this set of patients are at less risk of oxyhemoglobin desaturation during intubation, and that they should be easier to preoxygenate, be less challenging to support with bag-valve mask ventilation in the peri-intubation phase, and have a longer time threshold for desaturation during prolonged laryngoscopy attempts. However, published data comparing these phenomena between care areas do not currently exist. Data from pediatric EDs have demonstrated that, irrespective of underlying pathophysiology, laryngoscopy times exceeding 30 seconds in duration are associated with a five-fold increase in the odds of clinically significant oxyhemoglobin desaturation.[4]

If a child is being intubated in an ED, there are several empiric considerations that have a potential direct bearing on the performance of the procedure. First, all children who require intubation in an ED are severely ill or injured, and can be assumed to be ASA class 3 or greater simply by definition. Second, all patients of all ages in an ED either have, or should be presumed to have, a full stomach and a greater risk of vomiting and aspiration. Third, more than 50% of children requiring intubation in the ED have a presumed or actual cervical spinal injury and require appropriate precautions during intubation. While the truly "difficult pediatric airway" (defined as difficulty with achieving glottic visualization using a laryngoscope) is likely exceedingly rare in the ED, these aforementioned characteristics should be incorporated into planning and decision-making with regard to airway management.

The Challenge of the Infrequent Fundamental Procedure

Despite the fact that tracheal intubation is a fundamental, essential skill for emergency providers, pediatric tracheal intubation is an uncommon occurrence when measured at the level of an individual provider. A recent survey of pediatric ED directors found that the annual incidence of tracheal intubation in the pediatric ED (PED) ranged from 12 to 64 cases per year.[5] Sixty-two percent of surveyed PED directors believed that their faculty did not encounter sufficient exposure to tracheal intubation in their clinical duties to maintain competence at this essential procedure. Additionally, the same survey found that there was a negligible difference in the median number of tracheal intubation cases per faculty at the PEDs where their directors thought exposure was insufficient (five cases per faculty per year) and those where their directors thought exposure was sufficient (seven cases per faculty per year). Data from tertiary PEDs published in the past few years have shown low-frequency exposure to tracheal intubation for PED faculty, with fewer than half of PED faculty performing tracheal intubation during a year of typical clinical experience, and supervising tracheal intubation performance a median of four times per year.[6,7]

Published data on exposure to pediatric tracheal intubation among trainees in pediatrics and pediatric emergency medicine (PEM) also show scant – and possibly diminishing – experience. Multiple studies have shown that pediatric residents are exposed to opportunities for attempting tracheal intubation less often.[8–10] A study of video-recorded tracheal intubation attempts from a tertiary PED demonstrated success rates of 33% for residents and 50% for PEM fellows; this same study demonstrated equivalent first-attempt success rates for PEM attendings and anesthesiologists.[1] Multihospital registry data on pediatric TI in the ICU have shown a significant positive association between residents attempting tracheal intubation and the occurrence of adverse events.[11] In 2013, the Accreditation Council for Graduate Medical Education removed non-neonatal tracheal intubation from the core competencies for house-staff training in pediatrics.

Finally, while historically reported as infrequent, physiological deterioration during intubation may be more common than previously appreciated in children. In the previously mentioned study of video-recorded cases of pediatric emergency intubation, oxyhemoglobin desaturation (defined as pulse oximetry of < 90%) has been shown to occur in up to one-third of cases of emergency tracheal intubation in the PED. Cardiovascular instability (bradycardia, hypotension) has been noted to occur in up to 8% of patients, with cardiac arrest from asphyxia occurring in 2%.[1] This combination of high clinical risk, infrequent occurrence, and dwindling exposure among trainees has led to widespread reconsideration of what operators are appropriate to perform tracheal intubation in the PED. Careful attention should be paid to training exposure and cumulative clinical experience among personnel in the PED who may be required to perform tracheal intubation on children.

Medications

Sedatives

Sedatives used for intubation should render the patient rapidly unconscious. They should ideally have minimal side effects on hemodynamics or intracranial pressure, but all sedatives have adverse effects and efficacy limitations. A thorough understanding of the side effects of various drugs is essential so that the best option for a given patient's situation can be determined.

Etomidate is the most commonly used sedative for intubation in the ED. Its advantages are rapid onset, reliable pharmacokinetics, and minimal cardiovascular or cerebrovascular side effects. Etomidate is an inhibitor of 11-beta hydroxylase and is known to suppress adrenal corticosteroid synthesis. The clinical significance of this side effect is not clear from published studies; nonetheless, routine use of etomidate for facilitating intubation in children has been

Table 18.1 Sedatives

Medication	Dose
Benzodiazepines (midazolam, lorazepam)	0.1–0.2 mg/kg
Narcotics (fentanyl)	1–2 mcg/kg
Ketamine	1–3 mg/kg
Etomidate	0.3 mg/kg
Propofol	1–4 mg/kg

questioned by some groups. Of particular note, the current recommendations of the American Heart Association Pediatric Advanced Life Support guidelines state that etomidate should be avoided in children being intubated as a result of septic shock.[12]

Ketamine is a dissociative anesthetic with rapid onset; most often in a single arm-heart-brain circulation. It has the effects of increasing heart rate, right atrial pressure, and systemic vascular resistance, making it the theoretical drug of choice for patients who are hypotensive and/or in shock. Published studies in adults and children have found varying effects on intracranial pressure (see below).

Propofol is a potent vasodilator and myocardial depressant; even a single dose of propofol frequently results in hypotension, which makes it unsuitable for hypovolemic patients, children in shock, or patients in whom maintenance of cerebral perfusion is essential. While propofol is widely used as an intravenous induction agent for children in the operating room, its use in the ED should be limited based on the uncertain and evolving pathophysiology that is generally present in children requiring intubation in the ED.

Benzodiazepines are generally considered safer with anticonvulsant and amnestic effects, reversibility (with flumazenil), and less cardiovascular depression. However, dosing is variable in that a standard dose (e.g., 0.1 mg/kg) does not reliably result in unconsciousness in a child. Higher doses are often required, which have a slower onset and place the patient at higher cardiovascular risk.

Neuromuscular Blocking Agent (NMBA) (Paralyzing Agent)

Succinylcholine is the most rapid-onset NMBA. It has an onset time of 30 to 60 seconds and a duration of 3 to 8 minutes. It is a "depolarizing" paralyzing drug, causing muscle fasciculation prior to the onset of paralysis. This can cause muscle pain, myoglobin release, potassium release (hyperkalemia), histamine release, and a higher risk of malignant hyperthermia. It also frequently results in transient bradycardia; atropine premedication is often recommended to minimize this effect (see below). Succinylcholine carries a "black-box" warning pertaining to the risk of hyperkalemic cardiac arrest in children; this was the result of a series of cases of children with undiagnosed skeletal muscle myopathies receiving succinylcholine. The incidence of this severe side effect in routine use in the pediatric ED is exceedingly rare, and succinylcholine remains in widespread use in pediatrics.

Nondepolarizing NMBAs do not cause fasciculations and their attendant side effects. While several different medications in this class are available, rocuronium and vecuronium are the most frequently used in emergency airway management. Rocuronium has an onset time of 1 to 3 minutes and a duration of 30 to 45 minutes. Larger doses have faster onset times, but longer durations. Vecuronium has been observed to have a slightly longer onset time, but with a similar dose dependency (i.e., higher doses shorten the onset time and lengthen the duration of effect).

The longer duration of action of nondepolarizing NMBAs may be perceived to be a disadvantage. However, in most instances, maintenance of the paralysis is preferable for imaging, ventilator management, vascular access, and so on. Succinylcholine requires repeated doses or conversion to a longer-acting agent (generally a nondepolarizing NMBA) to maintain paralysis when needed. Paralyzing drugs with longer durations require maintenance of sedation as well to avoid conscious paralysis.

Adjunctive Agents
Atropine

Atropine is a vagolytic medication, which reduces the risk of bradycardia resulting from laryngoscopy or succinylcholine use; a physiologic phenomenon more commonly observed in infants and younger children. Atropine reduces oral secretions if ketamine is going to be given. Data on atropine premedication during pediatric intubation in the ED have not clearly demonstrated a benefit in terms of reducing the incidence of bradycardia during laryngoscopy. In 2015, American Heart Association Pediatric Advanced Life Support (AHA PALS) guidelines stated that premedication with atropine for emergency airway

Table 18.2 Neuromuscular blocking agents (paralytics)

Medication	Dose
Succinylcholine	1–2 mg/kg
Rocuronium	0.6–1.2 mg/kg
Vecuronium	0.1–0.2 mg/kg
Cisatracurium	0.1–0.2 mg/kg

management in children was no longer routinely recommended.[13]

Lidocaine

Lidocaine is administered to blunt the autonomic effects of laryngoscopy on hemodynamics and intracranial pressure during laryngoscopy. Historically, it has been recommended for patients undergoing intubation as a result of traumatic brain injury. Meta-analyses in adults have failed to demonstrate a benefit of lidocaine premedication during intubation, and have shown a higher incidence of hypotension and bradycardia. Analogous data in pediatric patients do not exist in published literature.

Approach to ED Airway Management in Specific Pathophysiologic States

Traumatic Brain Injury

Known or suspected traumatic brain injury (TBI) accounts for more cases of pediatric intubation in the ED than all other diagnoses combined.[2] Advantages to placement of an advanced airway in TBI patients include control of minute ventilation – permitting normoventilation and/or hyperventilation as is clinically appropriate – minimization of cerebral metabolic oxygen consumption through sedation or anesthesia, and facilitation of other necessary procedures. Risks associated with intubation in TBI patients include the potential for hypotension during induction, the autonomic physiologic response to laryngoscopy, and the potential for clinically significant hypercarbia in the event of prolonged laryngoscopy times.

The choice of induction agent for intubation in TBI patients has been a subject of controversy. Historically, ketamine has been considered relatively contraindicated for intubation in the setting of intracranial hypertension; review of the literature that serves as the basis for this recommendation, however, has demonstrated that the data are very limited. More recently, an increasing number of studies in adults have shown that ketamine has an inconsequential influence on intracranial pressure (ICP) in TBI patients, and its use has not been associated with worsened outcomes. Data in pediatric patients are limited. One study of pediatric TBI patients with measured ICPs > 25 mmHg, despite first-tier therapy, found that a single dose of ketamine lowered ICP by a median of 30% while maintaining or increasing cerebral perfusion pressure.[14] Etomidate has also been shown to lower ICP in pediatric TBI patients without a concomitant decrease in mean arterial pressure.[15] While satisfactory sedation may also be achieved with benzodiazepines, narcotics, or propofol, all of these classes of agents may be more likely to cause clinically significant hypotension during intubation; clinical data on children with TBI have demonstrated that even brief periods of hypotension in the acute management phase have been associated with worsened outcomes.[16]

Postintubation management is of particular importance in TBI patients prior to their disposition to the operating room or ICU. Cerebral vascular resistance is highly responsive to arterial carbon dioxide levels, with hypercarbia resulting in cerebrovascular dilatation and increased cerebral blood flow; conversely, hypocarbia results in cerebrovascular constriction, limiting cerebral blood flow. Continuous quantitative capnometry is essential in the intubated TBI patient, and a goal of normocarbia (exhaled carbon dioxide levels of 35–40 mmHg) is usually recommended. Controlled hyperventilation may be considered in a child with signs of impending herniation, or as transient presumptive therapy while additional therapies (e.g., hyperosmolar therapy) are being instituted. Sustained hyperventilation may risk diminishing perfusion to injured brain and the penumbral regions of TBI and is not recommended.

Septic Shock

When a child is being treated for septic shock, intubation may become necessary due to a decline in their mentation, refractory acidosis, impending respiratory failure, or to facilitate establishment of central venous and arterial vascular access to optimize hemodynamic support. Advantages to intubating a child with septic shock are numerous. Sedation and neuromuscular blockade result in a reduction in oxygen demand, both by reducing cerebral metabolic consumption and the "unloading" of respiratory muscles associated with increased spontaneous work of breathing, which can amount to up to 40% of cardiac output in children. Additionally, the transition to positive-pressure ventilation and the associated increase in intrathoracic pressure results in a reduction in afterload to the left ventricle, which can be beneficial in septic shock with elevated systemic vascular resistance.[17]

Disadvantages to intubation in the setting of septic shock include the impact of induction medications on the cardiovascular system, where most classes of medications (i.e., narcotics, benzodiazepines, propofol) cause myocardial depression and/or vasodilatation. The transition to positive-pressure ventilation and the associated increase in intrathoracic pressure also impairs venous return to the right atrium and can lessen preload, which can worsen cardiac output.

Current guidelines published by the American College of Critical Care Medicine (ACCM) state that, in pediatric septic shock, "the decision to intubate and ventilate is based on clinical assessment of increased work of breathing, hypoventilation, or impaired mental status."[17] Additional recommendations from the ACCM guidelines include volume administration both before and during induction and intubation, along with support from vasoactive infusion(s) either peripherally or centrally.

The correct medications to use to intubate a septic patient remain a point of controversy. ACCM guidelines recommend ketamine as the induction agent of choice, along with atropine premedication as indicated. Etomidate is the most controversial medication in the setting of sepsis; due to its inhibitory influence on endogenous corticosteroid synthesis, it has come under scrutiny for its potential association with worse outcomes in septic patients. Clinical data on this phenomenon are mixed: evidence establishing a clear causal association between etomidate use and increased mortality in septic children or adults is lacking in published literature.[18] Nonetheless, both the American Heart Association and the ACCM recommend avoiding routine use of etomidate to facilitate intubation in children with septic shock.[12,17]

Status Asthmaticus

Tracheal intubation is uncommonly indicated in acute asthma exacerbations. Intubation of a child with asthma may become necessary based on declining mental status, severe hypoxemia, or cardiovascular instability. A recent study from a pediatric ICU collaborative found that invasive mechanical ventilation was performed in only 10% of asthma patients in PICUs during the study period.[19] Studies have also shown that intubation of children with asthma exacerbations occurs more commonly at non-pediatric centers, and that children intubated for asthma (without cardiac arrest) outside of an ICU have shorter duration of mechanical ventilation.[20,21] These data may be interpreted as suggesting that intubation may occur more often than is necessary in children with asthma and that noninvasive support techniques are sufficient for the large majority of children.

The advantages of intubation and assisted ventilation in a child with status asthmaticus include the relief of the metabolic stress of excessive respiratory muscle use, as well as the ability to manipulate mechanical ventilation settings in such a way as to guarantee a given minute ventilation while accurately monitoring plateau pressure. However, the disadvantages of positive-pressure ventilation in an asthmatic child center around the pathophysiologic phenomenon of dynamic hyperinflation; this is believed to be associated with an increased risk of clinically significant barotrauma. However, in the aforementioned multicenter PICU study, clinically appreciable barotrauma was only present in 6% of children undergoing mechanical ventilation for status asthmaticus.

Acute asphyxial asthma refers to a specific pattern of symptoms and pathophysiology in acute asthma, marked by very rapid progression of symptoms to a near-cardiac arrest state.[22] This life-threatening form of acute asthma exacerbation is distinct from typical status asthmaticus in that early intubation is frequently necessary, but the subsequent duration of assisted ventilation is significantly shorter than children with more typical progression of asthma symptoms.

Ketamine has classically been recommended as the induction agent of choice for intubating a patient with bronchospastic disease: this is based primarily on case reports, and robust clinical data supporting this effect do not exist. A recent systematic review found only a single randomized trial in non-intubated asthmatics, which did not demonstrate any improvement in symptoms or need for additional therapies, nor did it show any significant side effects of ketamine use.[23] Irrespective of its influence on airway resistance, ketamine may still be a favorable induction agent for an asthmatic, given the hemodynamic changes that frequently occur after intubation (see below).

Postintubation management of a child with status asthmaticus poses more significant challenges than the procedure of intubation itself. As described above, assisted ventilation of an asthma patient requires an unusual strategy of low ventilation rates with extended expiratory time to facilitate exhalation and carbon dioxide elimination; this can be challenging to achieve with manual bag-valve mask ventilation, and the use of a ventilator can be advantageous. Additionally, the elevated intrathoracic pressure in intubated asthmatics, compounded with vasodilation from beta-agonists and hypovolemia from increased insensible fluid losses, can lead to hypotension. Vascular access and equipment for rapid fluid administration should be available when preparing to intubate an asthmatic patient.

Cardiopulmonary Arrest

Most children receiving cardiopulmonary resuscitation (CPR) in the ED have suffered an out-of-hospital cardiac arrest. Cardiac arrests that actually occur in the ED comprise approximately 10% of all cases of pediatric in-hospital cardiac arrest.[24] In absolute terms, children receiving CPR account for approximately 25% of patients who undergo attempted intubation in tertiary pediatric EDs; the national or worldwide frequency of intubation during pediatric CPR is difficult to define as a result of wide variation in prehospital care teams' capabilities and training as well as variability in pediatric preparedness in the EDs of non-pediatric hospitals. Few published data have focused specifically on success rates for intubation during CPR in children.

The primary advantages of the presence of a secured airway during CPR are two-fold: first, ensuring the optimal method for controlling assisted oxygenation and ventilation; and second, permitting the use of quantitative end-tidal carbon dioxide measurement to titrate chest compression quality, as well as to provide a potential early sign of return of spontaneous circulation. Additionally, resuscitation medications such as epinephrine can be delivered intratracheally in an intubated patient, but this method of administration has become essentially obviated with the ubiquitous availability of intraosseous access devices in hospital and prehospital care.

Placement of an advanced airway can lead to significant interruptions in chest compressions.[25,26] A recent study in a pediatric ED utilizing video recording during resuscitations reported that chest compressions were paused in 54% of intubation attempts, and that 78% of the interruptions exceeded 10 seconds in duration.[27] Another recent analysis of a multihospital cardiac arrest database, looking specifically at events occurring in the ED, found that intubation was attempted during CPR more frequently in pediatric patients than in adult patients. Additionally, this study found that ED patients receiving CPR in whom intubation was never attempted had increased odds of survival.[24]

The role of tracheal intubation during CPR remains unclear in both adults and children. A recent consensus statement from the American Heart Association on optimizing CPR quality aptly stated that "the optimal time for insertion of an advanced airway during management of cardiac arrest has not been established."[28] The aforementioned study of video-recorded events in a pediatric ED found that intubation attempts done with chest compressions paused were no more likely to be successful than attempts made with ongoing CPR.[27] Intubation during CPR should be done with attention paid to minimizing interruptions in chest compressions as much as possible; ideally, it should be performed with ongoing, uninterrupted chest compressions.

References

1. Kerrey BT, Rinderknecht AS, Geis GL, Nigrovic LE, Mittiga MR. Rapid Sequence Intubation for Pediatric Emergency Patients: Higher Frequency of Failed Attempts and Adverse Effects Found by Video Review. *Annals of Emergency Medicine* 2012; **60**(3): 251–9.

2. Sagarin MJ, Chiang V, Sakles JC, Barton ED, Wolfe RE, Vissers RJ, et al. Rapid Sequence Intubation for Pediatric Emergency Airway Management. *Pediatric Emergency Care* 2002; **18**(6): 417–23.

3. Nishisaki A, Turner DA, Brown CA, 3rd, Walls RM, Nadkarni VM, National Emergency Airway Registry for C, et al. A National Emergency Airway Registry for Children: Landscape of Tracheal Intubation in 15 PICUs. *Critical Care Medicine* 2013; **41**(3): 874–85.

4. Rinderknecht AS, Mittiga MR, Meinzen-Derr J, Geis GL, Kerrey BT. Factors Associated with Oxyhemoglobin Desaturation during Rapid Sequence Intubation in a Pediatric Emergency Department: Findings from Multivariable Analyses of Video Review Data. *Academic Emergency Medicine* 2015; **22**(4): 431–40.

5. Losek JD, Olson LR, Dobson JV, Glaeser PW. Tracheal Intubation Practice and Maintaining Skill Competency: Survey of Pediatric Emergency Department Medical

Directors. *Pediatric Emergency Care* 2008; **24**(5): 294–9.

6. Donoghue AJ, Ades AM, Nishisaki A, Deutsch ES. Videolaryngoscopy versus Direct Laryngoscopy in Simulated Pediatric Intubation. *Annals of Emergency Medicine* 2013; **61**(3): 271–7.

7. Mittiga MR, Geis GL, Kerrey BT, Rinderknecht AS. The Spectrum and Frequency of Critical Procedures Performed in a Pediatric Emergency Department: Implications of a Provider-Level View. *Annals of Emergency Medicine* 2013; **61**(3): 263–70.

8. Donoghue AJ, Durbin DR, Nadel FM, Stryjewski GR, Kost SI, Nadkarni VM. Effect of High-Fidelity Simulation on Pediatric Advanced Life Support Training in Pediatric House Staff: a Randomized Trial. *Pediatric Emergency Care* 2009; **25**(3): 139–44.

9. Falck AJ, Escobedo MB, Baillargeon JG, Villard LG, Gunkel JH. Proficiency of Pediatric Residents in Performing Neonatal Endotracheal Intubation. *Pediatrics* 2003; **112** (6 Pt 1): 1242–7.

10. Leone TA, Rich W, Finer NN. Neonatal Intubation: Success of Pediatric Trainees. *The Journal of Pediatrics* 2005; **146**(5): 638–41.

11. Sanders RC, Jr., Giuliano JS, Jr., Sullivan JE, Brown CA, 3rd, Walls RM, Nadkarni V, et al. Level of Trainee and Tracheal Intubation Outcomes. *Pediatrics* 2013; **131** (3): e821–8.

12. Kleinman ME, de Caen AR, Chameides L, Atkins DL, Berg RA, Berg MD, et al. Part 10: Pediatric Basic and Advanced Life Support: 2010 International Consensus on Cardiopulmonary Resuscitation and Emergency Cardiovascular Care Science with Treatment Recommendations. *Circulation* 2010; **122**(16 Suppl. 2): S466–515.

13. de Caen AR, Berg MD, Chameides L, Gooden CK, Hickey RW, Scott HF, et al. Part 12: Pediatric Advanced Life Support: 2015 American Heart Association Guidelines Update for Cardiopulmonary Resuscitation and Emergency Cardiovascular Care. *Circulation* 2015; **132**(18 Suppl. 2): S526–42.

14. Bar-Joseph G, Guilburd Y, Tamir A, Guilburd JN. Effectiveness of Ketamine in Decreasing Intracranial Pressure in Children with Intracranial Hypertension. *Journal of Neurosurgery: Pediatrics* 2009; **4**(1): 40–6.

15. Bramwell KJ, Haizlip J, Pribble C, VanDerHeyden TC, Witte M. The Effect of Etomidate on Intracranial Pressure and Systemic Blood Pressure in Pediatric Patients with Severe Traumatic Brain Injury. *Pediatric Emergency Care* 2006; **22**(2): 90–3.

16. Vavilala MS, Bowen A, Lam AM, Uffman JC, Powell J, Winn HR, et al. Blood Pressure and Outcome after Severe Pediatric Traumatic Brain Injury. *The Journal of Trauma: Injury, Infection, and Critical Care* 2003; **55**(6): 1039–44.

17. Brierley J, Carcillo JA, Choong K, Cornell T, Decaen A, Deymann A, et al. Clinical Practice Parameters for Hemodynamic Support of Pediatric and Neonatal Septic Shock: 2007 Update from the American College of Critical Care Medicine. *Critical Care Medicine* 2009; **37**(2): 666–88.

18. Sprung CL, Annane D, Keh D, Moreno R, Singer M, Freivogel K, et al. Hydrocortisone Therapy for Patients with Septic Shock. *The New England Journal of Medicine* 2008; **358**(2): 111–24.

19. Bratton SL, Newth CJ, Zuppa AF, Moler FW, Meert KL, Berg RA, et al. Critical Care for Pediatric Asthma: Wide Care Variability and Challenges for Study. *Pediatric Critical Care Medicine* 2012; **13**(4): 407–14.

20. Carroll CL, Smith SR, Collins MS, Bhandari A, Schramm CM, Zucker AR. Endotracheal Intubation and Pediatric Status Asthmaticus: Site of Original Care Affects Treatment. *Pediatric Critical Care Medicine* 2007; **8**(2): 91–5.

21. Newth CJ, Meert KL, Clark AE, Moler FW, Zuppa AF, Berg RA, et al. Fatal and Near-Fatal Asthma in Children: the Critical Care Perspective. *Journal of Pediatrics* 2012; **161**(2): 214–21 e3.

22. Maffei FA, van der Jagt EW, Powers KS, Standage SW, Connolly HV, Harmon WG, et al. Duration of Mechanical Ventilation in Life-Threatening Pediatric Asthma: Description of an Acute Asphyxial Subgroup. *Pediatrics* 2004; **114**(3): 762–7.

23. Jat KR, Chawla D. Ketamine for Management of Acute Exacerbations of Asthma in Children. *Cochrane Database of Systematic Reviews* 2012; **11**: CD009293.

24. Donoghue AJ, Abella BS, Merchant R, Praestgaard A, Topjian A, Berg R, et al. Cardiopulmonary Resuscitation for In-Hospital Events in the Emergency Department: A Comparison of Adult and Pediatric Outcomes and Care Processes. *Resuscitation* 2015; **92**: 94–100.

25. Wang HE, Brown SP, MacDonald RD, Dowling SK, Lin S, Davis D, et al. Association of Out-of-Hospital Advanced Airway Management with Outcomes after Traumatic Brain Injury and Hemorrhagic Shock in the ROC Hypertonic Saline Trial. *Emergency Medicine Journal* 2014; **31**(3): 186–91.

26. Wang HE, Szydlo D, Stouffer JA, Lin S, Carlson JN, Vaillancourt C, et al. Endotracheal Intubation versus Supraglottic Airway Insertion in Out-of-Hospital

Cardiac Arrest. *Resuscitation* 2012; **83**(9): 1061–6.

27 Donoghue A, Hsieh TC, Nishisaki A, Myers S. Tracheal Intubation during Pediatric Cardiopulmonary Resuscitation: A Videography-Based Assessment in an Emergency Department Resuscitation Room. *Resuscitation* 2016; **99**: 38–43.

28 Meaney PA, Bobrow BJ, Mancini ME, Christenson J, de Caen AR, Bhanji F, et al. Cardiopulmonary Resuscitation Quality: [corrected] Improving Cardiac Resuscitation Outcomes Both Inside and Outside the Hospital: a Consensus Statement from the American Heart Association. *Circulation* 2013; **128**(4): 417–35.

Section 3

Special Topics

Chapter 19

Airway Management of the Neonate and Infant: the Difficult and Critical Airway in the Intensive Care Unit Setting

Janet Lioy, Erin Tkach, and Luv Javia

Characteristics of the Neonatal Airway

Airway Resistance and Physiology

The size of the neonatal airway in relation to older children and adults is especially important for understanding its functioning and pathophysiology (Figure 19.1). There are two basic types of airflow through an airway: laminar, or relatively smooth flow, and turbulent, or rough flow. Poiseuille's law, $R \propto 1/r^4$ (where R is resistance and r is radius) describes laminar airflow. By this equation, the resistance to airflow increases exponentially (to the fourth power) as the radius decreases. This effect is to the fifth power for turbulent flow, such as with a crying child. Due to this relationship, even minor narrowing of the airway can cause significant increases in resistance in neonates (Figure 19.2).

Other unique physiologic aspects of the neonatal airway must be taken into consideration during management. At birth, neonatal lungs are less compliant than adult lungs, but the chest wall is more compliant due to a higher cartilage composition. This combination results in a lower functional lung capacity than adults. Neonates have higher oxygen consumption rates, small lung volumes, and a reduced FRC. These factors result in quick, dramatic declines in PaO_2 with airway occlusion.[1–3]

Neonatal Airway Anatomy

Upper Airway

Nasal Cavity/Nasopharynx

On birth, neonates are preferential nasal breathers and are dependent on patent nares for adequate ventilation.[4,5] This is what makes choanal atresia an easy diagnosis in the otherwise healthy neonate as the task of suck, swallow, and breath are initiated during early feeding. Additionally, the nasal passages are very small, so even a slight decrease in diameter due to secretions or inflammation can lead to inadequate ventilation and obstructive apnea.[6,7]

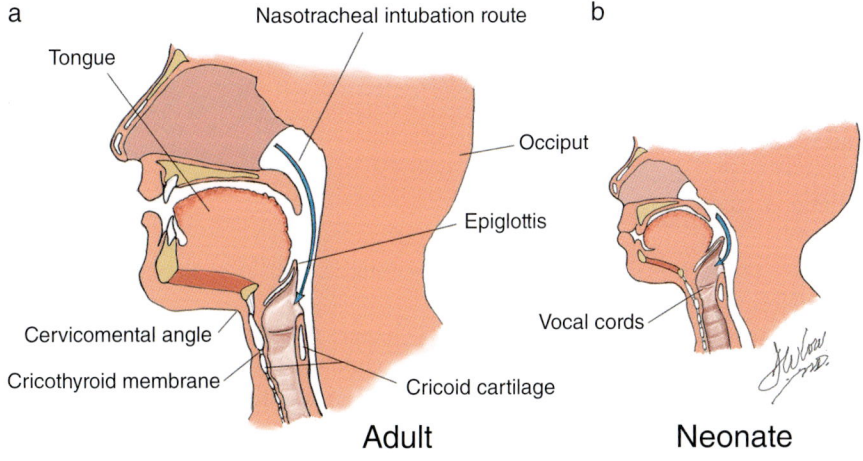

Figure 19.1 Sagittal view of the adult versus neonatal airway. Note the reduced nasopharyngeal space and larger occiput that may lead to airway obstruction in the neonate. (Adapted from Lioy and Sobol. *Disorders of the Neonatal Airway: Fundamental for Practice.* 2015.)

Section 3: Special Topics

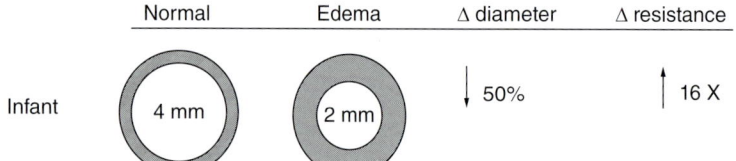
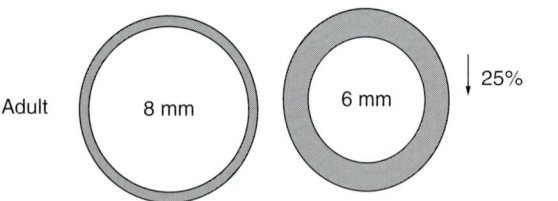

Figure 19.2 Differences in luminal size and airway resistance with 1 mm of circumferential edema: adult versus infant. (Adapted from Lioy and Sobol. *Disorders of the Neonatal Airway: Fundamental for Practice*. 2015.)

Oral Cavity/Oropharynx

The neonate's tongue and palate make up the oral cavity and oropharynx. The tongue is proportionally larger than in an adult and therefore potentially more obstructive.[8] Certain malformations can affect the tongue and cause airway obstruction requiring hemiglossectomy and ultimately tracheostomy. Birth defects, such as lymphatic malformations of the tongue, palatal tumors such as epignathus or epulis, and overgrowth syndromes such as Beckwith–Weidemann syndrome are all causes of macroglossia causing complete airway obstruction.

Hypopharynx and Larynx

The hypopharynx is the lowest part of the pharynx that lies behind the larynx down to the level of the cricoid, including areas like the pyriform sinus. The larynx is the entrance to the lower airway, and consists of the vocal cords, epiglottis, arytenoids, and subglottis. It is higher in the neck in neonates compared to adults.[1,2] It is also proportionally smaller, with relatively larger surrounding arytenoids and aryepiglottic folds[2,9–12] (Figure 19.3).

The neonatal epiglottis is proportionally narrower, larger, longer, and less flexible than in older children and adults. Sometimes, the epiglottis can be omega-shaped. These factors make it extremely susceptible to trauma during intubation and suctioning. The hypopharynx anatomy is more compact than in an adult and can be difficult to visualize, especially when secretions and edema are involved. During intubation, critical landmarks for exposure include the base of the tongue, the tip of the epiglottis, and the vallecula.

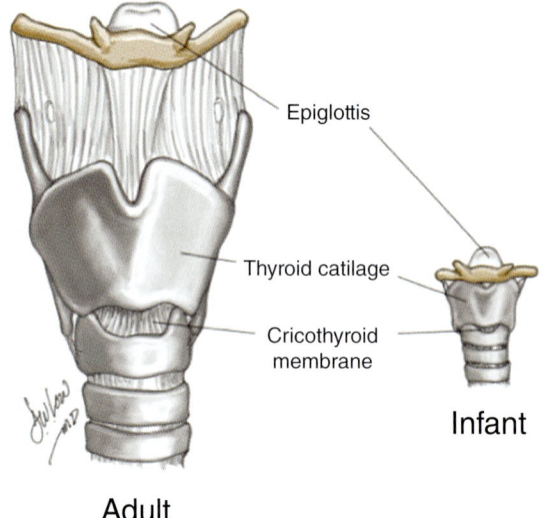

Figure 19.3 Differences in size and location of cricothyroid membrane, epiglottis, and thyroid cartilage in infants and adults. (Adapted from Lioy and Sobol. *Disorders of the Neonatal Airway: Fundamental for Practice*. 2015.)

The larynx changes over time. As a neonate grows into infancy and childhood, the larynx descends and becomes similar to an adult by 6 years of age. The larynx is cone- or funnel-shaped and is joined to the trachea by the cricoid cartilage. The cricoid cartilage is a complete cartilaginous ring and is the narrowest point in the airway of a young infant (in adults, the narrowest point is the glottic opening).[8] This narrowing is the reason uncuffed ETTs are generally used in neonates.

Lower Airway

Below the cricoid cartilage lies the trachea, the beginning of the lower airway. Compared to an adult, the neonatal trachea is proportionally shorter, narrower, more compact, located higher in the neck, and more anterior. There are cartilaginous rings anteriorly and a soft trachealis muscle posteriorly that provides flexibility during breathing (Figure 19.3).

Neck

One major difference between neonates and infants is the neck area. There are many differences in size, width, and dimension that differentiate the two. A neonate's neck is much shorter and composed of more subcutaneous fat and, almost always, different

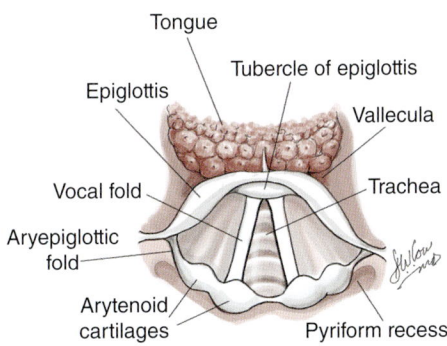

Figure 19.4 Detailed anatomical drawing of the neonatal airway showing all structures in relation to one another. (Adapted from Lioy and Sobol. *Disorders of the Neonatal Airway: Fundamental for Practice*. 2015.)

maneuvers are needed during intubation, such as cricoid pressure, neck rolls, and video laryngoscopy for difficult airways.

Common Neonatal Airway Disorders

Upper Airway

Nasal Cavity/Nasopharynx

Choanal stenosis/atresia is a posterior nasal obstruction, which is seen in 1 in every 5000–7000 births. While unilateral choanal atresia may not be diagnosed for years, the classic presentation of bilateral choanal atresia is acute respiratory distress and cyanosis, which improves with crying when the neonate is able to breathe orally. Inability to pass a catheter through the nares into the nasopharynx is suggestive of this disorder and fiberoptic nasal endoscopy and CT scan confirm the diagnosis.[9,13,14] With new high-definition ultrasounds, this can sometimes be diagnosed prenatally. This defect is found in several genetic syndromes, including CHARGE, and so a genetic workup is necessary with this diagnosis.[14,15] The most common surgical approach is an endoscopic repair with or without postoperative stenting. Subsequent balloon dilation may be required to keep the choanae patent. Surgical outcome is dependent on the degree of atresia, size of the neonate, and frequency of restenosis.[16]

Congenital pyriform sinus aperture stenosis is a rare condition, which also causes nasal obstruction. In this case, the obstruction is anterior at the nasal bony inlet resulting from overgrowth of the maxillary prominences.[9,10,17] On CT imaging, patients with congenital pyriform sinus aperture stenosis have a nasal inlet less than 11 mm. It requires a genetic

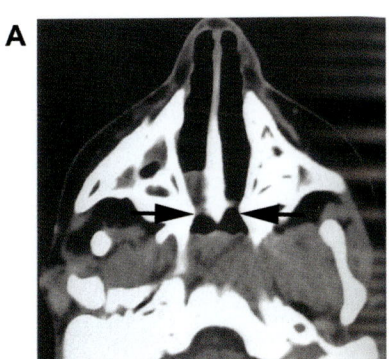
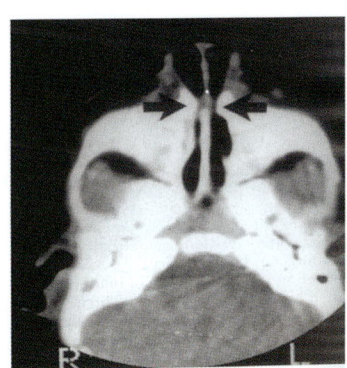

Figure 19.5A, B CT scan of head showing (A) choanal atresia and (B) pyriform aperture stenosis: seemingly similar defects, but embryologically in different anatomical locations.

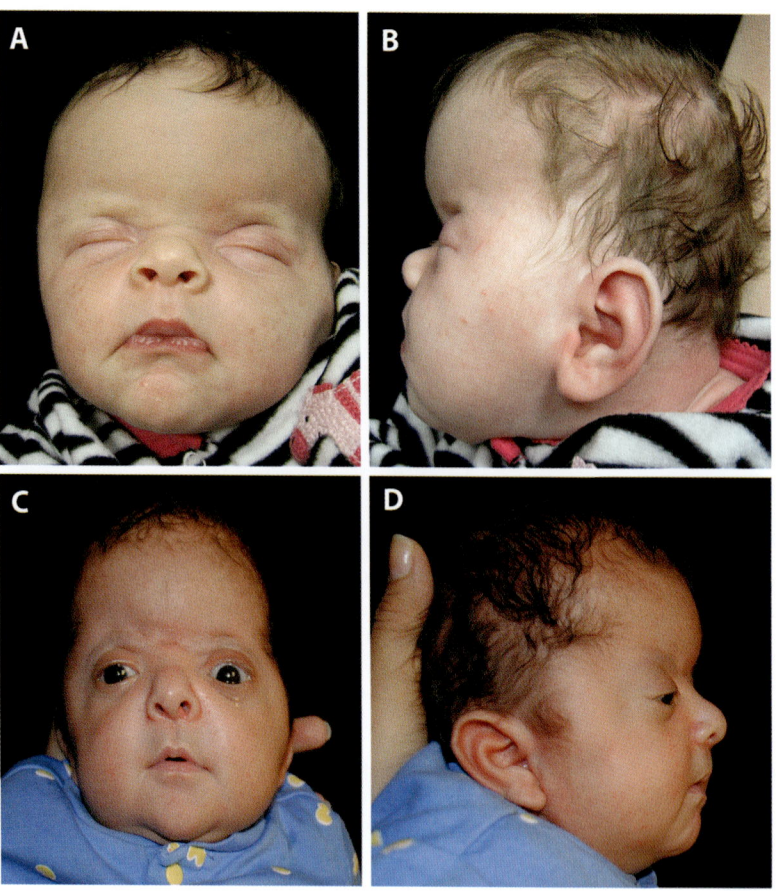

Figure 19.6 Crouzon and Apert syndromes. Note the brachycephaly, frontal bossing, hypertelorism, and maxillary hypoplasia. Some craniofacial malformations can have mandibular hypoplasia and tracheal stenosis with airway obstruction. (Adapted from Lioy and Sobol. *Disorders of the Neonatal Airway: Fundamental for Practice.* 2015.)

workup as well since it is associated with other midline defects such as central mega incisor, holoprosencephaly, hypopituitarism, and septo-optic dysplasia.[10,12,18,19]

An underdiagnosed entity that can be concurrent with pyriform aperture stenosis is nasal cavity stenosis. Congenital pyriform aperture stenosis is associated with narrowing of the anterior 75% of the nasal cavity.[20] Nasal cavity stenosis is a general narrowing of the midnasal cavity. Congenital pyriform sinus aperture stenosis is surgically managed via a sublabial drill-out procedure or more recent reports of dilation with rigid dilators.[21] Patients with nasal stenosis are managed with nasal cavity dilation as well. Stenting is also sometimes employed postoperatively.

Other nasal obstructions include masses in the nasal passages, such as nasolacrimal duct cysts, nasal encephaloceles, and nasopharyngeal tumors (i.e., teratomas).[22] Imaging studies can help delineate the extent of the lesion and are paramount for effective planning for surgical resection. Children with Crouzon, Apert, or Pfeiffer syndromes can have nasopharyngeal obstruction due to midface hypoplasia. This may require tracheostomy to establish a stable airway and then subsequent midface advancement surgeries for a more definitive, patent airway. Nasal septum deviation can cause obstruction as well.

Oropharynx

Retrognathia or micrognathia can displace the tongue to the rear of the oropharynx, causing obstruction. These findings are often associated with genetic craniofacial syndromes like Pierre Robin sequence or Stickler syndrome.[12] Obstruction can be relieved with tongue-lip adhesion, tracheostomy, or, the newer therapeutic option, mandibular distraction osteogenesis.[23] Prior to surgery, the airway obstruction can be partially alleviated with prone positioning or placement of an oral airway or nasal trumpet.

Chapter 19: Airway Management of the Neonate and Infant

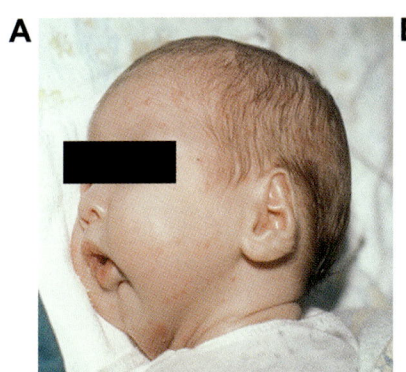
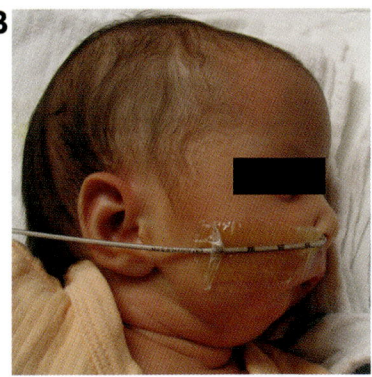

Figure 19.7A, B Severe micrognathia in a neonate. (Adapted from Lioy and Sobol. *Disorders of the Neonatal Airway: Fundamental for Practice.* 2015.)

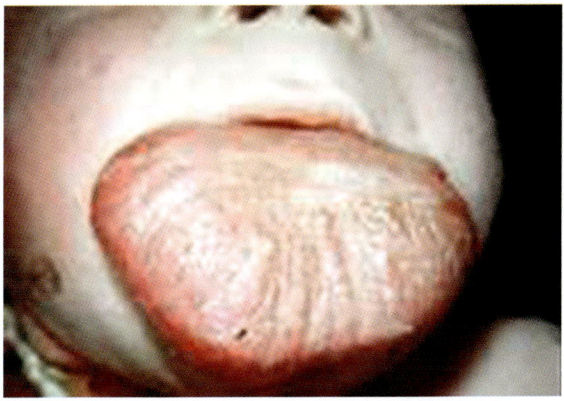

Figure 19.8 Infant with Beckwith–Wiedemann syndrome and severe macroglossia. (Adapted from Lioy and Sobol. *Disorders of the Neonatal Airway: Fundamental for Practice.* 2015.)

Macroglossia occurs frequently in neonates with genetic conditions such as trisomy 21 and Beckwith–Wiedemann syndrome. The majority of these patients may benefit from video laryngoscopy where the tongue-based obstruction can be easily seen on a large screen. However, there is a subset of macroglossia neonates with very critical airway requiring fiberoptic intubation. In severely obstructive cases, a tracheostomy may be required. The macroglossia in Beckwith–Wiedemann can worsen over time and occasionally partial resection of the tongue is required.[24] During an emergency, insertion of an oral airway is important; if intubation is not possible and the baby is spontaneously breathing, a nasopharyngeal trumpet should be considered.

An LMA can either give you ventilator access in an acute situation or serve as a starting point for performing a fiberoptic intubation, whereby an ETT loaded onto a flexible endoscope can be advanced through the LMA for intubation purposes.

Palatal structures do not tend to cause airway obstruction by themselves unless there is a congenital malformation. Rarely, tumors can arise and cause obstruction. Cleft palates can sometimes make visualization of the airway difficult if the defect is large.

Hypopharynx and Larynx

Laryngomalacia is the collapse of supraglottic structures resulting in airway obstruction. Laryngomalacia is the most common cause of stridor in children and presents with stridor of varying degrees, often worse with crying, supine positioning, and feeding. Laryngomalacia can worsen gastroesophageal reflux disease, and in its severe form can result in failure to thrive, cyanosis, pulmonary hypertension, or obstructive sleep apnea.[25] Diagnosis is made with awake fiberoptic laryngoscopy, but microlaryngoscopy and bronchoscopy may be needed to evaluate for secondary airway lesions. Supraglottoplasty can alleviate the obstruction in severe cases, but if unsuccessful, the infants may require tracheostomy.[26] Patients with concurrent neurological disease, cardiac disease, or grade II–III subglottic stenosis often fail supraglottoplasty and require tracheostomy. Aspiration can be present and often improves with surgery. Usually, however, the condition is self-limited and resolves with growth.

Rarely, vallecular cysts can cause a similar presentation as laryngomalacia, but careful flexible laryngoscopy can distinguish this entity. Treatment consists of resection or marsupialization.

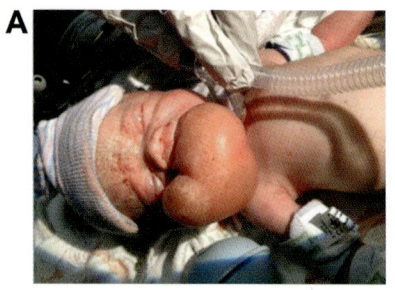
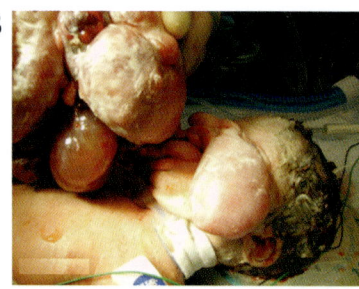

Figure 19.9A, B Complete oropharyngeal airway obstruction seen with oropharyngeal teratoma and epignathus. (Adapted from Lioy and Sobol. *Disorders of the Neonatal Airway: Fundamental for Practice*. 2015.)

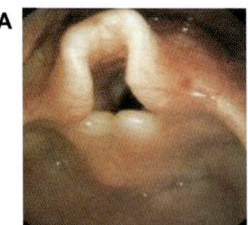
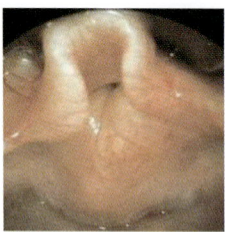
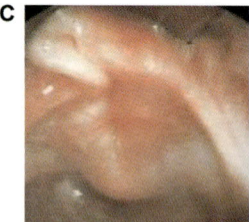

Figure 19.10A–C Two-month-old infant with severe laryngomalacia. Short aryepiglottic folds and arytenoid prolapse are notable. (Adapted from Lioy and Sobol. *Disorders of the Neonatal Airway: Fundamental for Practice*. 2015.)

Subglottic cysts are the result of obstruction of subglottic mucous glands by subepithelial fibrosis.[27] They are most commonly secondary to prematurity with a history of intubation and, if severe, can be addressed by marsupialization of the cyst under rigid bronchoscopy, either with Bugbee cautery or a laryngeal microdebrider. A quarter of patients may need more than one treatment due to recurrence. They have been described even after 2 days of intubation and present within 12 months of extubation.

Subglottic stenosis is acquired 95% of the time, often secondary to prolonged or traumatic intubation. As the cricoid ring is the narrowest part of the neonatal airway, the subglottis is at risk of intubation trauma and chondritis, with subsequent scarring from prolonged intubation or intubation with an oversized ETT. Congenital stenosis results from an elliptical cricoid and is rare, but can present a challenge during intubation. Usually, an ETT can be passed just through the vocal cords, but immediately encounters resistance. Subglottic stenosis is diagnosed with microlaryngoscopy and bronchoscopy in the operating room. Minor webs or thin stenoses can be managed with balloon dilation. Patients with more severe stenosis may require tracheostomy to provide a safe airway. Definitive airway reconstruction with laryngotracheal reconstruction or cricotracheal resection usually does not occur in the neonatal period and

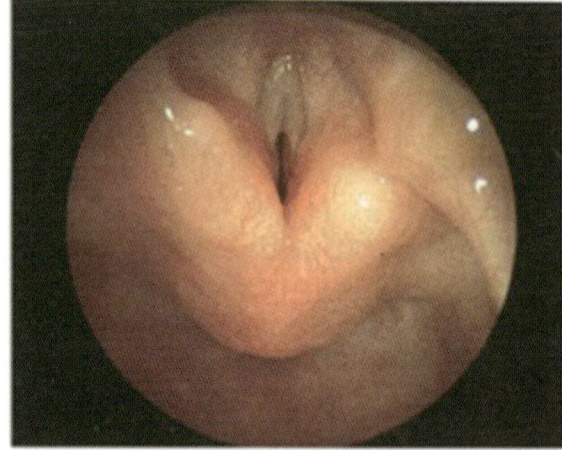

Figure 19.11 Bilateral vocal cord paralysis causing upper airway obstruction. (Adapted from Lioy and Sobol. *Disorders of the Neonatal Airway: Fundamental for Practice*. 2015.)

requires a multidisciplinary approach involving speech and swallow therapy, pulmonary and gastroenterology consultations, and management.

The second most common cause of stridor is bilateral vocal cord paralysis. This can present with severe inspiratory or biphasic stridor with a normal cry. Diagnosis is confirmed with flexible laryngoscopy. MRI scanning may be helpful. This is usually caused by CNS disorders like Arnold-Chiari malformation or hydrocephalus. Surgery, such as Chiari decompression or ventriculoperitoneal shunt, can help resolve the vocal cord paralysis. Many, but not all, children with bilateral vocal cord paralysis will require tracheostomy if symptoms do not improve. Subsequent surgical treatment after monitoring for possible spontaneous recovery can include vocal cord lateralization, cordotomy, or posterior cartilage graft laryngotracheal reconstruction.

Glottic webs or atresias can present with aphonia or hoarse cry and should elicit a workup for 22q11.2 deletion syndrome. These can be seen on flexible laryngoscopy and may require microlaryngoscopy with incision of web. More severe webs with subglottic extension may need laryngotracheal reconstruction.

Subglottic hemangiomas are rare, but can present with stridor and respiratory distress. This is diagnosed with microlaryngoscopy and bronchoscopy, and definitively treated with propranolol. Refractory cases may need laser excision or open surgical resection with laryngotracheal reconstruction.

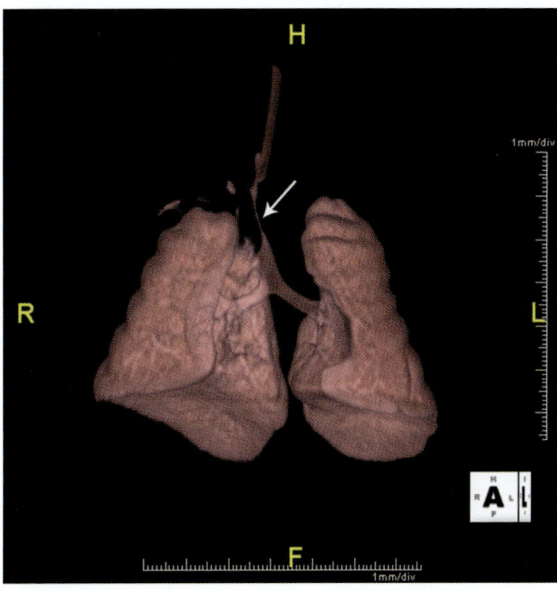

Figure 19.12 Long segment tracheal stenosis noted on CT angiogram. (Adapted from Lioy and Sobol. *Disorders of the Neonatal Airway: Fundamental for Practice.* 2015.)

Lower Airway

Tracheomalacia results from severe collapse of the soft trachealis muscle in the posterior trachea or external compression by a mass or cardiovascular structure.[8,28] Mucosal edema at the level of the cricoid ring will increase resistance to airflow by narrowing the tracheal lumen.[1,2] Cardiovascular anomalies that can result in tracheomalacia include double aortic arch and left pulmonary artery sling, and these may need cardiothoracic surgical intervention. Most cases of tracheomalacia can be monitored, but severe tracheomalacia may require tracheotomy and positive-pressure ventilation.

Long segment tracheal stenosis can result from complete tracheal rings and is a rare cause of stridor. Neonates with this issue can present with stridor, respiratory distress, recurrent pneumonias/respiratory infections, and "wet" breath sounds. If these children require intubation, usually the ETT will pass through the cords, but then resistance will be encountered, and the tube will not be able to be advanced to an expected depth. Microlaryngoscopy and bronchoscopy under anesthesia is required to make the diagnosis. Since many of these children have concurrent cardiovascular anomalies, an echocardiogram and CT angiogram of the chest with fine cuts through the trachea is warranted. While a minority of children can be observed conservatively, most children will require slide tracheoplasty by otolaryngology and cardiovascular surgery.

Delivery Room Management

The delivery room represents a unique opportunity for managing neonatal airways. Because the delivery room can be a chaotic environment, a predelivery huddle is useful to discuss what is known about the baby and what the plans are. Topics that should be discussed include the roles of each practitioner (e.g., head of bed/airway, heart rate, lead placement, emergency umbilical line placement, respiratory, IV placement), the airway equipment that is available, and important historical information (gestational age, pregnancy complications, estimated weight, anticipated neonatal concerns). If a neonate is known to have a syndrome with possible airway anomalies, this should be discussed, and an appropriate plan formed with inclusion of otolaryngology if indicated. Most full-service delivery hospitals provide an "airway box" or "airway cart," which is immediately available for deliveries and should be routinely checked.

Once the baby is born, the ease of resuscitation is variable. Premature neonates are notoriously more difficult to bag-mask-ventilate given their anatomy. Pressure on the eyes from the mask can cause a vagal response with bradycardia. To help with troubleshooting the airway if there are difficulties with ventilation, the Neonatal Resuscitation Program (NRP) suggests the use of the acronym MRSOPA (mask adjustment, reposition airway, suction mouth and nose, open mouth, increase pressure, alternative airway [such as ETT or LMA]).[29]

Fetal programs that deliver infants with birth defects affecting the airway (such as severe retrognathia/micrognathia, neck masses, venolymphatic malformations, oropharyngeal tumors, and CHAOS will have specialized equipment available in the delivery room. Management of these infants requires a high level of expertise and skill prior to or immediately following delivery and detailed communication among members of the team. Some of the infants may need a type of delivery called the EXIT procedure or a tracheostomy immediately following delivery. These mothers and neonates will be managed by a specialized group of surgeons, maternal-fetal medicine physicians, neonatologists, anesthesiologists, and otolaryngologists.

Airway Emergencies in the NICU

Timely and proper response to airway emergencies in the NICU is critical for successful management. Knowledge of normal neonatal airway anatomy, as well as common abnormalities that present in the neonatal period, is crucial for anticipating the needs of the baby. Useful guidelines for the management of neonatal airway emergencies do not exist as with pediatric and adult patients. Neonatal Resuscitation Program guidelines provide detailed guidance mostly for the depressed neonate at delivery.

Non-Intubated Emergencies

Oftentimes, airway emergencies are unanticipated and the baby is not known to have a difficult airway. The onset of acute illness, such as sepsis, can cause acute respiratory failure. Additionally, an emergency can develop with an attempt at anesthesia with apnea secondary to the medications. While attempting to establish an airway, there may be difficulty with bag-mask ventilation or placement of the ETT, and an airway problem will be revealed. Most commonly, though, the neonatal airway will be normal and the practitioner can successfully bag-mask-ventilate until an artificial airway is placed.

Unplanned Extubation

Unfortunately, unplanned extubations are not uncommon in the NICU. As part of Quality Improvement and Patient Safety initiatives, it is becoming more common to identify patients that are at especially high risk of unplanned extubation. The patients are at higher risk for a variety of reasons such as large amounts of secretions, activity, or tube position. By acknowledging the increased risk and making it a routine part of rounds, providers may be more cognizant of actions that may cause the extubation such as retaping of the tube.

Occasionally, a previously normal airway becomes designated as difficult on reintubation after an unplanned extubation. This often happens due to development of subglottic stenosis from prolonged intubation or airway edema from multiple extubations/reintubations.

Tracheostomy

Tracheostomies represent a particularly high risk for airway emergencies due to the tube itself and the underlying airway abnormalities that led to the initial need for tracheostomy. The highest risk is during the first week after the procedure when the wound is fresh and the stoma is not fully healed. Stay sutures placed on either side of the vertical incision in the trachea are placed to help facilitate insertion of the tube if it becomes dislodged. Otherwise, the tube can create a false track during replacement and end up positioned in the mediastinum, resulting in a pneumothorax, pneumomediastinum, or death.

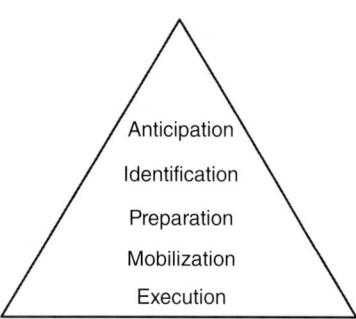

Figure 19.13 Pyramid of action and algorithm used for mobilizing the airway emergency team. (Adapted from Lioy and Sobol. *Disorders of the Neonatal Airway: Fundamental for Practice*. 2015.)

Difficulty with reinsertion can occur with a more mature tracheostomy as well. Routine cleaning occurs about every 7 days and occasionally the tube will have to be upsized as the child grows, so reinsertion is relatively common. Accidental decannulation can also occur, as can the need for emergent decannulation if the tube becomes obstructed. Though lower risk than with a fresh stoma, there is still the possibility of a false tract.

Critical versus Difficult Airway

Once a patient is known to have a challenging airway, communication of this diagnosis is key. It is crucial that, in the event of an emergency, providers can quickly ascertain the degree of difficulty they can expect to have with the airway so the proper equipment and specialists can be gathered. One way of categorizing these patients is labeling them as a difficult or critical airway, with signs placed at bedside clearly stating the category and reason. A *difficult* airway is a situation where bag-mask ventilation is successful, but the actual intubation can only be accomplished by a skilled, high-level clinician.[30,31] Alternatively, a *critical* airway is one in which bag-mask ventilation is unsuccessful and an advanced technique such as fiberoptic intubation by an experienced clinician is required. Critical airways can also include patients that cannot be intubated via normal tracheal intubation methods, such as a neonate with grade III or IV subglottic stenosis and a tracheostomy. Neonates with critical airways are at serious risk of decompensation.[32] Neonates with critical airway categorizations have diagnoses such as large pharyngeal teratomas that obstruct the airway, severe micrognathia, or acquired high-grade subglottic stenosis.

Effective Techniques and Devices for Neonatal Airway Management

Medications

The use of medications to assist with airway management is a relatively new concept in the field of neonatology. Research has now shown the utility of sedation and paralysis for intubation when possible. Typical drug regimens include a vagolytic (i.e., atropine) and an analgesic (i.e., morphine or fentanyl), with or without a paralytic (i.e., vecuronium or rocuronium). The AAP recommends that premedication should be used for all endotracheal intubations in newborns except in the case of emergent intubations during resuscitation. Their guidelines state that medications with rapid onset and short duration of action are preferred and an analgesic or an anesthetic dose of a sedative/hypnotic should be given. Vagolytics and paralytics should be considered.[33]

It is important to note, however, that there are specific airway circumstances in which premedication is not in the baby's best interest. In an emergent resuscitation, there may not be time to appropriately premedicate the baby. Fentanyl and other synthetic opioids have been associated with acute chest wall rigidity when administered too quickly in preterm and term infants. Also, the risk/benefit ratio of premedication should be considered in patients with known difficult or critical airways. Intubation of these infants is by definition difficult and the infant's own respiratory effort may be crucial for keeping an open airway. Depending on the clinical situation, a vagolytic and analgesic without paralysis may be possible

Table 19.1 Comparison of Difficult and Critical Airway Classification

Difficult airway	Critical airway
Non-life threatening History of difficult intubation	Life threatening Impossible visualization
Bag-mask ventilation/ LMA possible	Bag-mask ventilation/LMA impossible
Experienced intubator necessary	ENT required
Mild craniofacial micrognathia Midface hypoplasia Macroglossia Anterior larynx Subglottic narrowing Small mouth	Fresh tracheostomy < 1 week Laryngeal web Severe subglottic stenosis Tracheal clefts Severe craniofacial defect Severe micrognathia Severe macroglossia Oropharyngeal tumor Lymphangioma Obstructing neck mass

Adapted from Lioy and Sobol, *Disorders of the Neonatal Airway: Fundamental for Practice*. 2015 and helpful while managing a difficult airway. It is important for children with difficult and critical airways to continue spontaneous ventilation as this may be the only thing allowing for some degree of ventilation; paralysis or drug-induced apnea can turn a stable or urgent situation into an emergent or fatal situation. Even with a suspected normal airway, paralysis should only be used in the presence of an experienced airway provider.

Emergency Airway Cart

In order to effectively respond to an airway emergency, a well-equipped and mobile cart should be available, which contains all the important equipment. The drawers should be clearly labeled and the most important equipment (scopes, tubes, masks) should be in the upper drawers for easiest access. Basic emergency equipment should also be kept in a medium-sized box on the cart for quick use. Specialized equipment may be included for use by otolaryngology: this can include a microlaryngoscopy and bronchoscopy setup and a flexible laryngoscope/bronchoscope. Such equipment can be invaluable for helping with difficult or critical airways. A tracheostomy tray setup should always be part of the airway cart.

Oral Airway/Nasal Trumpet

Often overlooked, oral airways and nasal trumpets can be a quick method to bypass tongue obstruction. Hand ventilation and suctioning can occur through these tools. Combined with a good jaw thrust and mask ventilation, these tools can prove to be invaluable to maintaining an airway while equipment is set up for intubation.

LMAs

LMAs should be available at all airway emergencies, and airway providers should be instructed on their placement. There are situations where an LMA can provide critical ventilation temporarily while awaiting intubation or other airway management such as with acquired subglottic stenosis or retrognathia. If a patient has been designated as a difficult airway, it may be useful to have an LMA at bedside already in case of an emergency. An experienced provider can use a fiberoptic bronchoscope loaded with an ETT then to intubate through the LMA.

Nasal Intubation

Some ICUs use nasal intubation as their primary form of endotracheal intubation. Nasal ETTs are also useful for patients with excessive oral secretions or oral surgical wounds, prolonged intubation in older and active infants, and patients with facial malformations.[34] For routine intubation, however, more research is needed to determine whether nasal or oral intubation is preferable.[35]

Video Laryngoscopy

Recently, video laryngoscopy (such as the GVL or Storz C-MAC) has become extremely popular as an intubation tool for difficult and critical airways. Ultimately, video laryngoscopy will revolutionize intubation as a superb teaching tool, verification of ETT placement, and enhancing access of challenging intubations. Without a doubt, this type of equipment will be used at the bedside for most difficult and critical airway intubations by all skilled personnel. Future advances in airway management in neonates and infants will continue to grow as technology,

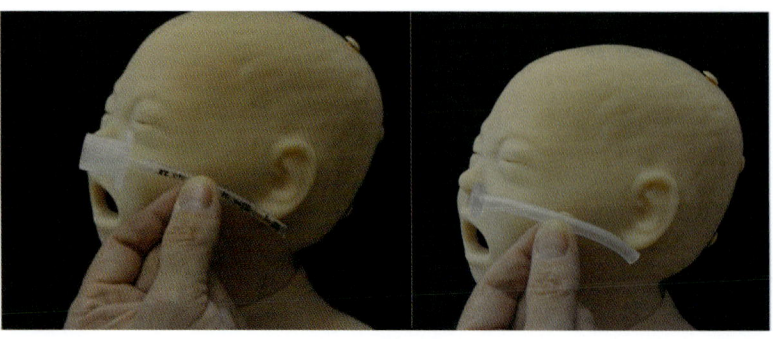

Figure 19.14 Nasopharyngeal airways. Guide to insertion, placement depth, and stabilization of nasopharyngeal airways in life-threatening oral obstruction. Note the nasal ETT is useful due to ease of bagging with connector. (Adapted from Lioy and Sobol. *Disorders of the Neonatal Airway: Fundamental for Practice.* 2015.)

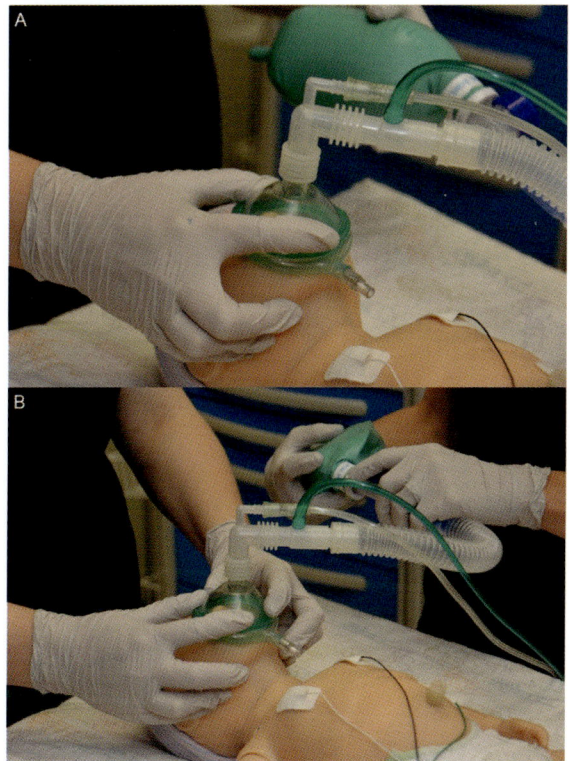
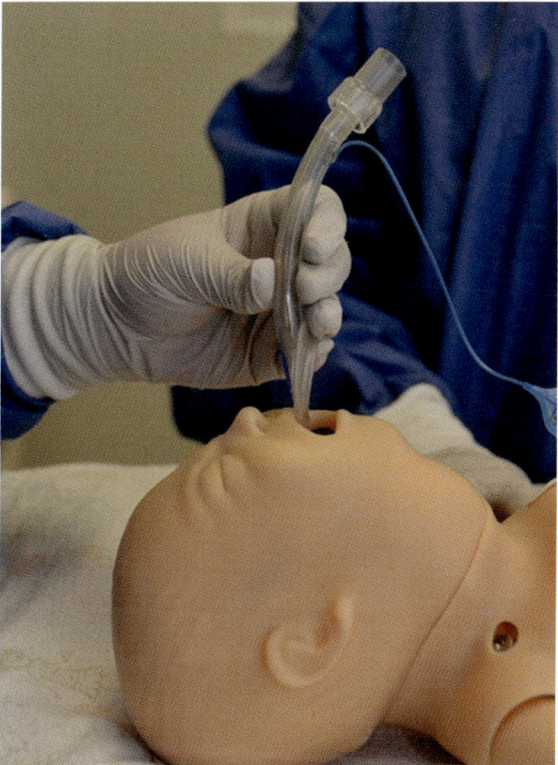
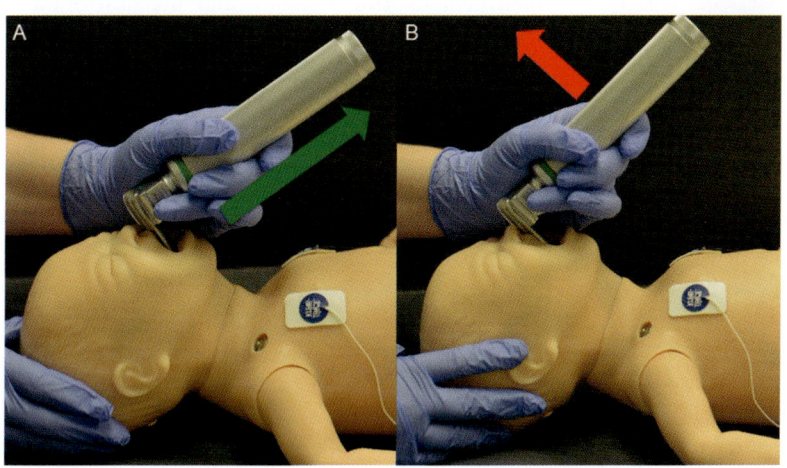

Figures 19.15–18 Bag-mask ventilation, LMA insertion, oral and nasal intubation techniques showing correct (green arrow) and incorrect (red arrow) placement.

(Adapted from Lioy and Sobol. *Disorders of the Neonatal Airway: Fundamental for Practice*. 2015.)

clinical care, and research dominate medical innovation and discovery.

Airway Challenges in the Micro Preemie

Currently, there are over 50 000 neonates with birth weights < 1500 g each year.[36] Medical advances in neonatology have resulted in survival of smaller and more immature infants than ever before. With survival, however, come long-term respiratory morbidities, especially in the very low birth weight (VLBW) and extremely low birth weight (ELBW) populations. These morbidities are most commonly acquired as a result of prematurity and its complications along with prolonged intubation and ventilation. Prematurity

Section 3: Special Topics

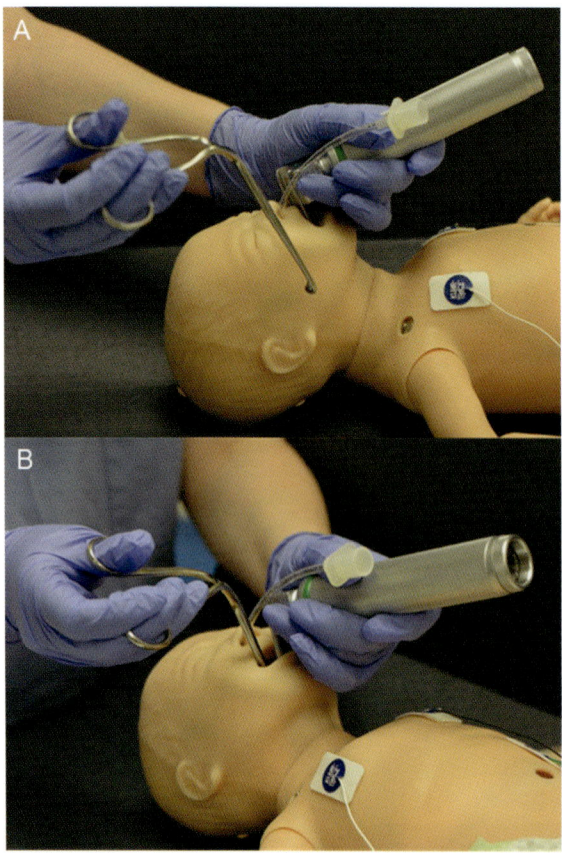

Figures 19.15–18 (cont.)

can bring challenges to anyone experienced in neonatal airway management. In the delivery room alone, practitioners may require the use of 00 or 0 laryngoscope blades and 2.5 mm ETTs (with some centers even using 2.0 mm tubes). The actual airway itself tends to be more anterior than older children and so may require a different approach than one is used to if they primarily intubate older patients. Once out of the delivery room, the challenges for the micro preemie have just begun.

Characteristics of the Micro Preemie Lung

The lungs of a micro preemie born between 22 and 28 weeks are immature in many ways. Distal capillaries of the pulmonary circulation are just starting to form. The lungs are in the saccular stage of lung development during which primitive air spaces are just starting to bud-off of terminal bronchioles. Each week is a critical period of development. For example, muscle cannot be identified in the airways distal to the small bronchi at 22 weeks, but can be seen at 24 weeks. Muscle cannot be measured in the airways of the terminal bronchioles until 26 weeks.[36]

When a baby is born prematurely, lung development is arrested. This results in fewer alveoli and increased interstitial collagen and elastin, and can have dramatic functional effects on the airways, despite an otherwise normal-appearing size and structure. Airway morbidities related to prematurity include vocal cord paresis or dysfunction, subglottic stenosis, and tracheobronchomalacia.[36] These topics will be discussed below, along with the major problem plaguing premature infants and their immature airways – BPD.

BPD/Chronic Lung Disease

The lungs of preterm infants are immature and therefore susceptible to damage from postnatal interventions. Because of the immaturity and the lack of surfactant, supplemental oxygenation and ventilation are often essential for survival. These therapies, however, can cause anatomical abnormalities resulting in impairment of lung function and the development of BPD.

Classic BPD was first described back in 1967 and occurred mainly in preterm infants born at 30–34 weeks' gestation.[37] These infants were treated at a time when ventilators were first being adapted for use in the newborn and the benefits of antenatal steroids and surfactant replacement were not yet known. The pathology of classic or "old" BPD is characterized by extensive injury with pulmonary fibrosis, peribronchial smooth muscle hypertrophy, pulmonary artery muscularization, necrotizing bronchiolitis, and large airway injury. As clinical practices have improved, BPD has also changed. Now, antenatal steroids for preterm labor, postnatal surfactant replacement therapy, specialized ventilators and gentle ventilation strategies, and research regarding appropriate oxygen saturations are commonplace. The BPD that is seen nowadays – the "new" BPD – affects smaller and more immature infants who often start with much less respiratory distress syndrome than previous generations. The signs of deterioration in lung function often begin to be displayed a few days to a few weeks after birth. Pathologically, this BPD is marked by delayed

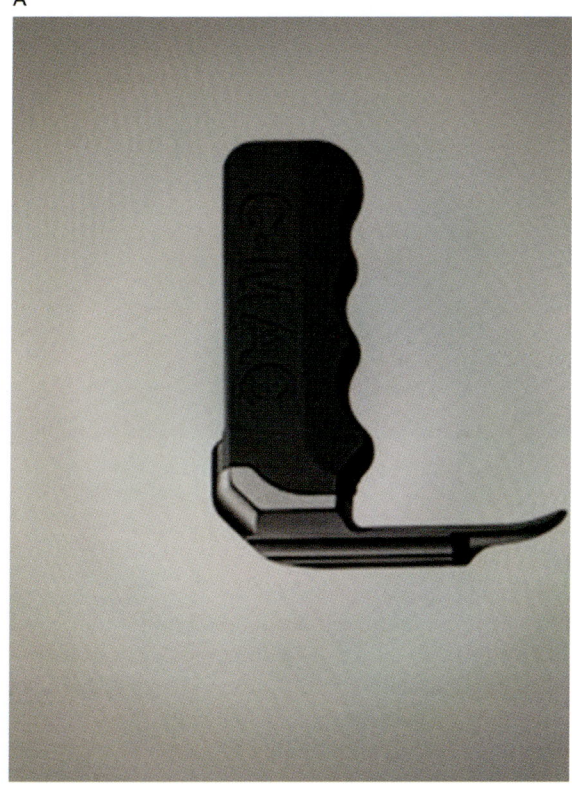
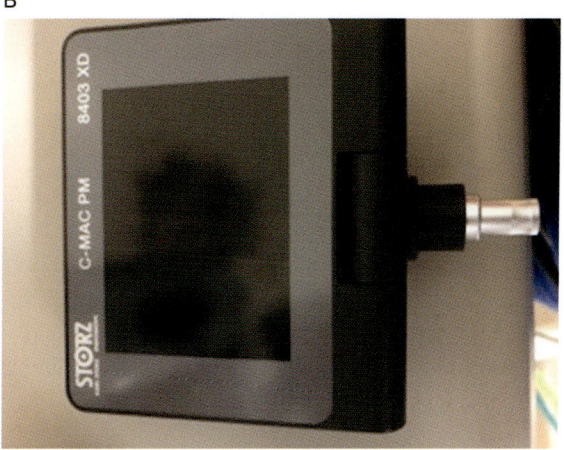

Figure 19.19A, B Video laryngoscopy for neonatal use with portable pocket monitor. Storz C-MAC used widely for neonatal and infant intubation. (Adapted from Lioy and Sobol. *Disorders of the Neonatal Airway: Fundamental for Practice.* 2015.)

alveolar and lung vascular development. Overall, the incidence of BPD in VLBW infants ranges between 15% and 65%, and it is thought that "new" BPD represents more than 80% of these infants.[36]

BPD patients can have episodic cyanotic spells, which are referred to as "BPD spells." The etiology is usually exacerbated ventilation/perfusion mismatch during agitation or pulmonary hypertension crisis and may require sedation to resolve. Some spells, however, are caused by airway collapse due to tracheobronchomalacia, which will be discussed in further detail below.

Tracheobronchomalacia

In premature infants with BPD, an incidence of tracheobronchomalacia between 16% and 50% has been reported.[36] Risk factors associated with the development of tracheobronchomalacia include lower gestational age, longer intubation time, higher mean airway pressures on the ventilator, infection, chronic inflammation, and extrinsic airway compression from structural anomalies such as vascular and skeletal malformations. It is thought that, as immature airways are exposed to positive-pressure ventilation, they can become deformed. These changes do not occur with adult airways because immature airways have a limited ability to generate tension with their smooth muscles to withstand barotrauma.[36]

Cyanotic spells in BPD that are caused by tracheobronchomalacia can result in severe desaturations and bradycardia. These episodes often require positive-pressure ventilation with high pressures to battle the malacia and resolve the vital sign changes. If not intubated, tracheobronchomalacia can also present as coughing, respiratory distress (sometimes with stridor), increasing oxygen requirement, increasing sedation needs, and inability to wean respiratory support.

Subglottic Stenosis

Babies with BPD may develop other issues related to prolonged intubation, such as subglottic stenosis. This is usually identified when an infant who was on minimum ventilator support ends up developing significant respiratory distress shortly after extubation.

Section 3: Special Topics

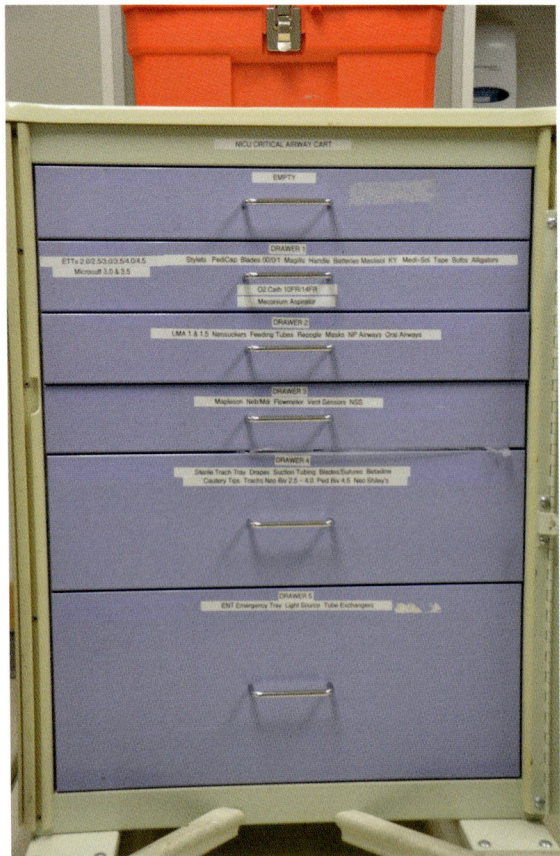

Figure 19.20 Airway cart carrying a variety of critical airway equipment; easily mobile and accessible during airway emergency.

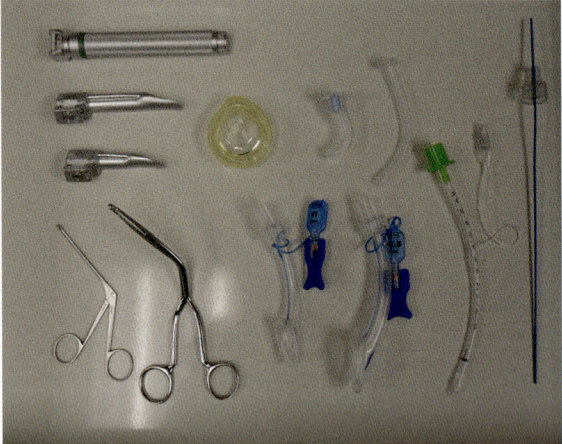

Figure 19.21 Various essential airways for noninvasive and intubation including two types of forceps for nasal intubation.

Visualization of the airway with direct laryngoscopy and bronchoscopy may show edema, granulation formation, and subglottic stenosis. Subglottic stenosis has been reported to have an incidence of up to 24.5% in VLBW infants who were intubated for more than 7 days.[38] Birth weight, gestational age, ETT size, oral versus nasal intubation, intubation trauma, number of intubations, infections, and duration of mechanical ventilation have all been shown to be associated with the development of subglottic stenosis.[36]

Vocal Cord Paralysis

A common problem in premature neonates is the patent ductus arteriosus (PDA). An open ductus arteriosus is normal in fetal circulation, but it should then close postnatally. If it does not close, it can cause issues with pulmonary overcirculation and may need to be surgically closed. The development of left vocal cord paralysis after surgical closure of a PDA has been well documented, with reported rates of as high as 67% in ELBW infants. Early symptoms may be stridor, hoarseness, weak cry, and feeding difficulties.[39] Interestingly, vocal cord paralysis may continue to impact these babies well into adulthood. A recent study found 54% of young adults between 23 and 27 years of age who were born ≤ 28 weeks' gestational age or ≤ 1000 g birth weight had left vocal cord paralysis as seen on flexible laryngoscopy.[36] Currently, in the hands of a few expert pediatric airway surgeons, there are newer, sophisticated techniques, such as anterior–posterior cricoid grafting/balloon dilation for disorders like vocal cord paralysis and subglottic stenosis.

Laryngomalacia

Although seen more frequently in the near-term or term neonate with a natural airway, laryngomalacia is the most common laryngeal anomaly and the cause of most stridor in the newborn.[40] Commonly noted omega-shaped epiglottis or particularly coiled epiglottis, such as seen in Figure 19.29, can also be encountered in premature infants, and can be more difficult to elevate when intubation is attempted. Frequently the process of intubation can be more challenging and requires higher-level expertise.

Chapter 19: Airway Management of the Neonate and Infant

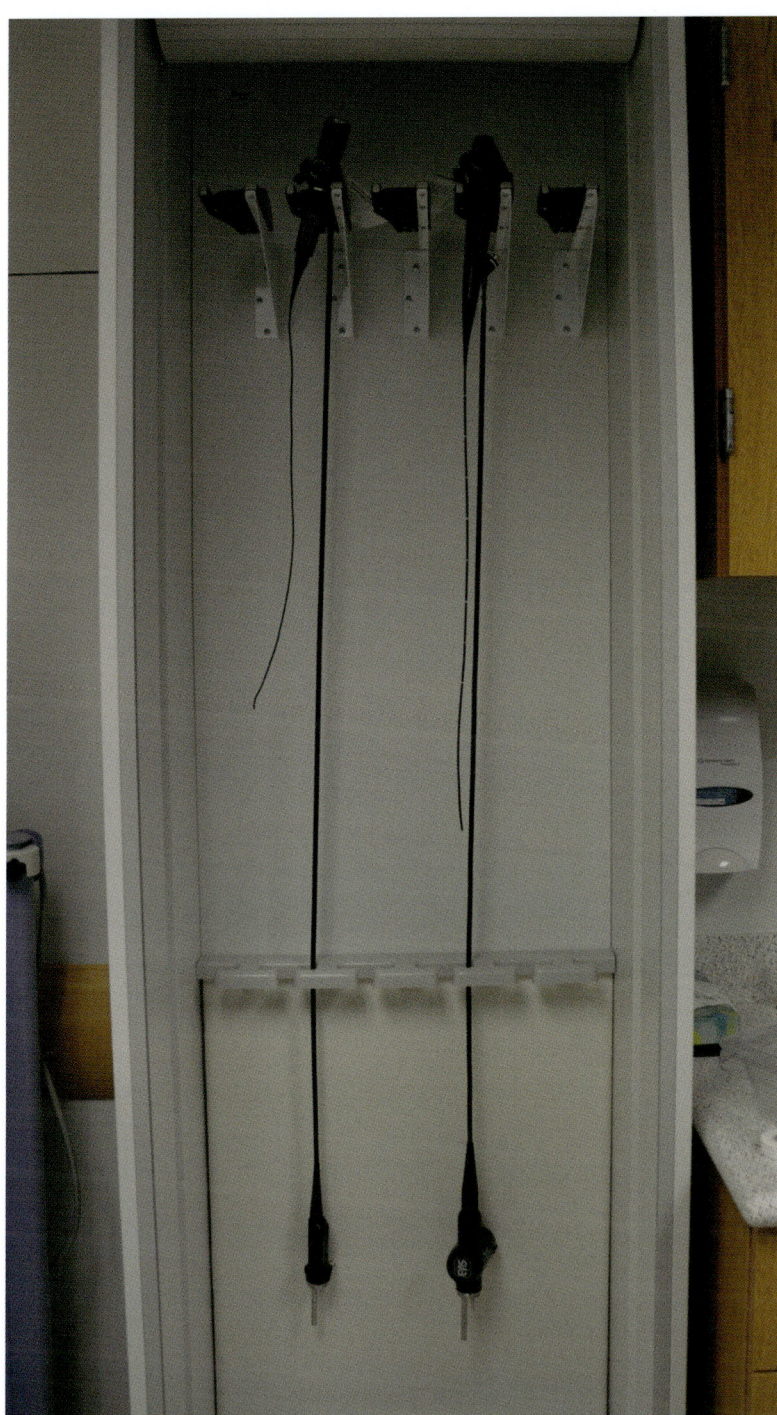

Figure 19.22 Fiberoptic laryngoscopes, which come in handy during airway emergencies needing intubation of difficult or critical airways.

Section 3: Special Topics

Tracheostomy

In micro preemies who require prolonged mechanical ventilation, including those who are able to be extubated but still require positive pressure, a tracheostomy is often the next step. Making that decision is challenging, however, and data are unclear regarding the optimal timing of tracheostomy and the long-term outcomes. DeMauro and colleagues retrospectively evaluated the 18–22-month outcomes of very preterm infants who received tracheostomies over a 10-year period. They found that tracheostomy was associated with a significantly increased risk of death or neurodevelopmental impairment, despite adjusting

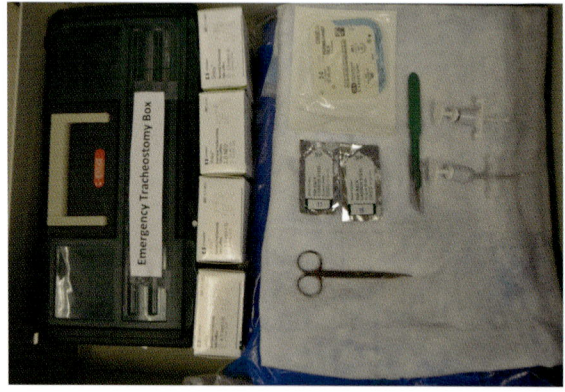

Figure 19.23 Tracheostomy tray used for emergent airway access.

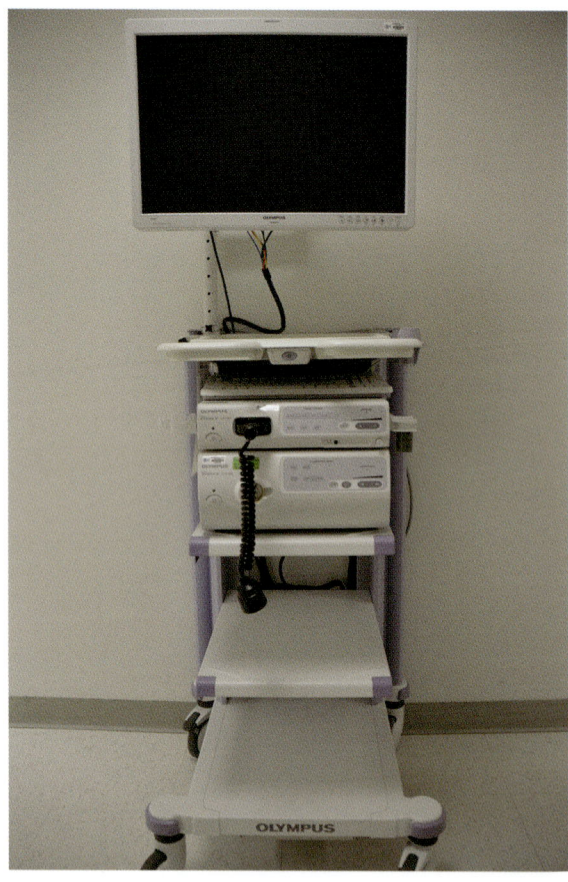

Figure 19.24 HD monitor for visualization of magnified airway images during fiberoptic intubation.

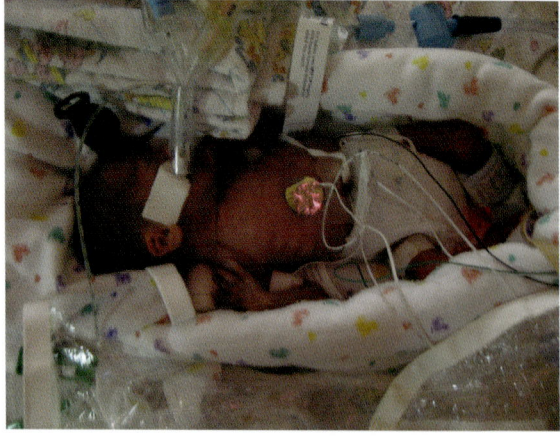

Figure 19.25 A 24-week extremely low birth weight neonate. (Courtesy of Dr. Janet Lioy, CHOP Neonatal Airway Program.)

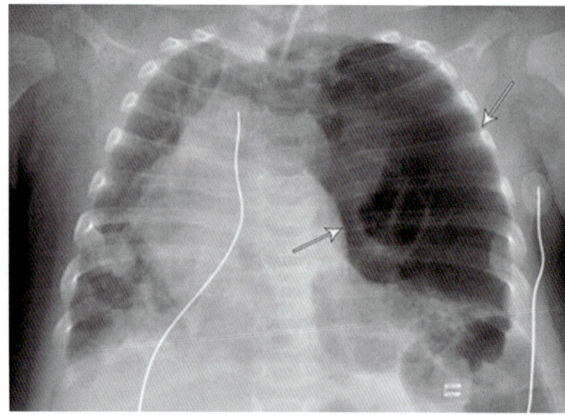

Figure 19.26 Chest X-ray of severe BPD. (Courtesy of Dr. Huayan Zang, CHOP Chronic Lung Disease Program.)

Chapter 19: Airway Management of the Neonate and Infant

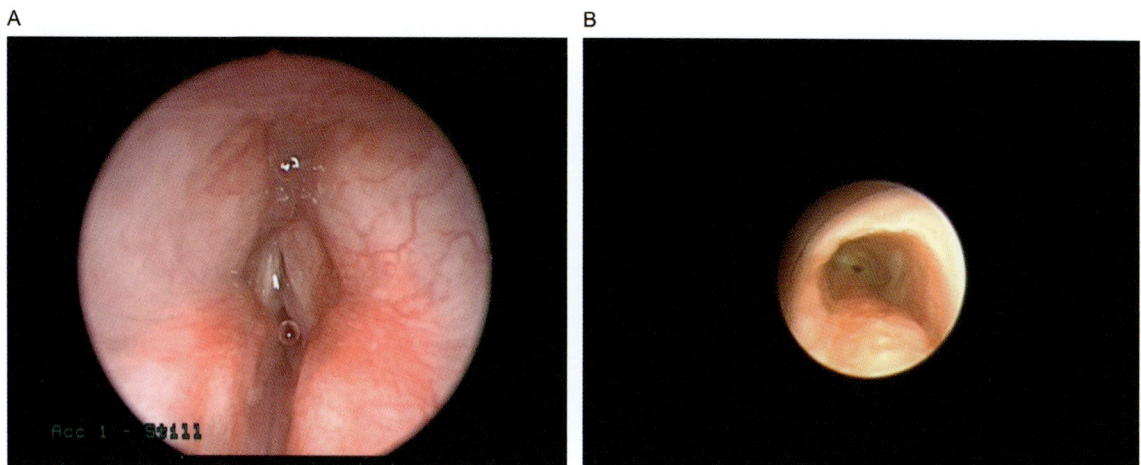

Figure 19.27A, B Subglottic stenosis in a 24-week micro preemie at the level of the vocal cords and below.
A. Level of vocal cords
B. Subglottis. (Courtesy of Dr. Ian Jacobs, CHOP Neonatal Airway Program.)

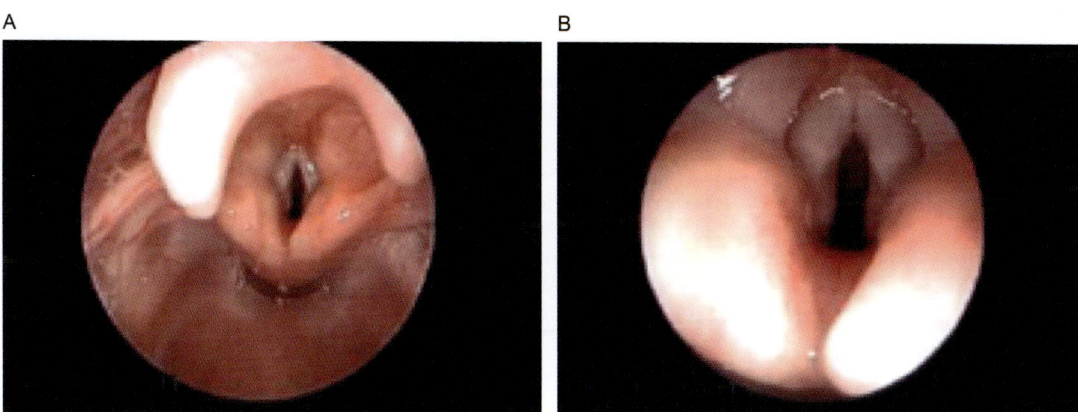

Figure 19.28A, B A. Before
B. After
Vocal cord paralysis in a preterm infant who underwent an anterior–posterior cricoid augmentation procedure with balloon dilation. (Courtesy of Dr. Ian Jacobs, CHOP Neonatal Airway Program.)

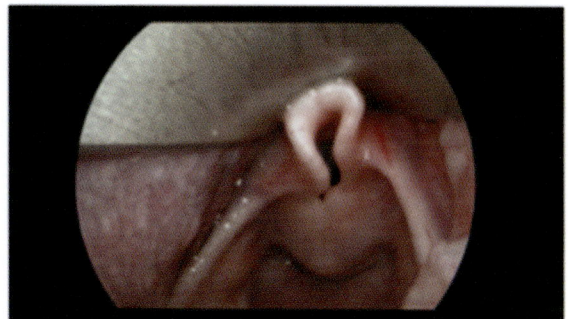

Figure 19.29 Laryngomalacia with notable omega-shaped epiglottis. (Courtesy of Dr. Steve Sobol, CHOP Neonatal Airway Program.).

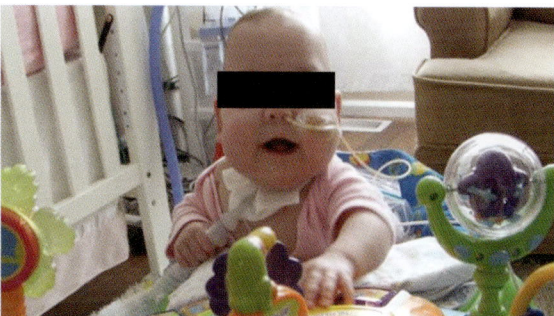

Figure 19.30 Happy with my tracheostomy. (Courtesy of Libby Schneeman, CHOP Center for Pediatric Airway Disorder parent.)

for 17 different factors. It was felt likely that there is another confounder that has not yet been identified causing the association. They also noted that there was a possible association between earlier (< 120 days) tracheostomy and better neurodevelopmental outcomes, possibly due to a shift in focus from mechanical ventilation weaning to developmental enrichment.[41]

Using the example of tracheobronchomalacia, tracheostomy may be the definitive management to give long-term positive-pressure ventilation and keep the airways open. A review by Jacobs and colleagues of 50 cases of tracheomalacia in 1994 showed that 75% of premature infants required tracheostomy; 71% were decannulated at an average age of 30 months. Other studies report tracheostomy in 12–62% of infants.[42] Despite the wide range in numbers, tracheostomy is a very real outcome for many micro preemies and impacts them for years to come. Most large Children's Hospitals have developed airway programs to deal with the increasing number of tracheostomies now being performed.

References

1. Luten R, Kissoon N. Approach to the Pediatric Airway. In Walls R, Murphy M, Luten R, eds. *Manual of Emergency Airway Management*. Philadelphia, PA: Lippincott, Williams, and Wilkins; 2004: 263–81.

2. Luten R, Mick N. Differentiating Aspects of Pediatric Airway. In Walls R, Murphy M, eds. *Manual of Emergency Airway Management*. 4th ed. Philadelphia, PA: Lippincott, Williams, and Wilkins; 2012.

3. Sarnaik A, Heidemann S. Respiratory Pathophysiology and Regulation. In Kleigman R, Rehrman R, Jenson H, eds. *Nelson's Textbook of Pediatrics*. 18th ed. Philadelphia, PA: Saunders; 2007.

4. Nguyen C, Javia L. Craniofacial Syndromes with Airway Anomalies: an Overview. In Lioy J, Sobol S, eds. *Disorders of the Neonatal Airway: Fundamentals for Practice*. New York, NY; Springer: 2015.

5. Scott. R. Shoem. Disorders of the Nasal Cavity. In Lioy J, Sobol S, eds. *Disorders of the Neonatal Airway: Fundamentals for Practice*. New York, NY: Springer: 2015.

6. Miller MJ, Carlo WA, Strohl KP, Fanaroff AA, Martin RJ. Effect of Maturation on Oral Breathing in Sleeping Premature Infants. *The Journal of Pediatrics* 1986; **109**(3): 515–91.

7. Bergeson PS, Shaw JC. Are Infants Really Obligatory Nasal Breathers? *Clinical Pediatrics* 2001; **40**(10): 567–9.

8. Santillanes G, Gausche-Hill M. Pediatric Airway Management. *Emergency Medicine Clinics of North America* 2008; **26**(4): 961–75, ix.

9. Lowinger D, Ohlms L. Otolaryngology: Head and Neck Surgery. In Hansen A, Pudler M, eds. *Manual of Neonatal Surgical Intensive Care*. 2nd ed. Shelton, CT: People's Medical Publishing House; 2009: 70–118.

10. Schaffer T, Wolfson M. Upper Airway: Structure, Function, and Development. In Abman S, Polin R, Fox W, eds. *Fetal and Neonatal Physiology*. 4th ed. Philadelphia, PA: Elsevier Saunders; 2011.

11. Litman RS, Weissend EE, Shibata D, Westesson PL. Developmental Changes of Laryngeal Dimensions in Unparalyzed, Sedated Children. *Anesthesiology* 2003; **98**(1): 41–5.

12. Pudler M. Cleft Lip/Palate and Robin Sequence. In Hansen A, Pudler M, eds. *Otolargnyology: Head and Neck Surgery*. 2nd ed. Shelton, CT: People's Medical Publishing House; 2009.

13. Maniglia AJ, Goodwin WJ. Congenital Choanal Atresia. *Otolaryngologic Clinics of North America* 1981; **14**(1): 167–73.

14. Harris J, Robert E, Källén B. Epidemiology of Choanal Atresia with Special Reference to the CHARGE Association. *Pediatrics* 1997; **99**(3): 363–7.

15. Keller JL, Kacker A. Choanal Atresia, CHARGE Association, and Congenital Nasal Stenosis. *Otolaryngologic Clinics of North America* 2000; **33**(6): 1343–51, viii.

16. De Freitas RP, Berkowitz RG. Bilateral Choanal Atresia Repair in Neonates – a Single Surgeon Experience. *International Journal of Pediatric Otorhinolaryngology* 2012; **76**(6): 873–8.

17. Brown OE, Myer CM, Manning SC. Congenital Nasal Pyriform Aperture Stenosis. *Laryngoscope* 1989; **99**(1): 86–91.

18. Hui Y, Friedberg J, Crysdale WS. Congenital Nasal Pyriform Aperture Stenosis as a Presenting Feature of Holoprosencephaly. *International Journal of Pediatric Otorhinolaryngology* 1995; **31**(2-3): 263–74.

19. Tavin E, Stecker E, Marion R. Nasal Pyriform Aperture Stenosis and the Holoprosencephaly Spectrum. *International Journal of Pediatric Otorhinolaryngology* 1994; **28**(2–3): 199–204.

20. Reeves TD, Discolo CM, White DR. Nasal Cavity Dimensions in Congenital Pyriform Aperture Stenosis. *International Journal of Pediatric Otorhinolaryngology* 2013; **77**(11): 1830–2.

21. Wine TM, Dedhia K, Chi DH. Congenital Nasal Pyriform Aperture Stenosis: is There a Role for Nasal Dilation? *JAMA Otolaryngology – Head & Neck Surgery* 2014; **140**(4): 352–6.

22. Katona G, Hirschberg J, Hosszú Z, Király L. Epipharyngeal Teratoma in Infancy. *International Journal of Pediatric Otorhinolaryngology* 1992; **24**(2): 171–5.

23. Goldstein J, Taylor J. Impact of Micro- and Retrognathia on the Neonatal Airway. In *Disorders of the Neonatal Airway.* New York, NY: Springer; 2015: 43–50.

24. Kacker A, Honrado C, Martin D, Ward R. Tongue Reduction in Beckwith–Weidemann Syndrome. *International Journal of Pediatric Otorhinolaryngology* 2000; **53**(1): 1–7.

25. O'Connor TE, Bumbak P, Vijayasekaran S. Objective Assessment of Supraglottoplasty Outcomes Using Polysomnography. *International Journal of Pediatric Otorhinolaryngology* 2009; **73**(9): 1211–16.

26. Powitzky R, Stoner J, Fisher T, Digoy GP. Changes in Sleep Apnea after Supraglottoplasty in Infants with Laryngomalacia. *International Journal of Pediatric Otorhinolaryngology* 2011; **75**(10): 1234–9.

27. Mudd P, Andreoli S, Sobol S. Malformations, Deformations, and Disorders of the Neonatal Airway: a Bullet Point Review. In Lioy J, Sobol S, eds. *Disorders of the Neonatal Airway.* New York, NY: Springer; 2015.

28. Berg E, McClay J. Tracheobronchomalacia. In Lioy J, Sobol S, eds. *Disorders of the Neonatal Airway.* New York, NY: Springer; 2015.

29. *Textbook of Neonatal Resuscitation.* 6th ed. American Academy of Pediatrics and American Heart Association; 2012.

30. Apfelbaum JL, Hagberg CA, Caplan RA, et al. American Society of Anesthesiologists Task Force on Management of the Difficult Airway. *Anesthesiology* 2003; **98**(5): 1269–77.

31. Apfelbaum JL, Hagberg CA, Caplan RA, et al. Practice Guidelines for Management of the Difficult Airway: an Updated Report by the American Society of Anesthesiologists Task Force on Management of the Difficult Airway. *Anesthesiology* 2013; **118**(2): 251–70.

32. Zur K. The Critical Airway. In Mattei P, ed. *Fundamentals of Pediatric Surgery.* New York, NY: Springer; 2011.

33. Kumar P, Denson SE, Mancuso TJ. Premedication for Nonemergency Endotracheal Intubation in the Neonate. *Pediatrics* 2010; **125**(3): 608–15.

34. Gray M, French H. Use of Simulation Training in Preparation for Neonatal and Infant Airway Emergencies. In Lioy J, Sobol S, eds. *Disorders of the Neonatal Airway: Fundamentals for Practice.* New York, NY: Springer; 2015.

35. Spence K, Barr P. Nasal versus Oral Intubation for Mechanical Ventilation of Newborn Infants. *Cochrane Database of Systematic Reviews* 2000 (2): CD000948.

36. Zhang H. Effects of Prematurity, Prolonged Intubation, and Chronic Lung Disease on the Neonatal Airway. In Lioy J, Sobol, S, eds. *Disorders of the Neonatal Airway: Fundamentals for Practice.* New York, NY: Springer Science+Business; 2015: 243–61.

37. Northway WH, Jr., Rosan RC, Porter DY. Pulmonary Disease Following Respirator Therapy of Hyaline-Membrane Disease. Bronchopulmonary dysplasia. *New England Journal of Medicine* 1967; **276**(7): 357–68.

38. Downing GJ, Kilbride HW. Evaluation of Airway Complications in High-Risk Preterm Infants: Application of Flexible Fiberoptic Airway Endoscopy. *Pediatrics* 1995; **95**(4): 567–72.

39. Engeseth MS, Olsen NR, Maeland S, Halvorsen T, Goode A, Roksund OD. Left Vocal Cord Paralysis after Patent Ductus Arteriosus Ligation: a Systematic Review. *Paediatric Respiratory Reviews* 2018; **27**: 74–85.

40. Laundry A, Thompson DM. Congenital Laryngomalacia: Disease Spectrum and Management. In Lioy J, Sobol, S, eds. *Disorders of the Neonatal Airway: Fundamentals for Practice.* New York, NY: Springer; 2015.

41. DeMauro SB, D'Agostino JA, Bann C, et al. Developmental Outcomes of Very Preterm Infants with Tracheostomies. *The Journal of Pediatrics*, **164**(6): 1303–10. e1302.

42. Jacobs IN, Wetmore RF, Tom LW, Handler SD, Potsic WP. Tracheobronchomalacia in Children. *Archives of Otolaryngology – Head & Neck Surgery* 1994; **120**(2): 154.

Section 3 **Special Topics**

Chapter 20

Airway Management in EXIT Procedures

Debnath Chatterjee and Timothy M. Crombleholme

Introduction

Advances in prenatal imaging, including ultrasonography and fetal MRI, have allowed more accurate diagnosis of several structural fetal anomalies that put the newborn at risk for airway compromise immediately after birth. The EXIT procedure has enabled securing the airway and performing other fetal interventions in a controlled fashion, while still on placental support, thereby preventing life-threatening airway compromise after birth. This chapter will focus on the newer evolving indications, preoperative planning, anesthetic management, and strategies for fetal airway management during an EXIT procedure.

Indications

The EXIT procedure was initially developed to secure the airway in fetuses with severe congenital diaphragmatic hernia (CDH) who had undergone in utero fetal tracheal clipping to promote lung growth.[1] While still on placental support, a variety of procedures – including orotracheal intubation, bronchoscopy, tracheostomy, central-line placement, and administration of surfactant – were performed before cutting the umbilical cord and delivering the newborn. Over the years, the indications for an EXIT procedure have evolved and now include securing the airway in fetuses with large oropharyngeal and/or neck masses, CHAOS, severe micrognathia, and resection of large lung or mediastinal masses compromising the intrathoracic airway[2-5] (Table 20.1).

EXIT-to-Airway

The most common indication for an EXIT procedure is to secure the airway in fetuses who are at risk for life-threatening airway compromise after birth, which can be secondary to either extrinsic compression by mass effect or intrinsic obstruction secondary to laryngeal atresia or stenosis. Fetal neck masses include cervical teratoma, oropharyngeal teratoma (epignathus), epulis, lymphatic malformation, hemangioma, and goiter. They can cause significant distortion of the airway anatomy, making airway management after birth very challenging.[2,3,5,6] Additionally, compression of the fetal esophagus impedes

Table 20.1 Indications for EXIT Procedures

Type	Source of obstruction	Fetal malformations
EXIT-to-airway	Extrinsic compression	Cervical teratoma, lymphatic malformation epignathus, epulis, hemangioma
	Intrinsic obstruction	CHAOS, laryngeal atresia/stenosis, laryngeal web/cyst
	Iatrogenic	Prior fetal endoscopic tracheal occlusion for CDH
	Miscellaneous	Severe micrognathia (jaw index < 5th percentile)
EXIT-to-resection	Persistent mediastinal compression	Congenital pulmonary airway malformation, bronchogenic cyst, thoracic or mediastinal tumors
	High output heart failure	Sacrococcygeal teratoma
EXIT-to-ECMO		CDH with poor prognostic indicators Hypoplastic left heart syndrome with intact/restrictive atrial septum
EXIT-to-separation	Bridge to separation	Conjoined twins

fetal swallowing, resulting in polyhydramnios, which may predispose to preterm labor. Among fetal neck masses, cervical teratomas are large, bulky tumors in the anterior neck with representation of all three germ layers. They are usually solid, with some cystic areas and have well-defined borders.[3,6] Cervical teratomas can be massive and have the potential to cause significant airway obstruction after birth. Lymphatic malformations, on the other hand, have poorly defined borders and tend to be more infiltrative of surrounding structures; sometimes even infiltrating the fetal airway. The natural history of cervical lymphatic malformations depends on the gestational age (GA) at diagnosis. Lymphatic malformations diagnosed early in the second trimester have a more cystic appearance and are usually located in the posterior triangle of the neck.[3,6] They are frequently associated with chromosomal or structural anomalies, and have a poor prognosis, with over 90% of fetuses dying in utero. In contrast, lymphatic malformations diagnosed in the late second or third trimester, or postnatally, are usually located in the anterior triangle of the neck. They are rarely associated with chromosomal or structural anomalies, and have a good prognosis. Epignathus is a rare oropharyngeal teratoma arising from the sphenoid bone, palate, or pharynx, which usually presents as a large exophytic mass protruding through the mouth and obstructing the upper airway (Figure 20.1).[6] They can grow very rapidly in large proportions, dislocating the mandible and causing complete airway obstruction. Fetal hydrops may result from high output cardiac failure secondary to increased blood flow through the tumor. Epulis are tumors that arise from the gingival mucosa and present as an oral mass that may protrude through the mouth.

CHAOS is due to near-complete or complete intrinsic obstruction of the fetal airway from laryngeal or tracheal atresia, laryngeal web or cyst, and tracheal stenosis.[3] CHAOS is characterized by bilaterally enlarged echogenic lungs, flat or inverted diaphragms, and dilated tracheobronchial tree, resulting in massive ascites and fetal hydrops. The EXIT-to-airway approach has been successfully used in the setting of CHAOS to perform a tracheostomy.[7] Severe micrognathia can also cause complete airway obstruction from posterior displacement of the tongue (glossoptosis), and occlusion of the oropharyngeal airway. This can result in polyhydramnios and preterm labor (Figure 20.2). The indications for an

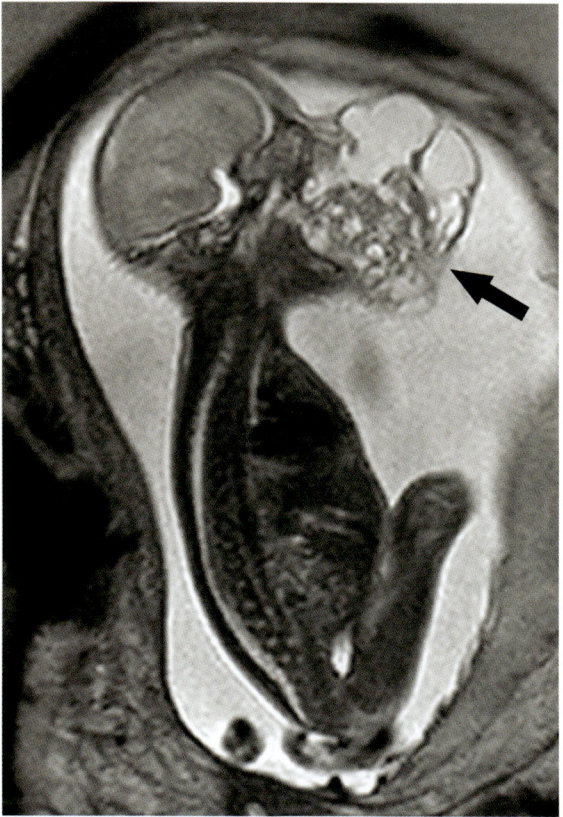

Figure 20.1 Fetal MRI showing large exophytic oropharyngeal teratoma (black arrow).

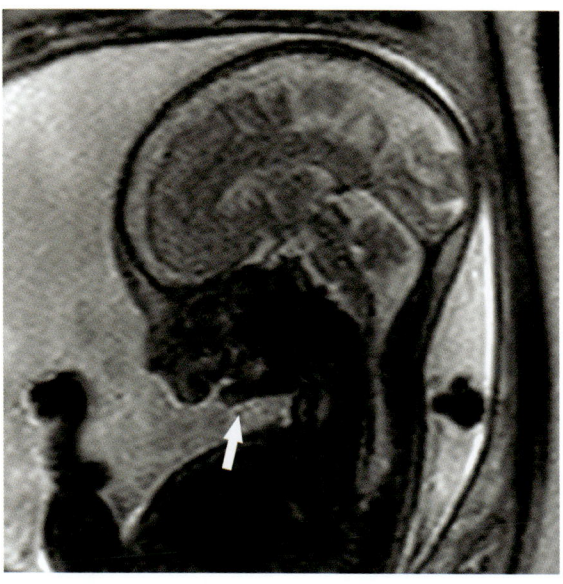

Figure 20.2 Fetal MRI showing severe micrognathia (white arrow).

EXIT-to-airway procedure in fetuses with severe micrognathia include a jaw index of less than the fifth percentile associated with signs of aerodigestive obstruction (glossoptosis, polyhydramnios, and absence of stomach bubble).[8] Fetuses with severe CDH and poor-prognostic indicators (liver herniation and observed-to-expected lung to head ratio [O/E LHR] < 1.0) may benefit from fetal endoscopic tracheal occlusion (FETO) to promote lung growth.[9] FETO involves fetoscopic placement of an endoluminal balloon in the fetal trachea between 27 and 29 weeks' (GA), followed by elective fetoscopic removal of the balloon at 34 weeks' (GA). Fetoscopic removal of the balloon is often possible, even in the face of preterm premature rupture of membranes, and there is survival benefit if the pregnancy can be maintained for ≥ 24 hours following removal of the tracheal balloon. However, if the mother is in active labor, it may be necessary to perform an EXIT procedure to allow removal of the balloon under bronchoscope guidance.

EXIT-to-Resection

Fetal lung masses may be solid or cystic and include congenital pulmonary airway malformation (CPAM), bronchopulmonary sequestration, bronchogenic cyst, and pericardial and mediastinal teratoma. The prenatal natural history of fetal lung masses is variable and depends on its size and the degree of compression from the mass on mediastinal structures.[10,11] Most CPAMs grow between 18 and 26 weeks' (GA), and reach a plateau, staying proportional to or decreasing in size relative to the size of the growing fetus. However, a small subset of fetal lung masses continues to grow, causing mediastinal shift and compression of the great vessels and heart. Esophageal compression results in maternal polyhydramnios. Compression of the vena cava impairs right atrial blood return, resulting in fetal hydrops. In other cases, intrathoracic compression of the airway by a bronchogenic cyst or pericardial or mediastinal teratoma may make neonatal resuscitation nearly impossible (Figure 20.3).

Fetuses that do not develop hydrops are managed conservatively with serial ultrasounds, planned delivery at term, postnatal evaluation, and elective resection of the lung mass. Fetal interventions are typically reserved for fetuses that develop hydrops despite steroid administration. In the presence of a macrocyst

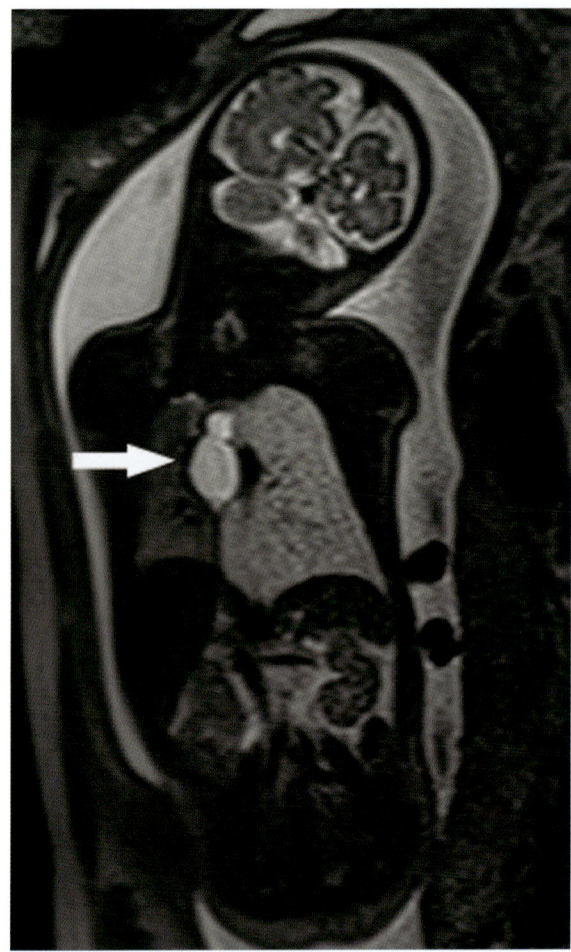

Figure 20.3 Fetal MRI showing large bronchogenic cyst (white arrow) at the level of the carina with complete obstruction of the left mainstem bronchus, resulting in hyperinflation of the left lung and rightward mediastinal shift.

amenable to drainage, an ultrasound-guided thoracocentesis or thoracoamniotic shunt placement is performed. If the lung mass is multicystic or predominantly solid in nature, the treatment options depends on the (GA). For fetuses less than 32 weeks' (GA), open fetal surgery with fetal lobectomy is recommended for solid lesions, while fetal thoracoscopic fenestration is recommended for multicystic lesions followed by placement of a thoracoamniotic shunt. For fetuses more than 32 weeks' (GA) with large lung masses and persistent mediastinal compression causing hydrops, an EXIT-to-resection is performed while still on placental support.[10–12] After securing the fetal airway and obtaining fetal intravenous access, a fetal thoracotomy is performed on placental support, followed by resection of the lung mass. The EXIT-to-resection approach has also been used for other space-occupying thoracic lesions, such as mediastinal teratoma and lymphangioma.

Other Indications

The role of EXIT-to-ECMO in the management of CDH remains controversial.[4] Fetal ECMO cannulation while on placental support has been shown to improve survival in a small series of fetuses with severe CDH with poor-prognostic indicators (liver herniation, O/E LHR < 1.0, O/E LHR ≤ 25%, percentage of predicted lung volume < 15%, and total lung volume ≤ 18 mL) and/or associated congenital heart disease.[13] However, a more recent follow-up study by the same group showed no benefit and, therefore, a recommendation for EXIT-to-ECMO for severe CDH could not be made.[14] The EXIT procedure has also been used for emergency separation for thoraco-omphalopagus conjoined twins, where both twins were intubated and umbilical catheters were placed, before separating the abnormal parasitic twin with a rudimentary heart.[15]

Preoperative Planning

Technological advances in prenatal imaging have allowed more accurate diagnosis of several fetal anomalies that can cause life-threatening airway compromise after birth. A detailed anatomical ultrasound survey and amniocentesis for karyotype and microarray should be performed to rule out associated fetal anomalies. In addition, an ultrafast fetal MRI should be performed to accurately delineate the anatomical relationship of the mass to the airway, assess the degree of airway compression and identify fetuses that would benefit from an EXIT procedure.[6] If significant fetal airway obstruction is suspected, the mother should ideally be referred to a fetal treatment center with experience in performing EXIT procedures. A multidisciplinary team of specialists, including fetal or pediatric surgery, maternal-fetal medicine, ENT surgery, anesthesiology, neonatology, radiology, nursing, and social work should be actively involved in the counseling of the mother and her family. All management options including EXIT procedure, neonatal resuscitation, expectant management, palliative care, or pregnancy termination should be discussed. Risks and benefits of each option should be discussed and the parents must be given realistic expectations for their baby's prognosis and postnatal course.[6] The timing of the EXIT procedure is often dictated by the severity of polyhydramnios and preterm labor. The mean (GA) of fetuses with neck masses undergoing EXIT procedures is 34 weeks.[3] The entire EXIT team should participate in a preoperative walk-through in the operating room to discuss responsibilities of each team, carefully plan out the critical steps during the EXIT procedure and address logistical concerns. Additionally, a "telephone tree" should be put in place with the goal of rapid communication and assembly of the team to perform the EXIT procedure in less than one hour of notification. Emergency EXIT is more often the case than elective scheduled delivery by an EXIT procedure.

Anesthetic Management

Maternal safety is always our foremost concern and the risk of maternal complications must be weighed against potential benefits to the fetus. A detailed preoperative anesthetic evaluation must be performed to rule out the presence of maternal comorbidities that increase anesthetic risk. Maternal preoperative lab testing should include a complete blood cell count and type and cross-match. In addition, leukocyte reduced, irradiated O negative blood, cross-matched to the mother, should be readily available for the fetus. Fetal evaluation should include a detailed assessment of all diagnostic and imaging studies, including ultrasonography, fetal MRI, fetal echocardiography, and, when indicated, karyotype analysis. Relevant information for the anesthesiologist includes placental location, fetal airway anatomy, baseline fetal heart rate and function, presence of fetal hydrops, results of fetal karyotyping, and estimated fetal weight for drug dosing.

Unlike most cesarean sections, EXIT procedures are typically performed under general anesthesia. Preoperatively, a lumbar epidural catheter is placed for postoperative analgesia. The patient is positioned supine on the operating table, with left uterine displacement. After adequate preoxygenation, a rapid-sequence induction is performed to facilitate endotracheal intubation. In addition to standard ASA monitors, a second large-bore intravenous access is obtained and an arterial line is inserted for close hemodynamic monitoring. General anesthesia is maintained with either volatile agents or intravenous anesthetic agents, such as propofol and remifentanil infusions. To ensure adequate uteroplacental blood flow, maternal hemodynamics are closely monitored and supported with phenylephrine and ephedrine, if necessary. Continuous fetal echocardiography is performed to monitor fetal heart rate, ventricular function, and ductal patency. Fetal bradycardia (fetal heart rate < 100 bpm) is a sign of fetal distress that warrants immediate attention.

After maternal laparotomy, the uterus is exposed, and the placental borders are mapped with a sterile ultrasound probe. Achieving profound uterine relaxation is one of the central tenets of the EXIT procedure.[3] Traditionally high doses (2–3 MAC) of volatile agents have been used to achieve profound uterine relaxation.[16] However, use of high doses of volatile agents has been associated with significant fetal cardiac dysfunction.[17] Alternatively, supplementing volatile agents with intravenous anesthetic agents (propofol and remifentanil infusions) has allowed lowering the dose of volatile agents required for uterine relaxation, thereby minimizing fetal cardiac dysfunction.[18,19] Subsequently, a hemostatic hysterotomy is performed using a specialized absorbable uterine stapler (Medtronic). The hysterotomy site is dictated by the location of the placenta and the lower uterine segment is used if at all possible. Maintaining uterine volume is critical during an EXIT procedure to prevent cord compression and placental separation.[3] To maintain uterine volume, warm lactated ringers solution is continuously infused into the uterine cavity and then the fetal head, arms, and upper torso are partially delivered through the hysterotomy. To ensure adequate fetal analgesia and immobilization, an intramuscular fetal cocktail of fentanyl (20 mcg/kg), vecuronium (0.2 mg/kg), or rocuronium (2 mg/kg) and atropine (20 mcg/kg) is administered into the fetal shoulder. In addition to continuous fetal echocardiography, a pulse oximeter probe is placed on a fetal hand to monitor fetal oxygen saturation. The normal range for fetal oxygen saturation is 30–70%.

Regardless of the indication for the EXIT procedure, the fetal airway should be secured first, should the EXIT procedure be abandoned early secondary to placental abruption, excessive uterine tone compromising uteroplacental gas exchange or evidence of prolonged fetal distress. Additional equipment for alternative airway management techniques should be readily available on the sterile surgical field (Table 20.2). Direct laryngoscopy and endotracheal intubation is usually the first option for securing the

Table 20.2 Equipment for Fetal Airway Management

Disposable sterile laryngoscope handle with Miller 1, 0, and 00 blades

Endotracheal tubes (uncuffed): 2.0, 2.5, 3.0, and 3.5 with stylets

Armored ETTs: 3.0 and 3.5

Tracheostomy tubes: 2.5 and 3.0 Neonatal Bivona, 3.0 Neonatal Shiley

Sterile Mapleson D bag and circuit

SGA devices: conduit for flexible bronchoscopic-guided tracheal intubation

Sterile tubing for oxygen administration

Flexible bronchoscope: 2.5 mm

Rigid telescope: 1.9 mm and 2.5 mm

HD camera and light cord

ETT tube changer for retrograde intubation

Feeding tubes: 2.5 fr and 3.0 fr for surfactant administration

Major neck tray for tracheostomy or mass excision

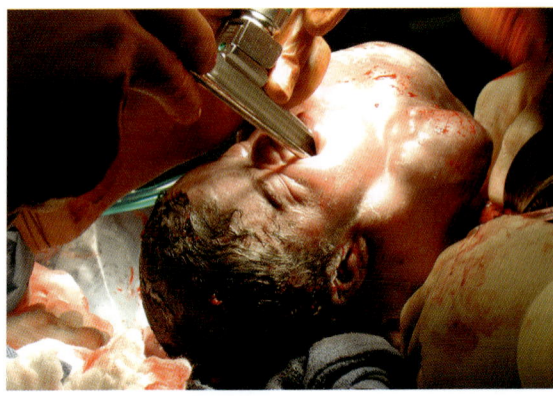

Figure 20.4 Direct laryngoscopy in a fetus with a large cervical teratoma during an EXIT-to-airway procedure.

fetal airway (Figure 20.4).[2,3] However, the algorithm for fetal airway management depends on the underlying diagnosis (Figure 20.5). In a fetus with severe micrognathia, direct laryngoscopy is unlikely to be successful and a formal tracheostomy is the preferred option. In a fetus with CHAOS, a bronchoscopy should be performed first to rule out a laryngeal web or cyst, which can be decompressed before proceeding with orotracheal intubation. If the

Chapter 20: Airway Management in EXIT Procedures

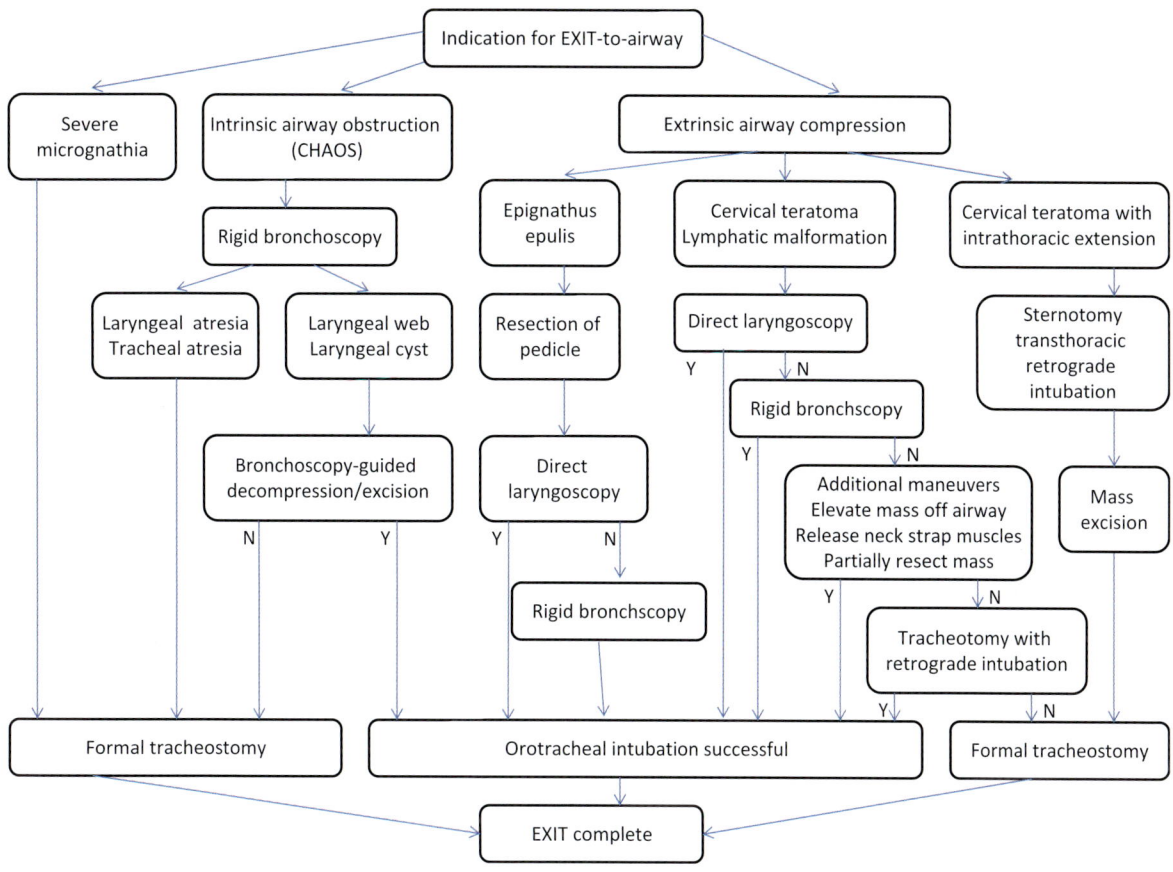

Figure 20.5 Fetal airway management algorithm for EXIT procedures (CHAOS: congenital high airway obstruction syndrome).

bronchoscopy reveals laryngeal or tracheal atresia, a tracheostomy is performed. In fetuses with oral or neck masses causing extrinsic compression of the airway, direct laryngoscopy and endotracheal intubation is attempted first. Additional maneuvers including rigid bronchoscopy, elevating the mass off the airway, release of neck strap muscles, partial or complete mass resection, or retrograde wire intubation may be necessary for securing the airway.[2,3] For cervical teratomas that extend into the mediastinum and cause superior vena cava syndrome, a median sternotomy and transthoracic retrograde intubation (TRI-EXIT) is performed to secure the airway before attempting excision of the mass and tracheostomy.

After securing the fetal airway, the position of the endotracheal or tracheostomy tube is confirmed using flexible bronchoscopy and surfactant is administered, if clinically indicated. To prevent accidental dislodgement, the ETT is usually sutured to the maxillary gingival ridge. Ventilation of the lungs is not initiated until just prior to delivery as that would initiate the process of transitional circulation and placental separation. Subsequently, other planned fetal interventions are performed. A fetal peripheral intravenous line is inserted for administration of drugs and blood products. For EXIT-to-resection of fetal lung and thoracic masses, a fetal thoracotomy is performed while still on placental support. Similarly, EXIT-to-ECMO involves placement of ECMO cannulas while still on placental support. In addition, umbilical arterial and venous cannulas may be inserted before terminating the EXIT procedure.

On completion of the fetal procedure, the volatile agent is discontinued to allow return of uterine tone. Close communication between the surgeons and anesthesiologists is critical at this stage to coordinate care.[3] Immediately after cutting the umbilical cord and delivering the newborn, oxytocin is administered and manual uterine massage is initiated. Additional uterotonic drugs should be readily available for excessive maternal hemorrhage. The neonatology team usually performs the initial resuscitation of the newborn. A separate team of surgeons, anesthesiologists, and nurses should be readily available in an adjoining operating room for completion of surgery on the newborn should the EXIT procedure be aborted early. After dosing the epidural catheter with local anesthetic, and reversing neuromuscular blockade, the mother's trachea is extubated when fully awake. Postoperative analgesia is achieved using an epidural infusion with patient-controlled rescue doses and additional intravenous analgesics, as needed.

Summary

The EXIT procedure has enabled performing lifesaving procedures on fetuses at risk for severe airway compromise and hypoxia after birth. The indications for an EXIT procedure have evolved and now include securing the airway in fetuses at risk for airway obstruction, resection of fetal lung and thoracic masses, and ECMO cannulation, while still on placental support. Patients requiring an EXIT procedure should be referred to an experienced fetal treatment center for optimal planning and management of the delivery and neonatal resuscitation. Appropriate patient selection is critical and a multidisciplinary team-based approach is strongly recommended. The anesthetic management should focus on maintaining adequate uteroplacental blood flow by supporting maternal hemodynamics, achieving profound uterine relaxation prior to hysterotomy, maintaining uterine volume, and minimizing fetal cardiac dysfunction. Fetal airway management should be the first step during all EXIT procedures and being prepared with alternative airway management strategies is critical.

References

1. Mychaliska GB, Bealer JF, Graf JL, Rosen MA, Adzick NS, Harrison MR. Operating on Placental Support: the Ex Utero Intrapartum Treatment Procedure. *Journal of Pediatric Surgery* 1997; **32**(2): 227–31.
2. Walz PC, Schroeder JW Jr. Prenatal Diagnosis of Obstructive Head and Neck Masses and Perinatal Airway Management. *Otolaryngologic Clinics of North America* 2015; **48**(1): 191–207.
3. Marwan A, Crombleholme TM. The EXIT Procedure: Principles, Pitfalls, and Progress. *Seminars in Pediatric Surgery* 2006; **15**(2): 107–15.
4. Liechty KW. Ex-Utero Intrapartum Therapy. *Seminars in Fetal and Neonatal Medicine* 2010; **15**(1): 34–9.
5. Moldenhauer JS. Ex Utero Intrapartum Therapy. *Seminars in Pediatric Surgery* 2013; **22**(1): 44–9.
6. Ryan G, Somme S, Crombleholme TM. Airway Compromise in the Fetus and Neonate: Prenatal Assessment and Perinatal Management. *Seminars in Fetal and Neonatal Medicine* 2016; **21**(4): 230–9.
7. Crombleholme TM, Sylvester K, Flake AW. Salvage of a Fetus with Congenital High Airway Obstruction Syndrome by Ex Utero Intrapartum Treatment (EXIT) Procedure. *Fetal Diagnosis and Therapy* 2000; **15**(5): 280–2.
8. Morris LM, Lim FY, Elluru RG, Hopkin RJ, Jaekle RK, Polzin WJ, et al. Severe Micrognathia: Indications for EXIT-to-Airway. *Fetal Diagnosis and Therapy* 2009; **26**(3): 162–6.
9. Jani JC, Nicolaides KH, Gratacós E, Valencia CM, Doné E, Martinez JM, et al. Severe Diaphragmatic Hernia Treated by Fetal Endoscopic Tracheal Occlusion. *Ultrasound in Obstetrics and Gynecology* 2009; **34**(3): 304–10.
10. Cass DL, Olutoye OO, Cassady CI, Zamora IJ. EXIT-to-Resection for Fetuses with Large Lung Masses and Persistent Mediastinal Compression Near Birth. *Journal of Pediatric Surgery* 2013; **48**(1): 138–44.
11. Hedrick HL, Flake AW, Crombleholme TM. The Ex Utero Intrapartum Therapy Procedure for High-Risk Fetal Lung Lesions. *Journal of Pediatric Surgery* 2005; **40**(6): 1038–43.
12. Chatterjee D, Hawkins JL, Somme S. Ex Utero Intrapartum Treatment to Resection of a Bronchogenic Cyst Causing Airway Compression. *Fetal Diagnosis and Therapy* 2014; **35**(2): 137–40.
13. Kunisaki SM, Barnewolt CE, Estroff JA, Myers LB. Ex Utero Intrapartum Treatment with Extracorporeal Membrane Oxygenation for Severe Congenital Diaphragmatic Hernia. *Journal of Pediatric Surgery* 2007; **42**(1): 98–104.
14. Stoffan AP, Wilson JM, Jennings RW. Does the Ex Utero Intrapartum Treatment to Extracorporeal Membrane Oxygenation Procedure Change Outcomes for High-Risk Patients with Congenital Diaphragmatic Hernia? *Journal of Pediatric Surgery* 2012; **47**(6): 1053–7.
15. Bouchard S, Johnson MP, Flake AW, Howell LJ. The EXIT Procedure: Experience and Outcome in 31 cases. *Journal of*

Pediatric Surgery 2002; **37**(3): 418–26.

16 Lin EE, Moldenhauer JS, Tran KM, Cohen DE, Adzick NS. Anesthetic Management of 65 Cases of Ex Utero Intrapartum Therapy. *Anesthesia & Analgesia* 2016; **123**(2): 411–17.

17 Rychik J, Cohen D, Tran KM, Szwast A, Natarajan SS, Johnson MP, et al. The Role of Echocardiography in the Intraoperative Management of the Fetus Undergoing Myelomeningocele Repair. *Fetal Diagnosis and Therapy* 2014; **37**(3): 172–8.

18 Boat A, Mahmoud M, Michelfelder EC, Lin E, Ngamprasertwong P, Schnell B, et al. Supplementing Desflurane with Intravenous Anesthesia Reduces Fetal Cardiac Dysfunction during Open Fetal Surgery. *Pediatric Anesthesia* 2010; **20**(8): 748–56.

19 Ngamprasertwong P, Vinks AA, Boat A. Update in Fetal Anesthesia for the Ex Utero Intrapartum Treatment (EXIT) Procedure. *International Anesthesiology Clinics* 2012; **50**(4): 26–40.

Section 3 **Special Topics**

Chapter 21

One-Lung Ventilation

T. Wesley Templeton and Eduardo Goenaga-Diaz

Introduction

One-lung ventilation in children undergoing non-cardiac surgery presents unique challenges that frequently require specialized equipment and creative solutions to achieve success. At the time of writing, the infrequency of these cases at any one institution limits our ability to perform prospective trials to compare different devices and approaches. As a result, most of the primary literature on this topic is based on individual experience and cases series.[1–4] Despite this issue, this area of practice still continues to brim with innovation and creativity with multiple approaches leading to success.

Indications for Lung Isolation

Traditionally, the indications for lung isolation have been categorized as absolute or relative. In absolute indications, there is a need to wholly isolate one lung from the other to either prevent contamination of one lung from the other or to maintain gas exchange in the non-diseased lung. The first absolute indication for lung isolation is for conditions in which failure to isolate would lead to damage to healthy lung tissue. Damage to healthy lung tissue may occur in conditions such as empyema and pulmonary hemorrhage of a single lung, where blood or purulent contaminants may spill over into the healthy lung. In these cases, lung isolation preserves function of the unaffected lung and prevents disease progression. An analogous but different situation occurs in patients with alveolar proteinosis. In these patients, unilateral lung lavage is often routinely performed on each lung sequentially on different days to remove proteinaceous debris that accumulates in the airway, interfering with normal gas exchange. In these cases, lung isolation prevents spillage of the irrigant and debris from the lung being lavaged into the lung being ventilated during the procedure.[5,6]

Other absolute indications include bronchial disruption, bronchopleural fistula, and sometimes bullous disease, which may lead to ineffective gas exchange. The common feature in these patients is a difference in effective compliance between the two lungs. In the case of bullous or emphysematous disease, the intrinsic compliance of the diseased lung is increased, whereas in the case of airway disruption, tidal volume is lost into the pleura or fistula through a defect. In both these cases, positive-pressure tidal

Table 21.1 Common Indications for One-Lung Ventilation in Pediatric Patients[8]

Lung resection
    Lung biopsy
    Congenital lung malformation resection
        CPAM
        Pulmonary sequestration
        Bronchial atresia
        Congenital lobar emphysema
Vascular surgery
    PDA ligation
    Vascular ring division
    Repair of coarctation of the aorta
Surgery in the mediastinum
    Esophageal atresia repair
    Tracheoesophageal fistula
    Mediastinal mass resection
Orthopedic surgery
    Anterior spinal fusion
Other
    Congenital diaphragmatic hernia
    Chest wall mass resection

volume will flow preferentially to the diseased lung. In severe cases, this may lead to minimal alveolar expansion and therefore minimal ventilation of the unaffected lung. In these situations, lung isolation and one-lung ventilation allow for ventilation of the healthy lung, allowing gas exchange without loss of tidal volume.[7]

In contrast, relative indications for one-lung ventilation revolve primarily around facilitating exposure for thoracic surgery. The impact of adequate lung isolation should not be understated as lung isolation and adequate one-lung ventilation can have a direct bearing on the quality and duration of surgery.

Physiology of One-Lung Ventilation in Children

In most cases, thoracic procedures are typically performed in a flexed, lateral decubitus position. In anesthetized patients, this position can cause significant changes in respiratory mechanics and physiology.[9] In adults, it has been shown that compliance and ventilation increase in the nondependent lung, while there is a loss of compliance and FRC in the dependent lung. This is due to external compression of the dependent lung from the mediastinum, increases in intraabdominal pressure transmitted to the chest via the diaphragm and a decrease in the compliance of the chest wall adjacent to the dependent lung. Pulmonary blood flow is also significantly affected in patients in the lateral decubitus position. This is because blood flow, which in the supine position is directed to the posterior segments of the lung, is transferred preferentially to the dependent lung as a result of gravity shunting blood away from the nondependent lung. Isolation of the nondependent lung leads to atelectasis and decreased compliance, thus shifting ventilation back to the dependent lung. Loss of nondependent lung volume also increases pulmonary vascular resistance through hypoxic pulmonary vasoconstriction and mechanical means. This results in a further redistribution of pulmonary blood flow to the dependent lung. The net effect of all of these is a shift of both ventilation and perfusion to the dependent or ventilated lung and more closely matched ventilation/perfusion ratios.

In young children, these compensatory effects are not as effective. In infants in particular, a more compliant chest wall leads to airway closing volumes at or below FRC, which can lead to atelectasis at normal tidal breathing in the supine patient. This is typically made worse in infants in the lateral position as their more compliant chest wall allows the dependent lung to be compressed to an even greater extent. As a result, the anesthetized infant in the lateral position may be prone to significant airway volume loss. Additionally, an absolute reduction in the hydrostatic gradient across both lungs in smaller patients reduces the degree of redistribution of pulmonary blood flow to the dependent lung. These factors, along with a higher metabolic oxygen requirement at baseline, can result in greater ventilation/perfusion mismatches, which can, in some cases, at least theoretically, lead to an increased risk of hypoxemia during one-lung ventilation.[10,11] In general, though, whether it is due to the relative health of their lung tissue or other compensatory mechanisms, hypoxemia refractory to basic recruitment strategies and PEEP on the ventilated lung is actually unusual in routine pediatric thoracic cases utilizing one-lung ventilation.

Techniques for One-Lung Ventilation in Children

At the time of writing, there are a number of approaches to one-lung ventilation in children. In many cases, the appropriate choice will depend on the size of the child and comfort level of the clinician with any given device or technique. Available techniques include double-lumen tubes, bronchial blockers, and endobronchial intubation. In younger patients, the use of mainstem intubation or an endobronchial blocker are the only currently available approaches for lung isolation. In children greater than 8 years of age, double-lumen tubes and bronchial blockers are the most commonly used techniques.

Table 21.2 One-Lung Ventilation Technique by Age

Age	Mainstem intubation	Bronchial blocker	Double-lumen tube
0–6 months	*	*	
6–12 months	*	*	
1–5 years	*	*	
5–8 years		*	
8–18 years		*	*

Endobronchial Intubation

In children less than 5 years of age, endobronchial intubation remains a very common approach to one-lung ventilation. One of the keys to achieving success with this technique is choosing an appropriately sized ETT. Due to the discrepancy in size between the trachea and mainstem bronchi, the clinician must sometimes use a smaller tube than would be indicated for routine intubation to successfully achieve isolation.[12]

The primary advantage of this technique is that, in most cases, it is technically easier to execute than many occlusive blocker techniques in young children.[10] In left-sided surgical cases, the favorable anatomy of the tracheal bronchial tree allows for the ETT to be advanced while simultaneously auscultating the left chest. Once breath sounds disappear on the left, the clinician can assume that the ETT has passed into the right mainstem bronchus. This blind approach is not appropriate when attempting to isolate the right side because of the more acutely angled takeoff of the left mainstem bronchus relative to the long axis of the trachea.

More generally, a flexible fiberoptic bronchoscope can be utilized to facilitate placement of the ETT within either mainstem bronchus.[10,12,13] It is typically a good idea to test fit the flexible fiberoptic bronchoscope within the planned ETT prior to beginning if the difference between the inner diameter of the ETT and the published outer diameter of the scope is less than 3 mm. Occasionally, prior repairs to a flexible fiberoptic scope will actually enlarge the outer diameter of a given scope. If not checked ahead of time, scope/ETT mismatches can potentially lead to binding and ultimately impede effective airway management.

Table 21.3 Endotracheal Tube Size for Endobronchial Intubation

Age	Endotracheal tube size
0–5 months	3.0 uc
6–12 months	3.5 uc, 3.0 c
1 year	3.5 c, 4.0 uc
2 years	3.5 c, 4.0 c
3 years	4.0 c
4 years	4.0 c

uc: uncuffed; c: cuffed

To execute this approach, an appropriately sized flexible fiberoptic scope is inserted into the ETT and is advanced into the right or left mainstem bronchus. The tube is then advanced over the fiberscope into the mainstem bronchus of the lung, which will be ventilated. Ideally, the tip of the bronchoscope should be placed 5–10 mm into the bronchus and the end of the tube should be advanced until it is barely visible within the field of view of the flexible fiberoptic bronchoscope. Care should be taken when advancing the ETT in right-sided cases given the frequency of a proximal takeoff of the right upper lobe bronchus. If the ETT is advanced too distally, ventilation of the upper lobe may be compromised, reducing the amount of lung tissue involved in gas exchange, potentially leading to even higher levels of retained carbon dioxide and potentially worsening oxygenation.[10,14] Additionally, the clinician should attempt to approximate the anticipated position of the head relative to the thorax during the procedure. This is important in young children because even small changes in flexion or extension of the patient's neck can lead to clinically significant changes in ETT position relative to the carina with attendant loss of lung isolation. Once correctly positioned, the ETT should be secured and a decrease in tidal volume and absent breaths sounds on the operative side should be confirmed.

Assuming adequate intravenous access, and an arterial line, if desired, has been placed, the patient should then be moved to the lateral decubitus position taking care again not to flex or extend the neck significantly. Once the patient is positioned, isolation should be reconfirmed by auscultation. If it appears that isolation has been lost, a fiberoptic bronchoscope should be inserted to assess the position of the tube relative to the carina. In many cases, it may be necessary for the clinician to unsecure the tube and repeat the above process in the lateral position. Importantly, the clinician should withdraw the fiberoptic scope and ETT enough to visualize the carina before repeating placement as it is sometimes easy to mistake segmental branching for the carina. Assuming lung isolation is now present, the patient should be continued on 100% oxygen to allow for absorption atelectasis and collapse of the lung on the operative side.[15]

The primary disadvantage of this technique remains an inability to rapidly change from one-lung ventilation to two-lung ventilation, especially while surgery is ongoing. Contributing to this is the fact

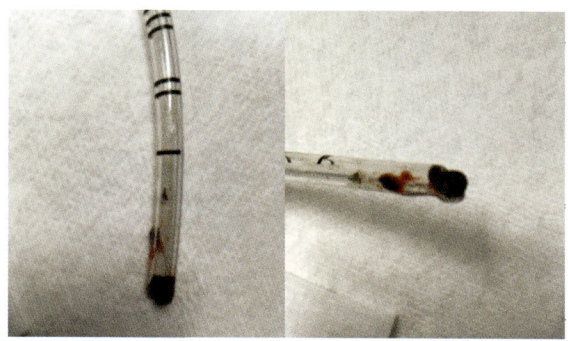

Figure 21.1 Near-complete occlusion of 3.5 uncuffed ETT used for endobronchial intubation in a 6-month-old for a left-sided thoracotomy. Frequent increases in ventilatory pressures, decreases in tidal volume, and interruptions of end-tidal carbon dioxide were observed throughout.

that any manipulation of the tube usually must be performed under the drapes with poor visualization of the exterior airway. This can make performing this safely very technically challenging as even small movements in a young infant may incur the risk of inadvertent extubation. Another significant frailty of this approach is the potential for an inadequate bronchial seal, leading to partial ventilation and aeration of the lung on the operative side. Lastly, it is possible that the ETT may become occluded with thickened secretions and/or clot from surgical trauma, thereby limiting gas exchange, especially as case duration increases. In many cases this can be remedied by suctioning with a flexible catheter, but not always.

Single-Balloon Catheter-Based Bronchial Blocker

Single-balloon catheter-based bronchial blockers remain one of the most well-documented approaches to one-lung ventilation in children. One of the key design improvements for these devices when compared to Fogarty catheters and other previously used devices has been the implementation of high-volume, low-pressure occlusive cuffs.[2] Although the inflation pressures in all these devices typically exceed mucosal perfusion pressures, the lower requisite inflation pressures in devices designed specifically for use in the airway at least theoretically reduce the potential for bronchial mucosal injury.[16]

Commercially available endobronchial blockers include the Arndt endobronchial blocker (Cook Medical), the Fuji Uniblocker (Ambu), and the Fogarty embolectomy catheter (Edwards Life Sciences). The Arndt endobronchial blocker remains the most well-documented bronchial blocker in children, with a number of groups having published their experience with this device.[1,3,4] Generally speaking, bronchial blockers are semirigid catheters with a high-volume, lower-pressure occlusive balloon at the distal end connected to a pilot balloon at the proximal end, which allows for inflation. When correctly placed, the inflated balloon at the distal tip should rest just distal to the carina, occluding the mainstem bronchus and preventing air movement in or out, thus isolating the lung on the operative side.[10]

Approaches to the placement of a bronchial blocker can be divided into two large groups: intraluminal and extraluminal. In larger children, the most common mode of placement remains intraluminal, but this is not to say that extraluminal placement needs to be limited to young children. In fact, in one recently published adult study, investigators demonstrated a significant decrease in time to perform correct Arndt blocker placement with an extraluminal approach compared to the manufacturer recommended intraluminal approach.[17]

In the intraluminal approach, the endobronchial blocker is inserted via a device-specific multiport adapter into the ETT lumen and, from there, is passed into the desired mainstem bronchus. In very young patients, due to the combined outer diameter of a bronchial blocker and a flexible fiberoptic scope, this is not possible. This is because there is simply not enough room inside the ETT to accommodate both the blocker and the flexible fiberoptic scope simultaneously. In these cases, the clinician must adopt an extraluminal approach to placement. In the extraluminal approach, the bronchial blocker is frequently placed into the glottis prior to placing the ETT, allowing it to remain extraluminal. The flexible fiberoptic scope can then be passed independently through the ETT to assist with and visualize placement. Details of various approaches to this will be covered later in this chapter.

Not surprisingly, choosing the appropriately sized endobronchial blocker remains one of the key factors in successfully achieving lung isolation with a blocker device in younger patients and can have a significant impact on what type of blocker placement technique is used.[1] For example, in patients 3–8 years of age, we have found the 5 fr Arndt bronchial blockers to be less effective because the occlusive balloon tends to be too

Table 21.4 Bronchial Blocker Sizing Related to Age and Intraluminal versus Extraluminal

Age	Bronchial blocker device							
	Fogarty 3 fr	Fogarty 4 fr	Arndt 5 fr	Arndt 7 fr	Arndt 9 fr	Fuji 5 fr	Fuji 9 fr	Cohen 9 fr
0–5 months	E	E	E			E		
6–12 months	E	E	E			E		
1–2 years	E/I	E/I	E			E		
3–7 years			E/I	E		E/I		
8–9 years				E/I	E		E	E
10–18 years					E/I		E/I	E/I

Fogarty: Fogarty embolectomy catheter; Arndt: Arndt endobronchial blocker; Fuji: Fuji Uniblocker; Cohen: Cohen endobronchial blocker; E: extraluminal; I: intraluminal

small to occlude the mainstem bronchus without significant overinflation. Therefore, at 3 years of age, we recommend transitioning to an extraluminal 7 fr Arndt endobronchial blocker. If the clinician prefers an intraluminal approach in this age group, they will have to use the 5 fr Arndt or 5 fr Uniblocker. It should be noted that some authors do support the use of a 5 fr blocker in this age group.[13,18]

Intraluminal Approaches to Bronchial Blocker Placement

Assuming a child is adequately sized, there are two different techniques for performing intraluminal placement of a bronchial blocker. In both techniques, the patient is first intubated with an appropriately sized single-lumen ETT, typically erring on the side of having an ETT with as large an internal diameter as possible that does not apply excessive pressure on the glottic mucosa. The tube is then secured at least 3–4 cm above the carina. In the case of the Arndt blocker, it is inserted into the proper port on the manufacturer-supplied multiport adapter. The included wire is then looped over the fiberoptic scope, which has also been inserted into another port on the multiport adapter, and both entities are then inserted into the lumen of the ETT. In children, prior to beginning an intraluminal approach, the clinician should check to make sure the bronchial blocker and the lassoed fiberoptic scope will fit through the 15 mm adapter as it narrows at the point of insertion into the ETT. Sometimes the combined profile of both devices will actually fit through the ETT, but not through the 15 mm adapter. These devices must fit through the adapter simultaneously to execute intraluminal placement of the blocker. Assuming everything is compatible from a size perspective, the fiberoptic scope is then manipulated into the desired mainstem bronchus and the Arndt endobronchial blocker is then threaded down and ultimately off of the fiberoptic scope into position.[13,17]

A second approach is to simply insert the Arndt blocker or other manufacture's blocker through the included multiport adapter into the ETT until it meets intermediate resistance at an appropriate depth of insertion. The fiberoptic scope is then inserted and the blocker position is adjusted under direct visualization. This approach tends be fairly straightforward in cases where the clinician desires to isolate the right side, but can be more challenging in left-sided cases. When attempting to perform this for a left-sided case, it may be necessary to place a bend in the Arndt to assist in steering the blocker and/or it may be necessary to rotate the ETT to attempt to direct the device into the left mainstem bronchus.

Although a reliable approach in larger children, the intraluminal approach has limited utility in smaller children. In fact, the smallest internal diameter tube for which this is possible is a 4.5 mm ETT in combination with a 5 fr blocker and a 2.2 mm

Chapter 21: One-Lung Ventilation

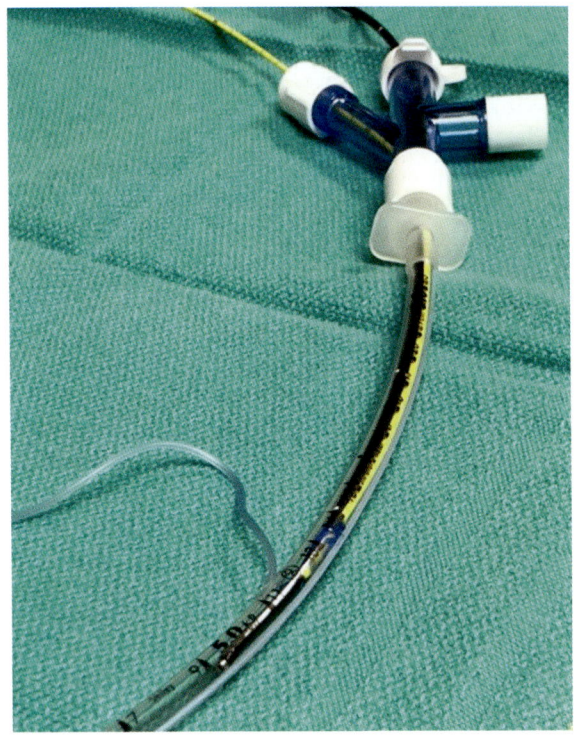

Figure 21.2 5 fr Arndt bronchial blocker and 2.8 mm flexible fiberoptic scope inserted through multiport adapter with 2.8 mm flexible fiberoptic scope lassoed by the bronchial blocker within a 5.0 cuffed ETT.

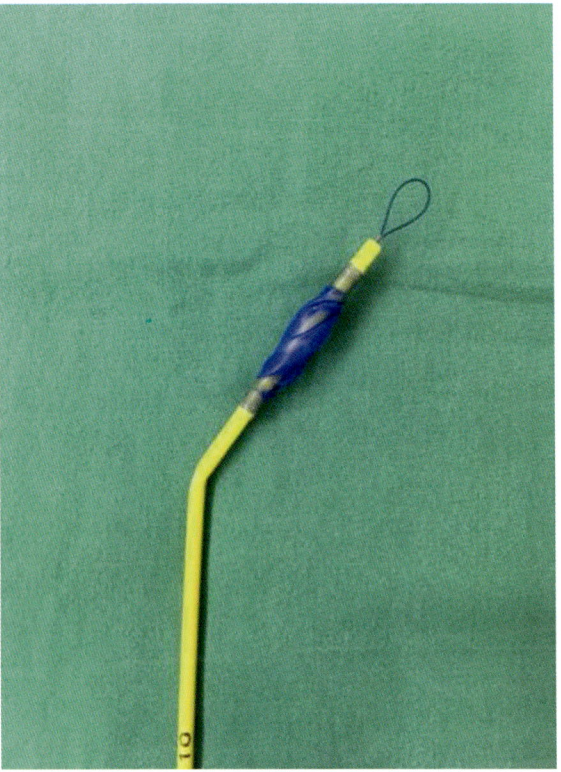

Figure 21.3 Arndt endobronchial blocker with bend placed at distal tip to facilitate placement.

fiberoptic scope. Other combinations of blocker and scope will require an even larger ETT. The most significant technical limitations of the intraluminal approach is frequent binding of the fiberoptic scope and the bronchial blocker within the ETT during placement.[17] One potential advantage to this technique, though, is that in patients where the blocker and flexible fiberoptic scope do not completely occlude the ETT lumen, the patient can be continuously ventilated during blocker placement.

Extraluminal Approaches to Bronchial Blocker Placement

Since the early part of the twenty-first century, a number of techniques for extraluminal placement of a bronchial blocker have been described in children.[1,3,4,12] In some cases, these techniques are device-specific, but some approaches can be applied to devices from different manufactures. In most extraluminal techniques in children, the bronchial blocker is inserted first with an appropriately sized ETT placed adjacent to it within the glottis. Although not essential, it has been our experience that it is preferable to place the ETT anterior to the bronchial blocker so that the mechanical force applied to the proximal portion of the blocker is more easily translated into motion at the tip. In some cases, we have noticed that anterior position of the blocker can lead to difficulties with motion of the distal tip secondary to deformation of the blocker within the hypopharynx, especially as it warms to body temperature.

Once both the ETT and blocker have been placed within the glottis, the ETT should be connected to the circuit. Great care should be exercised to ensure that the ETT is not placed too distally into the trachea. As with intraluminal approaches, it is important to maintain a certain amount of working room to visualize and manipulate the blocker.

At this point, it is important to assess vertical mobility of the blocker and the glottic leak pressure.[1] If the ETT is too large, the blocker may be pinned against the glottic mucosa preventing the necessary proximal and distal translation for appropriate placement. In this situation, the ETT should be changed to a half size smaller and/or the clinician may consider using a similarly sized uncuffed ETT if they originally began with a cuffed one. If the ETT is too small, and the leak therefore too large, it may not be possible to adequately ventilate the child during the procedure. In this situation, a larger outer-diameter tube must be used. In children less than 2 years of age, this compromise is even more important because of exponential increases in the level of resistance to airflow in smaller and smaller ETTs. In most cases, this compromise will occur at a leak pressure around 18 to 24 cm of water.[1] In general, it is acceptable to use either uncuffed or cuffed ETTs so long as the previously discussed issues of blocker mobility and leak pressure are in balance.

At this point in the technique, a flexible fiberoptic scope should be inserted into the ETT to begin optimizing placement. In patients less than 2 years of age, the 15 mm adapter will frequently have to be removed to allow for insertion of the scope. In larger children, if the scope can pass through the adapter, the manufacturer's multiport adapter can be used to allow for ventilation during bronchoscopy and blocker positioning. Unfortunately, ventilation may be less effective in situations where the scope nearly occludes the lumen of the ETT. In very young patients, blocker positioning will typically have to be performed under conditions of apnea. In situations where the respiratory pathophysiology of the child may be too significant to allow for any meaningful period of apnea, fluoroscopy can also be used to visualize and manipulate the bronchial blocker while ventilation is maintained.[3]

With the fiberoptic scope in the ETT, it is then important to identify anterior and posterior landmarks within the trachea. In some cases where there are secretions, or placement of the ETT is too deep, or the tracheal rings are less prominent, it may be initially difficult to assess the orientation of the anterior/posterior axis of the trachea and therefore difficult to tell right from left. In this situation, additional time should be spent to confirm tracheal anatomy. If the bronchial blocker appears to be positioned in the correct mainstem bronchus, the blocker depth should be adjusted to bring the proximal edge of the occlusive balloon just distal to the carina. In a majority of cases, the blocker will naturally head toward the right mainstem bronchus, but it can be withdrawn and redirected to the left by either turning the head to the right or by actually steering the blocker using a twisting motion on the proximal shaft. To further facilitate this, we have found it helpful to introduce a 35–45-degree bend relative to the long axis of the Arndt endobronchial blocker 1.0 cm proximal to the distal cuff.[1,19] This is not necessary with the Fuji blocker as it is manufactured with a bend at its distal tip. If vertical translation becomes difficult, it is sometimes necessary to use your index finger to press the blocker shaft against the posterior oropharynx, bracing it, to allow vertical translation of the device. Frequently, this process will require two sets of hands to simultaneously maintain visualization of the airway and effectively manipulate the blocker (see Video 11).

Table 21.5 Endotracheal Tube Size and Age Guidelines for Extraluminal Placement of a Bronchial Blocker

Some variation exists depending on the choice of blocker size.	
Age	Appropriate internal diameter endotracheal tube size
0–4 months	3.0 c, 3.0 uc, 3.5 uc
5–12 months	3.0 c, 3.5 c, 3.5 uc, 4.0 uc
1–3 years	3.5 c, 4.0 c, 4.0 uc, 4.5 uc
4–7 years	4.0 c, 4.5 c, 5.0 c
8–10 years	5.0 c, 5.5 c

c: cuffed; uc: uncuffed

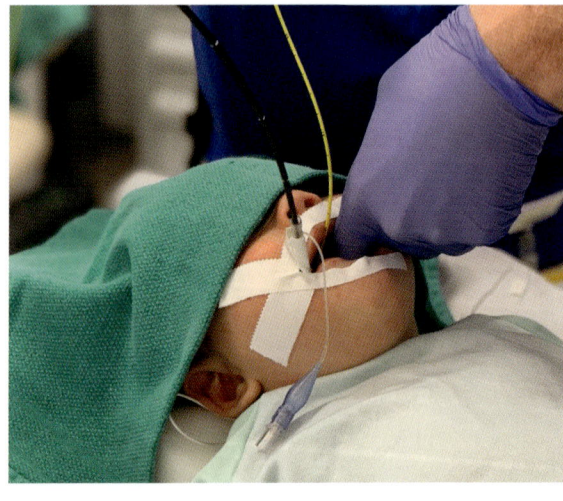

Figure 21.4 Clinician inserting index finger into oropharynx of a 7-month-old to pin 5 fr extraluminal bronchial blocker against posterior oropharyngeal wall to improve vertical translation.

Chapter 21: One-Lung Ventilation

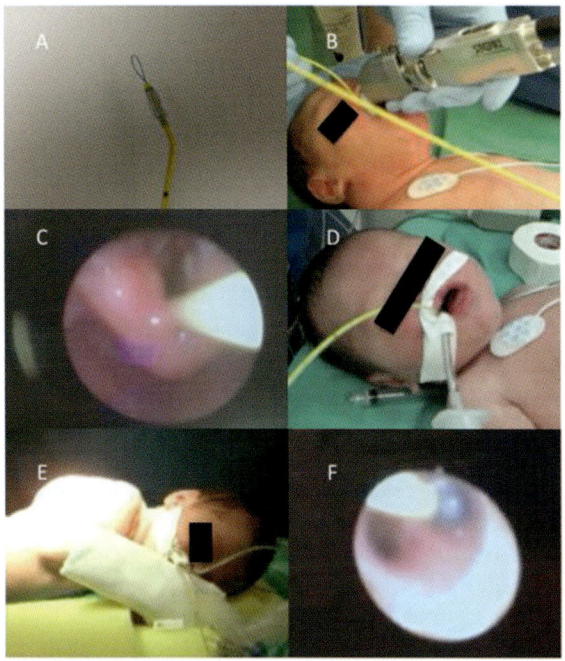

Figure 21.5 A. Arndt prepared with 35–45 degrees 1.0 cm proximal to cuff; B. Video laryngoscopy with placement of Arndt; C. 5 fr Arndt present within glottis before ETT; D. Arndt and ETT present orally in supine position; E. Patient in lateral position with Arndt and ETT; F. Arndt inflated in right mainstem bronchus to achieve isolation observed with video-assisted fiberoptic bronchoscopy.[1] (Adapted from Templeton, TW. *Bending the Rules*. 2016.)

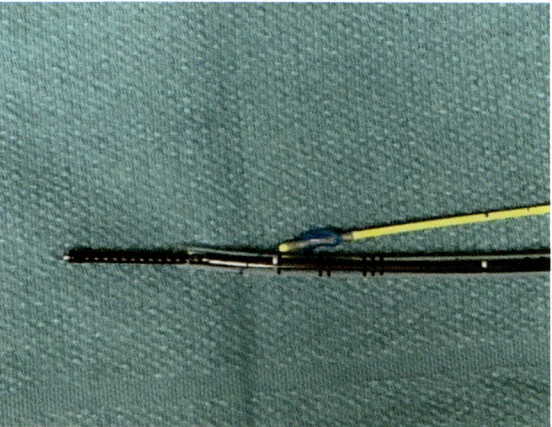

Figure 21.6 5 fr Arndt bronchial blocker lassoed to an ETT with a flexible fiberoptic scope driven through it. The blocker is then passed via the loop, off the ETT, onto the fiberoptic scope and down into the desired mainstem bronchus.

Another approach to extraluminal placement of the Arndt blocker uses the wire loop to guide the blocker from the ETT to the fiberoptic scope to ultimately guide the blocker into the desired mainstem bronchus.[20] In this approach, the wire loop of the Arndt endobronchial blocker is initially placed around the distal tip of the ETT. The now lassoed ETT and blocker are then placed as a single unit during laryngoscopy. Once present within the glottis, a flexible fiberoptic scope is introduced into the ETT and advanced into the desired mainstem bronchus. At this point, the blocker is threaded off the ETT on to the flexible fiberoptic scope and into the desired mainstem bronchus. Once the blocker is visualized passing over the end of the bronchoscope, the bronchoscope is withdrawn into the trachea, leaving the blocker in place distally. The depth of the blocker is then adjusted as necessary. If this fails, it is sometimes possible to pass the scope through the wire loop within the trachea and then repeat this process. However, in many cases, it may be necessary to remove all three devices and repeat the whole process again, starting with the laryngoscopy.

One final approach to extraluminal placement, which has been published recently, takes advantage of the technique of mainstem intubation to facilitate extraluminal blocker placement.[12] This technique can be applied to Fogarty catheters, the Arndt, and the Fuji blocker. In this technique, the patient is induced and intubated with a relatively small ETT. The tube is then advanced using a fiberoptic bronchoscope into the mainstem bronchus on the operative side. The fiberoptic scope is withdrawn and the bronchial blocker is then passed through the ETT to an appropriate depth just distal to the distal end of the ETT into the desired mainstem bronchus. If desired, the clinician can further confirm correct endobronchial placement of the ETT via auscultation prior to introducing the blocker. In some cases, this may actually break up the period of apnea required into smaller time epochs, potentially reducing the risk of desaturation during blocker placement. When placing a 5 fr Arndt blocker through a 3.0 internal diameter ETT, it is necessary to retract the blocker's wire loop slightly to get the blocker to enter into the ETT. Also, it may be necessary to apply a small amount of lubricant to the occlusive balloon to reduce binding.[12] Next, the ETT is withdrawn while holding the bronchial blocker in place. A second laryngoscopy is then performed, and an appropriately sized ETT is placed adjacent to the bronchial blocker. Following this, the

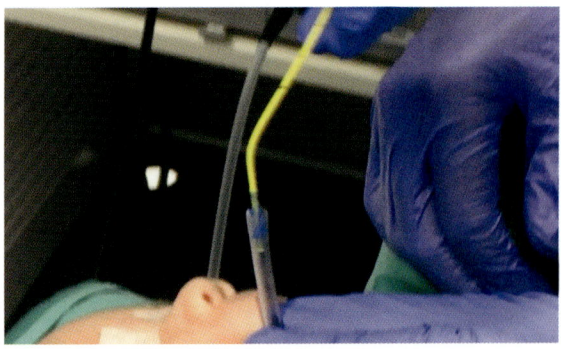

Figure 21.7 5 fr Arndt endobronchial blocker with distal bend being inserted into 3.0 ETT to be threaded into left mainstem following endobronchial placement of the ETT using a flexible fiberoptic scope.

flexible fiberoptic scope is inserted into the ETT to perform any final depth adjustments. In situations where visualization within the trachea is poor secondary to heme or secretions and/or the child has poor pulmonary reserve limiting the allowable period of apnea, fluoroscopy can be used to facilitate the initial endobronchial intubation in this technique (see Video 12).

The primary limitation of this technique, like many other techniques, is the period of apnea between initial placement of the fiberoptic scope and eventual placement of the second ETT. In cases of desaturation, though, the patient can be mask-ventilated between removal of the first ETT and the second laryngoscopy if necessary without disturbing the blocker's position.[12] The second limitation is simply that the first ETT must be small enough to pass into the desired mainstem bronchus. In infants less than 5 months of age this may often need to be a 3.0 uncuffed ETT.

The Blocker Just Won't Go Where I Want It To!

In situations in young children where initial blocker placement continues to be challenging and the clinician is unable to place the blocker within the desired mainstem bronchus, we recommend starting over with another placement technique. Over time, we have found that this may actually hasten successful positioning, rather than persisting with a technique that is failing. At some point, the clinician may also consider changing to an endobronchial approach.

Tips on Intraprocedural Single-Balloon Endobronchial Blocker Management

Once the blocker is correctly positioned in the supine patient, we recommend inflating the cuff under direct visualization to assess the presence of isolation prior to turning the patient lateral. Typically, it is better for the occlusive balloon to be slightly deep at this point rather than too shallow. Frequently inflation of the cuff to achieve occlusion of the mainstem bronchus with the 5 fr blockers may require as much as 2–4 cm^3 of air, with larger blockers requiring even more volume. Isolation should be confirmed by a fall in tidal volume, absence of breath sounds, or point-of-care lung ultrasound.[1,21,22] A lack of confirmation with any of these should lead the clinician to question the blocker's position and quality of isolation.

If isolation appears to be good, the occlusive balloon on the blocker can either be left inflated to allow increased time for absorption atelectasis or deflated until final positioning in the lateral decubitus position. The patient should be placed on 100% oxygen. If the patient desaturates below 91% on initiation of one-lung ventilation, we recommend performing two or three recruitment breaths on the ventilated lung and increasing the level of PEEP. If hypoxemia persists, it may be necessary to deflate the occlusive cuff and continue with two-lung ventilation, informing the surgeon that they may have to simply retract or pack away the nondependent lung during the procedure. In some cases, CPAP to the nondependent lung may improve oxygenation, but if this is necessary at this early stage of the procedure, it is likely that this maneuver will not be sufficient as the case proceeds. Therefore, it is prudent to advise the surgeon that one-lung ventilation may need to be abandoned at some point later in the procedure and this should be taken into account in planning the surgical approach to the procedure. Nevertheless, in some patients, oxygenation may actually improve in the lateral position and they may tolerate one-lung ventilation better because of improved ventilation perfusion matching. Unfortunately, it is difficult to predict ahead of time which patients will respond in a positive way to lateral positioning. As a result, the clinician must be prepared for both scenarios.

Following placement of any additional lines, the patient should now be carefully moved to the lateral position, attempting to avoid flexion or extension, as even small changes in head position can lead to dislodgement of the bronchial blocker. Once the patient is completely positioned laterally, the fiberoptic scope should be reinserted into the ETT to make a final assessment of correct blocker laterality and depth. Frequently, small adjustments to blocker depth may be necessary. More often than not, the blocker will tend to move proximally out of the bronchus and will have to be repositioned slightly more distally. In rare cases in small infants, the blocker can actually become displaced into the other mainstem bronchus or into the trachea. At this point, it may be necessary to return the patient to the supine position and completely reposition the blocker. In some situations, the blocker can be replaced in the lateral position, but this is often technically challenging as gravity is working against the clinician with the desired mainstem bronchus now being in a nondependent position.

Intraoperatively, bronchial blockers do tend to move out of position secondary to surgical manipulation. In one study, repositioning rates in children less than 2 years of age were as high as 46%, so the clinician must be prepared to reposition these devices.[1] In clinical situations where there is an abrupt loss of end-tidal carbon dioxide and a fall in tidal volume with a bronchial blocker in place, the clinician's first thought should be that the occlusive balloon has migrated into the trachea. The balloon should be deflated immediately. Following deflation, the blocker should be reassessed with fiberoptic bronchoscopy and repositioned more distally. In other situations where there is simply a loss of isolation, it may be that the balloon has simply migrated out of the mainstem bronchus slightly and needs to be pushed back in a few millimeters. Frequently, secretions and blood may hamper visibility, oftentimes making repositioning challenging. In these situations, airway suctioning with a flexible suction catheter may help improve visualization. In the case of the Arndt, the wire loop should be left in place when possible to help maintain rigidity of the blocker and facilitate blocker replacement.[1,4]

Although no large studies evaluating these procedures in children exist, intraprocedural hypoxemia is probably less common in children than adults. However, the clinician should be prepared to deal with this issue should it arise. If initial recruitment maneuvers, increases in PEEP, and/or aggressive manual ventilation to the ventilated lung do not improve oxygenation, CPAP can be applied to the non-ventilated lung via a central channel present in both the Arndt and the Fuji. However, it is unclear how therapeutic this maneuver is in young infants, given the length and diminutive caliber of a 5 fr blocker's hollow channel. It should be noted that, when using an Arndt blocker, the wire loop must be removed prior to instituting CPAP via this channel. If the patient does not respond or develops worsening hypoxemia refractory to these maneuvers, it may be necessary to return to two-lung ventilation temporarily.

At the end of the procedure, the blocker should be removed prior to extubation. In the case of the Arndt blocker, the wire loop should be removed prior to removing the bronchial blocker to prevent the possibility of lassoing the ETT and thus preventing independent removal of the blocker.[1]

One-Lung Ventilation in Children with the EZ-Blocker

The EZ-Blocker (Teleflex) is a relatively new bronchial blocker with two occlusive balloon cuffs coming off a central 7 fr catheter in a Y configuration, which is designed to rest on the carina.[23,24] The distal Y configuration separates into two 4 cm long limbs, each housing a separate occlusive balloon. Although originally designed for use in adults, it has been used successfully in children as young as 6 years of age.[25] At this time, it is only manufactured in one size.

The EZ-Blocker can be deployed either intraluminally or extraluminally.[23,25,26] Much like the Arndt bronchial blocker, when used intraluminally, the EZ-Blocker is inserted into the manufacturer's supplied multiport adapter and inserted into a previously placed ETT. The blocker is then advanced down the ETT and allowed to rest on the carina. Frequently, on insertion, both limbs of the EZ-Blocker will pass into the right mainstem bronchus. If this occurs, the blocker should be withdrawn under direct visualization, rotated, and reinserted to allow one limb to rest in each mainstem bronchus with the central 6.5 mm confluence resting on the carina. The occlusive balloon on the operative side should then be inflated with 4–10 cm³ of air under direct visualization. In larger patients, sometimes even more air may be necessary to completely occlude the bronchus. By report, the intraluminal approach has been used in children as young as 10 years of age using a size 7.0 ETT.[27]

In smaller children for which a 7.0 ETT is too large, the device must be used in an extraluminal fashion. Of course, the native Y conformation of the

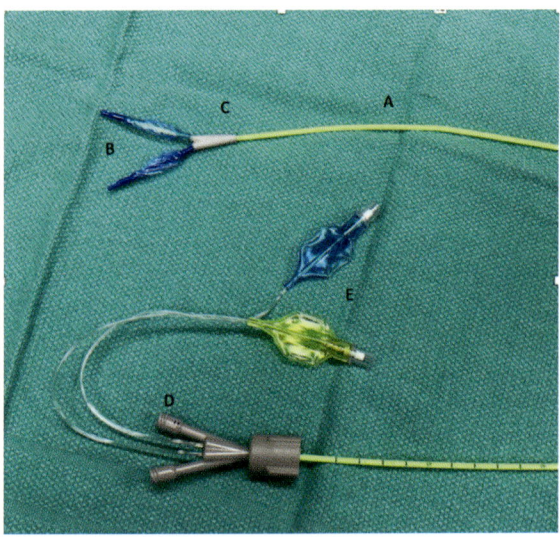

Figure 21.8 Anatomy of the EZ-Blocker: A. 7 fr shaft; B. Balloon cuffs; C. 6.5 mm central confluence; D. ports for CPAP or suctioning; E. Color-coded pilot balloons for balloon cuffs.

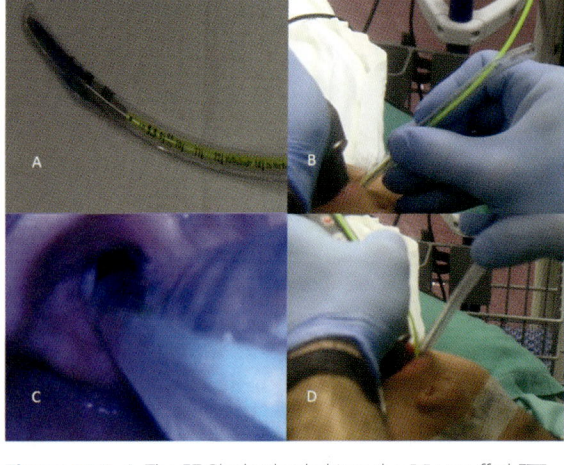

Figure 21.9 A. The EZ-Blocker loaded into the 5.5 uncuffed ETT introducer; B. Laryngoscopy and placement of the introducer with the EZ-Blocker within it; C. Laryngoscopic view of introducer and ETT in glottis; D. Peeling 5.5 ETT off the EZ-Blocker, leaving the blocker's distal end in the trachea.

device prevents introduction of the native blocker into the glottis. Instead, the device must actually be placed using an introducer.[26] In this approach, a 5.5 uncuffed internal diameter ETT is first cut lengthwise. The device limbs are then collapsed and the distal end of the blocker is fully inserted into the lumen of the 5.5 uncuffed ETT. Following induction of anesthesia, the 5.5 ETT introducer with the blocker fully enclosed is inserted during the initial laryngoscopy. The ETT is then peeled off the blocker, leaving the distal limbs within the trachea. The device is then typically advanced slightly and a cuffed ETT is then placed adjacent to it via a second laryngoscopy (see Video 13).

At this point, a flexible fiberoptic scope should be introduced through either a scope swivel adapter or directly into the ETT to visualize final placement. Frequently, the device will initially be positioned slightly distal with both limbs at least partially within one of the mainstem bronchi.[25] The device should be withdrawn, rotated using a twisting motion, and then reinserted to allow the two individual limbs to each rest in a single bronchus, with the central confluence atop the carina. As with previous techniques, it is important to try to secure the ETT as high as possible with it still safely within the glottis to allow for visualization of the distal trachea and the device. Once in place on the carina with a limb in each bronchus, the appropriate occlusive balloon should be inflated under direct visualization. In rare cases, it may not be possible to get the device to sit on the carina, but if both limbs are resting in the bronchus of the operative lung, it is possible to inflate one of them and still obtain isolation. Unlike other extraluminal bronchial blockers, the EZ-Blocker should not be removed prior to extubation. Instead, it should be removed simultaneously with the central confluence left distal to the end ETT to avoid vocal cord or glottic injury from the 6.5 mm central confluence and rigid ETT exiting the glottis with their combined diameter in a single moment.[28]

In our limited experience in children, the EZ-Blocker, when positioned correctly, may have the benefit of being more positionally stable than other blockers previously mentioned as a consequence of the distal limbs resting on each side of the carina. There are, however, no prospective trials in adults or children to confirm this assertion.[25] In general, the EZ-Blocker should probably be limited to use in children 6 years of age and older due to the 4 cm length of the distal limbs and size of the 6.5 mm central confluence. However, demonstration of adequate airway size via direct measurements from a recent high-resolution CT may allow for its use in slightly younger children. Additionally, it may represent a good alternative in cases where serial isolation of each side in a single case is necessary.[29]

One-Lung Ventilation in Children Using the Univent Tube

The Univent Tube (Fuji Systems) is an extraluminal bronchial blocker and ETT combined into a single unit, which can also be used to provide one-lung ventilation in children.[30,31] This device comes in three sizes 3.5, 4.5, and 5.5, which correspond to the internal diameter of the ventilating portion of the tube. The use of this device in children is primarily limited by the external diameter of the device. The 3.5 mm size has an external diameter of 8.0 mm. This corresponds to a size 6.0 cuffed ETT, suggesting that it probably should not be used in children younger than 7 years of age.

Following induction of anesthesia, the device is placed via standard laryngoscopic techniques into the glottis and trachea, with the blocker assembly sitting adjacent to the posterior portion of the larynx. Once inserted, the manufacturer suggests rotating the device 90 degrees so that the blocker channel is now ipsilateral to the intended surgical side. The blocker portion of the device should then be inserted, and proper depth should be confirmed with inflation of the cuff and auscultation of the operative side. Alternatively, the blocker can be placed under direct visualization using a flexible fiberoptic scope through the ventilating channel.[30] In some cases, it may be necessary to rotate the tube/blocker assembly to direct the distal tip of the blocker into the desired mainstem bronchus.

One potential advantage of this device may be positional stability because it is fixed relative to the ETT.[30] Disadvantages, however, include its low-volume, high-pressure cuff and the potential resistance to airflow incurred by the 3.5 mm internal diameter of the device when used in younger children.

Other extraluminal approaches with the Arndt or Univent blocker may allow for a larger ETT and therefore less resistance to air movement when used in the same patient.[31]

One-Lung Ventilation in Children Using a Double-Lumen Tube

The primary limitation of double-lumen tubes in children is their size, as the smallest double-lumen tube available is a 26 fr. Seefelder reports the external profile and dimension at the level of the tracheal cuff of the 26 fr double-lumen tube to be elliptical with a maximal diameter of 9.1 mm.[32] This corresponds to a size 6.5 cuffed ETT, thereby limiting its use to children who are 8 or 9 years of age and older. Double-lumen tube-size selection can be performed by evaluating a recent high-resolution CT of the chest to ensure that the trachea and mainstem bronchi will accommodate the device. The clinician can also estimate the diameter of the left mainstem bronchus from a measurement of the tracheal diameter via chest X-ray using the formula, left mainstem bronchus width = 0.69 × tracheal width.[33] It should be noted, though, that this relationship was derived in adults and should be used with some caution in children.

Methods for placement are similar in both adults and children.[10] Following induction, the tracheal lumen tube is inserted into the glottis and advanced slightly. The tube should then be rotated and a fiberoptic scope introduced into the tracheal lumen. Under direct visualization, the tube should be advanced until the proximal portion of the bronchial cuff is visualized at the level of the carina.[34] Although some reports would suggest that it is acceptable to advance a double-lumen tube blindly in adults, we highly recommend advancing these under direct

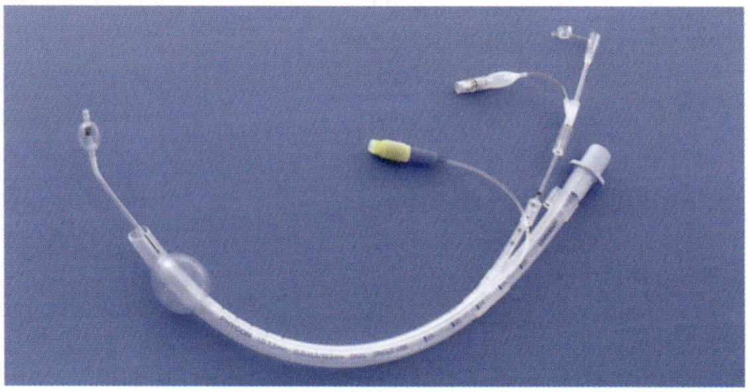

Figure 21.10 Univent Tube size 5.5 with enclosed ventilating lumen and enclosed endobronchial blocker. (Courtesy of Fuji System.)

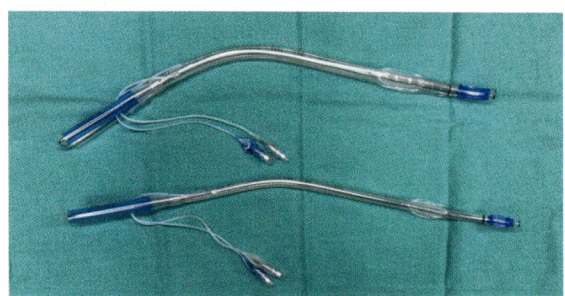

Figure 21.11 28 fr and 35 fr left-sided double-lumen tube with accompanying stylets. Tracheal cuff of 28 fr has an external diameter 10.2 mm versus 13.5 mm for the 35 fr.

Table 21.6 Summary of Double-Lumen Tube Size, Age, and Comparable Single-Lumen ETT

Age (years)	Double-lumen tube (fr)	OD of double-lumen tube (mm)	Comparable ID ETT size (mm)
9–10	26	8.7–9.3	6.5
10–12	28	9.3–10.2	7.0
12–14	32	10.5–11.2	7.5
>14	35	12.0–13.5	9.0

OD: outer diameter; ID: internal diameter; ETT: single-lumen ETT

visualization in children.[35,36] If there are issues with correct positioning and isolation, in many cases the provider has likely advanced the tube too distal.

Advantages of double-lumen tubes include their positional stability and their ability to isolate and ventilate both sides.[2,37] Additionally, it is possible to both suction as well as add effective CPAP to the isolated lung in the setting of incomplete collapse or intraprocedural hypoxemia.

One-Lung Ventilation in a Pediatric Patient with a Tracheostomy

In pediatric patients with a tracheostomy, lung isolation techniques are limited to those involving a bronchial blocker and endobronchial intubation.[20] In the case of endobronchial intubation, the tracheostomy is removed and an appropriately sized ETT is carefully inserted into the stoma and advanced into the desired mainstem bronchus using previously described techniques.

When using a bronchial blocker, a determination of whether to use an intraluminal or extraluminal approach should be made first. In smaller children in whom an extraluminal approach is the only viable option, both the ETT and bronchial blocker should be inserted adjacent to one another within the stoma following induction. If the stoma is too small to accommodate both, it is sometimes possible to insert the blocker through the glottis using laryngoscopy and then direct it down into the desired mainstem bronchus past the stoma and ETT. Either way, great care should be taken to minimize trauma to the stoma site to minimize the potential for blood in the airway. This is important as even moderate levels of secretions and small amounts of blood can have significantly deleterious effects on visualization of the airway. If this becomes an issue, fluoroscopy may be used to place the bronchial blocker.

In situations where the patient is large enough to accommodate an ETT compatible with an intraluminal blocker, previously discussed techniques can be used to facilitate placement following insertion of an ETT into the stoma. As with other techniques, though, the clinician should be careful to make sure the ETT is not inserted too far, thereby limiting visibility of the trachea and carina during blocker positioning. In patients with a tracheostomy, this is even more crucial because the entry point into the trachea is so much closer to the carina. In general, these techniques have been primarily described in adults, but certainly can be used in pediatric patients.[20]

One-Lung Ventilation Strategies in the Pediatric Patient with a Difficult Airway

There is very little literature to guide the clinician in terms of one-lung ventilation in children with a difficult airway. In children 8 years of age and older with a difficult airway, the airway should be secured carefully using techniques described elsewhere in the text with a standard single-lumen ETT and then an intraluminal bronchial blocker technique should be applied. In children less than 8 years of age, the clinicians should consider utilizing a mainstem intubation technique or, potentially, the intraluminal to extraluminal approach to extraluminal blocker placement described earlier in this chapter.[12]

In certain circumstances, if the clinician is comfortable, the Arndt bronchial blocker can be used intraluminally in combination with an SGA device.[38] This approach, however, may represent a significant imbalance in terms of risk versus benefit and should be undertaken with significant caution. In this technique, the patient is induced and an SGA device is placed. After confirming the SGA device position with a fiberoptic scope, the scope is withdrawn and

Table 21.7 Summary of Appropriate Age, Advantages and Disadvantages of Different One-Lung Ventilation Devices and Techniques

Method or device for one-lung ventilation	Age (years)	Advantages	Disadvantages
Endobronchial intubation	< 5	<ul><li>easy-to-execute technique</li><li>no special blocker or tube required</li><li>does provide good isolation in most circumstances</li></ul>	<ul><li>difficult to rapidly transition from one-lung ventilation to two-lung ventilation</li><li>limited options to manage intraprocedural hypoxemia</li><li>isolation can be incomplete, depending on position and bronchial seal</li></ul>
Single-balloon-based bronchial blocker	0–18	<ul><li>high quality of isolation when positioned correctly</li><li>easy to change from one-lung ventilation to two-lung ventilation</li><li>can be used in all ages, depending on size of blocker</li><li>can be used intra- or extraluminally</li></ul>	<ul><li>sometimes technically challenging to place</li><li>CPAP to non-ventilated lung may be ineffective</li><li>inability to suction non-ventilated lung</li></ul>
EZ-Blocker	6–18	<ul><li>high quality of isolation when positioned correctly</li><li>may be more positionally stable than other blockers secondary to design</li><li>easy to change from one-lung ventilation to two-lung ventilation</li><li>can sequentially isolate both lungs without repositioning</li><li>can be applied to greater range of ages</li><li>can be used intra- or extraluminally</li></ul>	<ul><li>can only be used in children 6 years and older</li><li>may be less positionally stable than double-lumen tube</li><li>CPAP and suctioning while available may be less effective due to size of channel</li></ul>
Univent Tube	6–18	<ul><li>high quality of isolation when positioned correctly</li><li>may be more positionally stable</li><li>easy to change from one-lung ventilation to two-lung ventilation</li></ul>	<ul><li>sometimes proper placement can be technically challenging</li><li>can only be used in children 6 years and up</li></ul>
Double-lumen tube	8–18	<ul><li>usually straightforward to place</li><li>high quality of isolation when positioned correctly</li><li>positionally very stable</li><li>easy to change from one-lung ventilation to two-lung ventilation</li><li>can apply CPAP to non-ventilated lung</li><li>can suction non-ventilated lung</li></ul>	<ul><li>large size makes it only applicable in children 8 years of age and up</li><li>potential for glottic and tracheal injury due to size</li></ul>

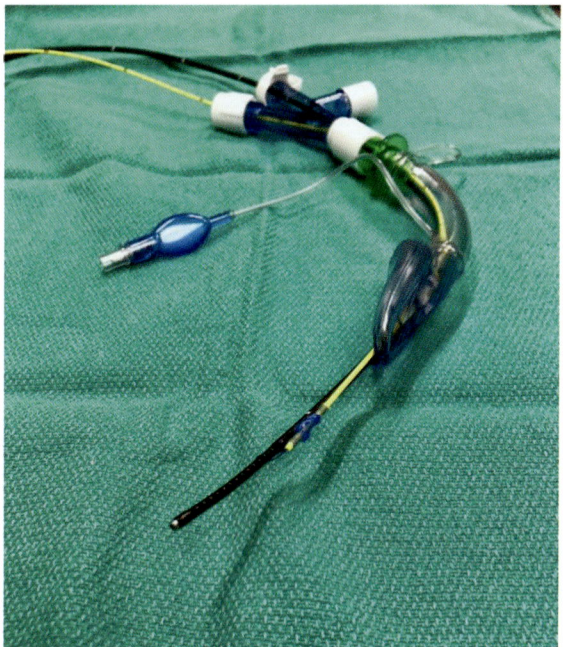

Figure 21.12 5 fr Arndt endbronchial blocker lassoed to 2.8 mm flexible fiberoptic scope passing through multiport adapter and air-Q size 1.5. Fiberoptic scope is driven down to desired mainstem bronchus and then bronchial blocker is threaded off scope and left in position.

the Arndt endobronchial blocker is lassoed to the scope following passage through the multiport adapter. The scope is then manipulated through the SGA device into the desired mainstem bronchus.[38,39] At this point, the loop is loosened and the scope withdrawn, leaving the blocker in place.

General Intraprocedural Management Principles for One-Lung Ventilation in Children

Once the lung has been isolated in any pediatric patient, there are several approaches to lung deflation. The most commonly employed technique is to simply allow for absorption atelectasis. In this approach, the lung is ventilated with 100% oxygen prior to initiating isolation in an attempt to mostly denitrogenate it, and then, once isolated, the oxygen is gradually absorbed by the pulmonary vasculature, causing the lung to deflate.[1,15] Because the lung has been isolated and no new gas reenters the lung, it will continue to deflate until positive pressure is reapplied to it. Another approach typically used with blocker techniques, although it could be used with a double-lumen tube, has been to actively deflate the desired lung by direct compression of the lung parenchyma by the surgeon in tandem with opening the anesthesia circuit to the atmosphere with the occlusive balloon down, followed by immediate inflation of the occlusive balloon or clamping of the appropriate lumen of the double-lumen tube.[1] For obvious reasons, this is not a great initial technique, but can be used to great effect following loss of isolation and device repositioning. Another variant of this is to simply open the circuit without direct compression by the surgeon and inflate the balloon after several seconds, allowing gas to passively exit the lung on the operative side prior to bronchial occlusion. In patients with a double-lumen tube, suction can also be applied to the nondependent lung to facilitate collapse as well. Lastly, in thoracoscopic procedures, the surgeon can insufflate carbon dioxide into the pleural cavity, leading to direct compression of the nondependent lung.[40] At the time of writing, no technique for collapse has been shown to be superior to another in pediatric patients.

In general, hypoxic vasoconstriction results in reasonable ventilation perfusion matching with few children becoming hypoxic to an extent that precludes single-lung ventilation.[1,4,41,42] There are cases, however, in children with significant respiratory disease where this may prove limiting, and good clinical judgment should be employed to prioritize adequate oxygenation over lung isolation. In general, a patient's oxygen saturations should be maintained at greater than 90%, although brief periods of desaturation down to 86% for less than 3–4 minutes may be acceptable in some patients.

Hypercarbia, and sometimes significant hypercarbia, should be expected in these cases.[1,41] Fortunately, respiratory acidosis appears to be well tolerated in pediatric patients with structurally normal hearts, and almost universally, patient's carbon dioxide levels will normalize rapidly following the reinstitution of two-lung ventilation. Significantly greater attention, however, should be applied to ongoing hemodynamics when performing one-lung ventilation in children with pulmonary hypertension and/or in children with cyanotic congenital heart disease where increases in pulmonary vascular resistance can lead to significant cardiovascular embarrassment.[43]

Summary

There are many techniques described here that have been used to successfully institute one-lung ventilation in children. All of them have advantages and disadvantages, and require some degree of practice and technical mastery to institute safely and effectively. Simulation can be an excellent resource for this. Care should be taken to weigh the risks and benefits of any one approach to one-lung ventilation in a given patient, realizing that perfect is oftentimes the enemy of good, and safety and safe airway management should always be the clinician's first priority.

References

1. Templeton TW, et al. Bending the Rules: a Novel Approach to Placement and Retrospective Experience with the 5 French Arndt Endobronchial Blocker in Children <2 Years. *Pediatric Anesthesia* 2016; **26**: 512–20.
2. Hammer GB, et al. Single-Lung Ventilation in Pediatric Patients. *Anesthesiology* 1996; **84**(6): 1503–6.
3. Marciniak B, et al. Fluoroscopic Guidance of Arndt Endobronchial Blocker Placement for Single Lung Ventilation in Small Children. *Acta Anesthesiology Scandanavia* 2008; **52**: 1003–5.
4. Stephenson, L. Routine Extraluminal Use of the 5F Arndt Endobronchial Blocker for One-Lung Ventilation in Children up to 24 Months of Age. *Journal of Cardiothoracic and Vascular Anesthesia* 2011; **25**(4): 683–6.
5. Wilson CA, Wilmhurst CA, AE Black. Anesthetic Techniques to Facilitate Lung Lavage for Pulmonary Alveolar Proteinosis in Children – New Airway Techniques and Review of the Literature. *Pediatric Anesthesia* 2015; **25**: 546–53.
6. Paquet C. Technique of Lung Isolation for Whole Lung Lavage in a Child with Pulmonary Alveolar Proteinosis. *Anesthesiology* 2009; **110**: 190–2.
7. Schmidt C, Bellensmann G, Van Aken H, Semik M, Bruessel T, Enk D. Single-Lung Ventilation for Pulmonary Lobe Resection in a Newborn. *Anesthesia & Analgesia* 2005; **101**: 362–4.
8. Haynes SR, Bonner S. Anesthesia for Thoracic Surgery in Children. *Pediatric Anesthesia* 2000; **10**: 237–51.
9. Dunn P. Physiology of the Lateral Decubitus Position and One-Lung Ventilation. *International Anesthesia Clinics* 2000; **38**: 25–53.
10. Hammer G. Single-Lung Ventilation in Infants and Children. *Pediatric Anesthesia* 2004; **14**: 98–102.
11. Neumann RP. The Neonatal Lung. *Pediatric Anesthesia* 2014; **24**: 10–21.
12. Templeton TW, et al. Inside Out: Repurposing Endobronchial Intubation to Facilitate Extraluminal Placement of a 5 Fr Arndt Bronchial Blocker in Young Infants. *Pediatric Anesthesia* 2018; **28**(7): 668–9.
13. Fabila TS. One Lung Ventilation Strategies for Infants and Children Undergoing Video Assisted Thoracoscopic Surgery. *Indian Journal of Anaesthesia* 2013; **57**(4): 339–44.
14. Kubota H, Toyoda Y, et al. Selective Blind Endobronchial Intubation in Children and Adults. *Anesthesiology* 1987; **67**: 587–9.
15. Ko R, Darling G, et al. The Use of Air in the Inspired Gas Mixture during Two-Lung Ventilation Delays Lung Collapse. *Anesthesia & Analgesia* 2009; **108**: 1092–6.
16. Letal M, Theam, M. Paediatric Lung Isolation. *British Journal of Anaesthesia Education* 2017; **17**(2): 57–72.
17. Templeton TW, Goenaga Diaz EJ, et al. A Prospective Comparison of Intraluminal and Extraluminal Placement of the 9-French Arndt Bronchial Blocker in Adult Thoracic Surgery Patients. *Journal of Cardiothoracic and Vascular Anesthesia* 2017; **31**: 1335–40.
18. Semmelmann A, Loop T, Anesthesia of Thoracic Surgery in Children. *Pediatric Anesthesia* 2018; **28**: 326–31.
19. Hsieh VC, Haberkern CM, Pediatric Endobronchial Blockers in Infants: a Refinement in Technique. *Pediatric Anesthesia* 2015; **25**: 438–9.
20. Tobias, J. Variation on One-Lung Ventilation. *Journal of Clinical Anesthesia* 2001; **13**: 35–9.
21. Nam JS, Seo H, Min HG. The Use of Lung Ultrasonography to Confirm Lung Isolation in an Infant who Underwent Emergent Video-Assisted Thoracoscopic Surgery: a Case Report. *Korean Journal of Anesthesia* 2015; **68**: 411–14.
22. Saporito A, Franceschini D, Tomasetti R, Anselmi L. Thoracic Ultrasound Confirmation of Correct Lung Exclusion before One-Lung Ventilation during Thoracic Surgery. *Journal of Ultrasound* 2013; **16**: 195–9.
23. Mungroop HE, Morei MN, Loef BG, Epema AH. Lung Isolation with a New Y-Shaped Endobronchial Blocking Device, the EZ-Blocker. *British Journal of Anaesthesia* 2010; **104**(1): 119–20.
24. Mourisse J, Verhagen A, van Rooji G, van der Heide S, Schuurbiers-Siebvers O, Van der Heijden E. Efficiency, Efficacy, and Safety of EZ-Blocker Compared with Left-Sided Double-Lumen Tube for One-Lung Ventilation.

Anesthesiology 2013; **118**(3): 550–61.

25. Templeton TW, Lawrence AE, et al. An Initial Experience with an Extraluminal EZ-Blocker: a New Alternative for One-Lung Ventilation in Pediatric Patients. *Pediatric Anesthesia* 2018; **2018**(28): 347–51.

26. Piccioni FV, Previtali P, et al. Extraluminal EZ-Blocker Placement for One-Lung Ventilation in Pediatric Thoracic Surgery. *Journal of Cardiothoracic and Vascular Anesthesia* 2015; **29**: e71–3.

27. Isil CT, Oba S. Paediatric Application of the EZ-Blocker for Thoracoscopic Sympathectomy. *British Journal of Anaesthesia* 2013; **111**: 845–6.

28. Templeton TW, Bryan YF. Outside is the New Inside. *Journal of Cardiothoracic and Vascular Anesthesia* 2017; **31**: e79.

29. Ueshima H, Otake H. Bilateral Pneumonectomy with Difficult Airway Managed by Using a Combination of i-gel and EZ-Blocker. *Journal of Clinical Anesthesia* 2016; **34**: 516.

30. Hammer GB, Redepath JH, Cannon WB. Use of the Univent Tube for Single-Lung Ventilation in Paediatric Patients. *Pediatric Anesthesia* 1998; **8**: 55–7.

31. Golianu B. Pediatric Thoracic Anesthesia. *Current Opinion in Anaesthesiology* 2005; **18**(1): 5–11.

32. Seefelder C. Use of the 26-French Double-Lumen Tube for Lung Isolation in Children. *Journal of Cardiothoracic and Vascular Anesthesia* 2014; **28**(3): e19–21.

33. Brodsky JB. Left Double-Lumen Tubes: Clinical Experience with 1170 Patients. *Journal of Cardiothoracic and Vascular Anesthesia* 2003; **17**(3): 289–98.

34. Slinger P. Fiberoptic Bronchoscopic Positioning of Double Lumen Tubes. *Journal of Cardiothoracic Anesthesia* 1989; **3**: 486–96.

35. Brodsky J. Con: Proper Positioning of a Double-Lumen Endobronchial Tube can Only be Accomplished with the Use of Endoscopy. *Journal of Cardiothoracic and Vascular Anesthesia* 1988; **2**: 105–9.

36. Brodsky JB, Mark JBD. A Simple Technique for Accurate Placement of Double Lumen Endobronchial Tubes. *Anesthesia Reviews* 1983; **10**: 26–30.

37. Clayton-Smith A, et al. A Comparison of the Efficacy and Adverse Effects of Double-Lumen Endobronchial Tubes and Bronchial Blockers in Thoracic Surgery: a Systematic Review and Meta-Analysis of Randomized Controlled Trials. *Journal of Cardiothoracic and Vascular Anesthesia* 2015; **29**: 955–66.

38. Li P, Gu H. One-Lung Ventilation Using Proseal Laryngeal Mask Airway and Arndt Endobronchial Blocker in Paediatric Scoliosis Surgery. *British Journal of Anaesthesia* 2009; **103**(6): 902–3.

39. Sun J. One-Lung Ventilation for Children with Pierre Robin Sequence Using Supreme LMA and Arndt Endobronchial Blocker: a Case Report. *International Journal of Clinical and Experimental Medicine* 2016; **9**(10): 20394–6.

40. Mack MJ, Acuff TE, Douthit MB, Bowman RT, Ryan WH. Present Role of Thoracoscopy in the Diagnosis and Treatment of Diseases of the Chest. *Annals of Thoracic Surgery* 1992; **54**: 403–9.

41. Sutton CJ, Puri S, Sprenker CJ, Camporesi EM. One-Lung Ventilation in Infants and Small Children: Blood Gas Values. *Journal of Anesthesia* 2012; **26**: 670–4.

42. Bird GT, et al. Effectiveness of Arndt Endobronchial Blockers in Pediatric Scoliosis Surgery: a Case Series. *Pediatric Anesthesia* 2007; **17**: 289–94.

43. Friesen RH. Anesthetic Management of Children with Pulmonary Arterial Hypertension. *Pediatric Anesthesia* 2008; **18**: 208–16.

Appendix: Airway Management Videos

Michelle Tsao, Anthony Tantoco, and Narasimhan Jagannathan

Video legends

Video 1: A neonate with Pierre Robin sequence. Note the severe upper airway obstruction and micrognathia present. This is a child who is likely to have an increased risk of complications during airway management. Refer to Chapters 1, 2, and 5 for further details.

Video 2: SGA device insertion techniques. Both standard midline and rotational insertion techniques are illustrated in this video. Refer to Chapter 5 for further details.

Video 3: Fiberoptic intubation of the trachea through the air-Q SGA device in a patient with Hunter syndrome. Refer to Chapters 5 and 8 for further details.

Video 4: Fiberoptic intubation of the trachea through the air-Q SGA device using a continuous ventilation technique. Refer to Chapters 5 and 8 for further details.

Video 5: Use of the King Vision video laryngoscope in patients with a potential difficult airway. Refer to Chapter 7 for further details.

Video 6: Use of the Storz C-MAC video laryngoscope for nasotracheal intubations.

Video 7: Use of the Storz fiberoptic bronchoscope for trans-oral tracheal intubation. Refer to Chapter 8 for further details.

Video 8: Use of the Storz fiberoptic bronchoscope for transnasal tracheal intubation. Refer to Chapter 8 for further details.

Video 9: Use of a hybrid technique using a GlideScope video laryngoscope with a fiberoptic bronchoscope to facilitate difficult tracheal intubation. Refer to Chapter 8 and Chapter 11.

Video 10: Use of the Supernova nasal mask for oxygenation and ventilation.

Video 11: Extraluminal placement of a 5 fr Arndt bronchial blocker in a 9-day-old infant with a chest wall cystic hematoma. Refer to Chapter 21 for further discussion of this technique.

Video 12: Extraluminal placement of a 5 fr Arndt bronchial blocker in 4-month-old using the intra- to extraluminal technique. Refer to Chapter 21 for further details.

Video 13: Extraluminal placement of an EZ-Blocker in a 6-year-old for schedule for resection of a mediastinal mass using the Piccioni approach. Refer to Chapter 21 for further details.

Index

acute asphyxial asthma 181
adenoids 3, 22
adverse events *see* complications of airway management
AECs *see* airway exchange catheters
age
   endobronchial tube size 214
   laryngoscope blade size 32
   one-lung ventilation 213–228
   rigid bronchoscope size 113
AincA Lighted Stylet 29–30
air bubbles, on US 144
air-Q SGA 44–46, 119–120
   self-pressurizing 41, 46
airflow resistance 61, 185
Airtraq SP video laryngoscope 83
airway exchange catheters (AECs)
   extubation 163–165
   intubation 29
   oxygenation 62, 164
airway obstruction 21–23, 132
   functional 14–15, 23, 95, 130, 132
   lower 15, 23, 191, 197
   upper *see* upper airway obstruction
algorithms for difficult airways 20–25
   EXIT procedure 209
   laryngospasm 14–17
   NICU emergencies 192
alveolar proteinosis 212
Ambu Aura-i SGA 47
Ambu AuraGain SGA 47
anatomy 1–3, 8
   craniofacial abnormalities 3–5, 8–10
   cricothyroid membrane 134
   neonates 2, 185–187
      premature lungs 196
anesthesia
   in the ED 178–181
   EXIT procedure 207–208
   flexible bronchoscopy 92–95, 174
   in neonates 193–194
   rigid bronchoscopy 114–115
   in trauma cases 172–173
      burns 174–175
   see also muscle relaxants
antisialagogues 94
Apert syndrome 5, 188
apneic oxygenation 13, 58

Arndt bronchial blocker 216–221, 224–226
articulating stylets 29
aspiration of gastric contents 15–16, 38, 172–173, 177
asthma 15
   acute exacerbations 181–182
atelectasis 56
   in one-lung ventilation 226
atropine 13–14, 94, 179–180
awake extubation 161, 163
awake intubation
   flexible bronchoscopy 63, 92–94, 174
   flexible bronchoscopy plus SGA 50, 121

B-mode ultrasonography 144
"Back" maneuver 33
bag-mask ventilation (BMV) 59–60, 172
Bailey's maneuver 165
balloon catheter bronchial blockers 215
   EZ-Blocker 221–222
   intraprocedural management 220–221
   placement 215–220
   size 215–216
   with a tracheostomy 224
barotrauma 59, 62, 65, 138, 181
BD Insyte cannula 158
Beckwith–Wiedemann syndrome 189
benzodiazepines 93, 179
bone, on US 144
Bonfils intubation endoscope (optical stylet) 30, 103–106
bovine spongiform encephalopathy (BSE) 28
BPD (bronchopulmonary dysplasia) 56, 196–200
bradycardia 8, 12, 55, 179–180
   fetal 208
Brambank Intubation Endoscope 30
branchial (pharyngeal) arches 1
branchial (pharyngeal) clefts 1–2
bronchial blockers 215, 225
   difficult airways 224–226
   EZ-Blocker 221–222
   intraprocedural management 220–221

placement 215–220
size 215–216
with a tracheostomy 224
Univent Tube 223
bronchopulmonary dysplasia (BPD) 56, 196–200
bronchoscopy *see* flexible bronchoscopy; rigid bronchoscopy
bronchospasm 15, 23
Bullard laryngoscope 61, 72–73
burns 170, 173–176
"BURP" maneuver 33

can't intubate, can't oxygenate (CICO) 132–140
   burns cases 175
   clinical governance 134
   cricothyrotomy 65, 134–138, 148–149, 158–159
   difficult airway carts 134, 158–159, 194
   oxygenation 137–140, 159
   problems with direct laryngoscopy 13, 133
   tracheostomy 24, 132–133, 135, 137
   US identification of structures 148–149
cannula cricothyrotomy 135, 137–138, 158–159
   oxygenation 63–65, 137–140, 159
cannulas, nasal
   high-flow O_2 58–59, 162
   low-flow O_2 58
carbon dioxide
   in head injuries 180
   in one-lung ventilation 226
carboxyhemoglobin 173
cardiac arrest 12, 20, 55, 182
CardioMed ETVC catheter 164
cardiopulmonary resuscitation (CPR) 182
cartilage, on US 144
caustic burns 170, 173
cervical area *see* neck
cesarean sections 207–208
CHAOS syndrome 205, 208–209
chemical burns 170, 173
chemotherapy 56–57

Index

chest trauma 169–172
chest wall 3, 185
choanal atresia 2, 185, 187
CICO *see* can't intubate, can't oxygenate
Clarus videoscope (Trachway) 107–108
Classic LMA/Unique LMA 42–43
cleft lip/palate/midface 4–5, 189
clinical examination 21
  trauma cases 171–172
clinical governance 134, 160
  see also training
Cobra Perilaryngeal Airway 48
complications of airway management 12–16
  of cricothyrotomy 137–138
  of flexible bronchoscopy 100
  of laryngoscopy 13, 60–61
  of oxygenation 55–57, 59–61
    barotrauma 59, 62, 65, 138, 181
  of rigid bronchoscopy 116–117
  of SGAs 40–41, 122
  of video laryngoscopy 83–85
  see also hypoxemia/hypoxia
computed tomography (CT) 169–172
congenital diaphragmatic hernia 65, 204, 206–207
conjoined twins 207
Cook airway exchange catheter 29, 163–164
CPR (cardiopulmonary resuscitation) 182
craniofacial abnormalities 3–5, 8–10, 60, 188
craniosynostosis 5
cricoid cartilage 3, 186–187
cricoid pressure 172–173
cricothyrotomy
  anatomy 134
  cannula versus scalpel 135–138, 158–159
  complications 137–138
  difficult airway carts 134, 158–159
  kits 65, 136
  oxygenation 137–138
  patient position 134–135
  US identification of structures 148–149
croup 15
Crouzon syndrome 5, 188
cyanotic spells in neonates with BPD 197
cysts 144, 189–190

DACs (difficult airway carts) 134, 155–160, 194
defogging methods 72, 99
delivery room management of neonates 191–192

EXIT procedure 65–66, 147–148, 204–210
dentition 2
  damage to 85, 114, 117
developmental anatomy *see* anatomy
dexmedetomidine 93
diaphragm
  congenital diaphragmatic hernia 65, 204, 206–207
  on ultrasound 152
difficult airway carts (DACs) 134, 155–160, 194
direct laryngoscopy (DL) 27–35
  and bronchoscopy
    flexible 97
    rigid 113, 115
  CICO scenario 13, 133
  complications 13, 60–61
  definition of difficult intubation 11–12
  equipment
    blades 27–28, 35
    exchange catheters 29
    introducers 29
    preparation 21, 30, 34
    stylets 28–30, 61
  EXIT procedure 208
  history 27, 31
  in infants 3, 27, 31
  oxygen delivery 28, 61–63
  techniques 31–33
    external laryngeal manipulation 33
    nasotracheal intubation 33–34
    paraglossal 33
    patient positioning 31–32
    retromolar 33
  see also video laryngoscopy
documentation, DACs 159–160
double-lumen tubes 223–225

ECMO, EXIT procedure 207, 209
embryonic development 1–2, 196
emergency airway management in the NICU 192–194
emergency department airway management 177–182
emergency front of neck access *see* front of neck access
endobronchial blockers 215, 225
  difficult airways 224–226
  EZ-Blocker 221–222
  intraprocedural management 220–221
  placement 215–220
  size 215–216
  with a tracheostomy 224
  Univent Tube 223

endobronchial intubation 214–215, 224–225
  in error 16
enhanced direct laryngoscopy 70, 82, 85
Enk oxygen flow modulator 64–65, 139
epiglottis 3, 186
epignathus 205
epinephrine 13–15, 23
epistaxis 34, 100
epulis 205
eschars 170, 174
Eschmann introducer 29
esophagus
  fetal, compression 204–206
  tracheal tube misplaced in 30, 151
etomidate 178–181
EXIT procedure 210
  indications 65–66
  intraoperative management 207–210
  preoperative period 147–148, 207
external laryngeal manipulation 33, 97
extubation 161–166
  unplanned in neonates 192
EZ-Blocker 221–222, 225

facemasks 10, 15, 21, 24
  bag masks 59–60, 172
  intubating 99
facial anatomy 2
  see also craniofacial abnormalities
facial burns 174
facial fractures 33–34, 169–170
Fastrach (intubating) LMA 44
fat tissue, on US 144
fentanyl 193
fetal development 1–2, 196
fetal endoscopic tracheal occlusion (FETO) 206
fetal interventions *see* EXIT procedure
fetal ultrasound 147–148
fiberoptic stylet scope (FSS) 105, 109
flexible bronchoscopy (fiberoptic, FOB) 90–101
  anesthesia 92–95, 174
  in burns 172–175
  complications 100
  endobronchial intubation 214
  equipment 90–91
    size 90–91, 95–96
  nasopharyngeal 94, 100
  oropharyngeal 94, 100
  oxygenation 63, 99
  preparation 91–92, 94
  retrograde 125–127
  SGA-assisted 48–50, 101, 118–122
  techniques 95–100, 119–126
  VL-assisted 122–125

231

Index

flexible fiberoptic endoscopy 170, 172–173
fluids, on US 144
FOB (fiberoptic bronchoscopy) *see* flexible bronchoscopy
foreign bodies 23, 148
 removal via rigid bronchoscopy 112, 114, 116
front of neck access (FONA)
 burns cases 175
 cricothyrotomy 65, 134–138, 158–159
 difficult airway carts 134, 158–159
 indications for 24, 132
 oxygenation 63–65, 137–140, 159
 tracheostomy 24, 133, 135, 137
 in neonates 192–193, 200–202
 one-lung ventilation 224
 US identification of structures 148–149
Frova intubating introducer 29
FSS (fiberoptic stylet scope) 105, 109
functional airway obstruction 14–15, 23, 132
 laryngospasm 14–15, 95, 130

gastric contents, aspiration 15–16, 38, 172–173, 177
gastric distension 22, 162
general anesthesia
 in burns cases 174–175
 in the ED 178–181
 EXIT procedure 207–208
 flexible bronchoscopy 92–93, 95
 rigid bronchoscopy 115
 in trauma cases 172–173
 see also muscle relaxants
GlideScope video laryngoscope 69, 71, 73–78, 85, 122
glottic webs/atresia 191
Goldenhar syndrome 4
gum elastic bougies (Eschmann introducer) 29

head injuries 33–34, 177, 180
heated humidified high-flow nasal cannula (HHHFNC) 58–59
heliox 166
help, calling for 22
hemangioma, subglottic 191
hemifacial microsomia 4
Hopkins telescope 113
hot water, softening tubes in 96
hybrid techniques 118
 retrograde-assisted FOI 125–127
 SGA-assisted FOI 48–50, 101, 118–122
 video laryngoscopy-assisted FOI 122–125

hydrops, fetal 206–207
hyoid bone 134
hypercarbia 180, 226
hyperventilation 180
hypopharynx 186, 189–191
hypoplasia, craniofacial 4
hypoxemia/hypoxia 13–14, 20, 55, 60
 children requiring intubation in the ED 177–178
 neonates 20, 56
 one-lung ventilation 220–221, 226

i-gel SGA 41, 46–47
iatrogenic injuries
 due to airway management 16, 170–171
 thermal 170, 174
incidence
 complications of airway management 12, 55
 difficult intubation 10–12, 60
 difficult mask ventilation 10
 difficult SGA 11
indirect laryngoscopy 69
 see also video laryngoscopy
infants
 awake intubation (using SGAs) 50, 121
 developmental anatomy 2–3
 direct laryngoscopy 3, 27, 31
 increased complication risk 13, 61
 micrognathia 11, 60
 video laryngoscopy 78, 80
inhalational injuries 170, 173
injured airways 169–176
 airway management (general) 171–173
 burns 170, 173–176
 iatrogenic 16, 170–171
introducers 29
intubating facemasks 99
intubating oral airways 99
intubation 21, 23–24
 and anatomy 3
 burns cases 173–176
 complications 12
 croup 15
 of flexible bronchoscopy 100
 of laryngoscopy 13, 60–61
 of rigid bronchoscopy 116–117
 of SGAs 122
 trauma 16, 170–171, 190
 tube misplacement 16, 30, 151
 of video laryngoscopy 83–85
 direct laryngoscopy 31–34
 in the ED 177–182
 endobronchial 214–215, 224–225
 in error 16
 EXIT procedure 208–209

fiberoptic intubation via SGA 48–50, 101, 118–122
fiberoptic intubation with VL 122–125
flexible bronchoscopy 95–100
incidence of difficult intubation 10–12, 60
nasal 33–34, 194
neonates
 anesthesia 193–194
 nasal 194
 US localization of tube 152–153
 video laryngoscopy 78, 80, 194–195
optical stylets 103–104, 107
oxygenation 13, 60–63
retrograde-assisted FOI 125–127
SGAs 44–49
trauma cases 173–177
ultrasonography (checking placement) 151–153
video laryngoscopy 69–72, 74–75, 79–80, 194–195
 see also extubation

jaw
 anatomy 2
 fractures 169, 172
 micrognathia 4, 11, 60, 188, 205–206, 208
jaw thrust 60, 97
jet ventilation 64–65, 139, 164

ketamine 93, 179–181

laryngeal anatomy 1, 3, 186–187
laryngeal braking 3
laryngeal manipulation 33, 97
laryngeal mask airways (LMAs) 43–44, 63, 118–119, 194
Laryngeal Tube/LT Suction II SGAs 47–48
laryngeal ultrasound 145–146
laryngomalacia 189, 198
laryngoscopy *see* direct laryngoscopy; indirect laryngoscopy; video laryngoscopy
laryngospasm 14–15, 95, 130
laryngotracheal injuries 170–171
Le Fort classification of facial fractures 169
LEMON (assessment of trauma cases) 171
Levitan scope (optical stylet) 105, 108
lidocaine 50, 94, 114, 121, 180
lighted stylets 29–30, 108–109
LMAs (laryngeal mask airways) 43–44, 63, 118–119, 194

232

Index

local anesthesia
  flexible bronchoscopy 92, 94
  laryngoscopy 180
  rigid bronchoscopy 114
  SGA in awake infant 50, 121
longitudinal (string of pearls) ultrasound technique 148–149
low birth weight neonates 195–202
  see also premature neonates
lower airway obstruction 15, 23, 191, 197
lung
  atelectasis 56, 226
  BPD 56, 196–200
  fetal masses (EXIT procedure) 206–207, 209
  neonates 185
    premature 56, 196–200
  ultrasonography 143, 145–147, 151–153
  pneumothorax 153
  see also one-lung ventilation
lymphatic malformations, cervical 205

M-mode ultrasonography 144–147
Macintosh laryngoscopy blade 27, 35
  insertion 32
  sizes 28, 32
macroglossia 186, 189
Magill forceps 34
Mallampati score 11
malleable stylets 28–29
malleable video stylets 108
mandible
  anatomy 2
  fractures 169, 172
  hypoplasia (micrognathia) 4, 11, 60, 188, 205–206, 208
Manujet III transtracheal jet ventilator 64–65, 139
mask ventilation 10, 15, 21, 24
  bag masks 59–60, 172
McCoy laryngoscopy blade 28
McGrath video laryngoscope 80–82
Melker cricothyrotomy/tracheotomy kit 158
micrognathia 4, 11, 60, 188
  EXIT procedure 205–206, 208
micro preemie neonates 195–202
  see also premature neonates
midline insertion of an SGA 41–42
Miller laryngoscopy blade 27, 35
  insertion 32–33
  size 28, 32
multidisciplinary approach 134, 160
muscle, on US 144
muscle relaxants 3–5, 95, 129–130
  in burns cases 174
  in the ED 179

functional airway obstruction 15, 23, 130
  reversal 95, 130

nasal cannulation
  high-flow O_2 58–59, 162
  low-flow O_2 58
nasal cavity stenosis 188
nasal trumpets 99, 194–195
nasal/nasopharyngeal obstruction 2, 185, 187–188
nasal/nasotracheal intubation 33–34, 194
  epistaxis 34, 100
nasopharyngeal flexible bronchoscopy 94, 100
neck
  burns 174–176
  fetal masses 204–206, 208–209
  neonatal 187
  trauma 169–170, 172, 177
neonates
  airway emergencies 192–194
  anatomy 2, 185–187
    premature lungs 196
    size (compared with adults) 185
  delivery room 191–192
  EXIT procedure 65–66, 147–148, 204–210
  intubation
    anesthesia 193–194
    nasal 194
    US localization of tube 152–153
    video laryngoscopy 78, 80, 194–195
  lower airway obstruction 191, 197
  nasopharyngeal airways 194–195
  oxygenation
    adverse effects 55–57, 196–200
    desaturation rates 57
    hypoxemia 20, 56
    physiology 61, 185
  premature 195–202
    adverse effects of O_2 therapy 56, 196–200
    extubation 166, 192
    hypoxemia 20
    pharyngeal collapse 2
    resuscitation 192
  resuscitation 51, 56, 192
  SGAs 51, 121, 194
  tracheostomy 192–193, 200–202
  upper airway obstruction 186–191, 197–198, 204–206
neuromuscular blockade see muscle relaxants
NICU emergencies 192–194
nose see entries at nasal

obese patients 30, 148
obstructive sleep apnea 3
oculoauriculovertebral spectrum 4
one-lung ventilation 227
  advantages and disadvantages of various devices 225
  and age 213–228
  bronchial blockers 215–223
  difficult airways 224–226
  double-lumen tubes 223–224
  endobronchial intubation 214–215, 224
  indications 212–213
  intraprocedural management 220–221, 226
  physiology 212–227
  with a tracheostomy 224
ontogeny 1–3
"open-box" algorithm 23–25
opioids 93, 166, 193
optical forceps 114, 116
optical stylets 103–109
  adult 107–109
  advantages and disadvantages of different devices 105–107, 109
  efficacy 104, 106–109
  intubation techniques 103–104, 107
  oxygenation 61, 106
  pediatric 30, 103–107
  specifications 105
Optiflow HHHFNC system 59
Optiscope optical stylet 108
oral airways 99, 163, 194–195
oropharyngeal anatomy 2–3, 186
oropharyngeal flexible bronchoscopy 94, 100
oropharyngeal injuries 85
oropharyngeal obstruction 22, 188–189, 205
oxidative stress 56
oxygenation 55–66
  adverse effects 55–57, 59, 196–200
  AECs 62, 164
  apneic 13, 58
  bag-mask ventilation 59–60, 172
  emergency FONA 63–65, 137–140, 159
  EXIT procedure 65–66, 147–148
  extubation 162, 164
  flexible bronchoscopes 63, 99
  heliox 166
  during intubation 13, 60–63
  during laryngoscopy 28, 61–63
  nasal cannula high flow 58–59, 162
  nasal cannula low flow 58
  nasal trumpets 99, 194–195
  one-lung ventilation 220–221
  optical stylets 61, 106

233

Index

oxygenation (cont.)
  preoxygenation 20, 57–58
  rigid bronchoscopes 62–63, 112
  SGAs 63
  video laryngoscopes 61–62, 82
  see also hypoxemia/hypoxia

palate 4–5, 189
papilloma (case history) 133
paraglossal laryngoscopy 33
Parker Flex-it articulating stylet 29
Parker Flex-Tip tracheal tube 96
patent ductus arteriosus 198
patient positioning
  cricothyrotomy 134–135
  direct laryngoscopy 31–32
  extubation 162
  one-lung ventilation 213–227
  rigid bronchoscopy 115
PEEP (positive end expiratory pressure) 57
Pentax AWS video laryngoscope 83
percutaneous cricothyrotomy kits 65, 136
perilaryngeal sealers 38–47
Pfeiffer syndrome 5, 188
pharyngeal anatomy 2–3, 8, 185–187
pharyngeal (branchial) arches 1
pharyngeal (branchial) clefts 1–2
pharyngeal pouches 1–2
pharyngeal sealers 39, 47–48
physiology 3, 8, 161
  neonates 61, 185
  one-lung ventilation 212–227
Pierre Robin sequence 4, 60, 121, 188
"pink" screen (red-out) 72, 98
pleura 146
pneumothorax 117, 138, 153
Poiseuille's equation 61, 185
positive end expiratory pressure (PEEP) 57
positive pressure ventilation (PPV)
  in extubation 166
  in septic shock 180–181
  and SGAs 40, 51
premature neonates 195–202
  adverse effects of O_2 therapy 56, 196–200
  extubation 166, 192
  hypoxemia 20
  lungs 196
  pharyngeal collapse 2
  resuscitation 192
preoxygenation 20, 57–58
propofol 23, 93–94, 179
ProSeal LMA 43
pyriform sinus aperture stenosis 187–188

RAFOI (retrograde-assisted fiberoptic intubation) 125–127
rapid-sequence induction 172–173
reactive airways 8, 13
  status asthmaticus 181–182
"red-out" (pink screen) 72, 98
reintubation (failed extubation) 164–166
remifentanil 166
respiratory acidosis 20, 58, 226
respiratory failure 171, 177
  see also hypoxemia/hypoxia
respiratory physiology 3, 8, 161
  hypoxemia 13–14, 55
  neonatal 185
  one-lung ventilation 212–227
resuscitation
  CPR in the ED 182
  of neonates 51, 56, 192
retinopathy of prematurity 56
retrograde-assisted fiberoptic intubation (RAFOI) 125–127
retromolar laryngoscopy 33
ribs 146
rigid bronchoscopy 62–63, 112–117
  complications 116–117
  equipment 112–114
  post-procedure care 116
  techniques 115–116
  uses 112, 116
risk factors
  for airway complications 12–13
  for difficult airway management 10–11
  for hypoxemia 55
Robertshaw laryngoscopy blade 28
rocuronium 179
rotational insertion of an SGA 41

scald injuries 170, 173
scalpel cricothyrotomy 136, 138, 158–159
scissors maneuver 32
sedatives/sedation
  in awake intubation 93–94, 174
  in the ED 178–181
  in extubation 166
Seldinger technique for tracheal access 136
Sellick's maneuver 172–173
SensaScope optical stylet 104–109
septic shock 180–181
Seward laryngoscopy blade 28
SGAs see supraglottic airways
Sheridan tube exchange catheter 164
Shikani optical stylet 30, 105–107
shock, septic 180–181
signposting the location of DACs 155
skull, anatomy 2, 8

sliding lung sign 147, 151–153
sniffing position 31–32
spinal injuries (cervical) 169, 172, 177
status asthmaticus 181–182
Storz video laryngoscope 78–80
stridor 161, 189–191, 198
string-of-pearls (longitudinal) ultrasound technique 148–149
stylet scope 105, 109
stylets
  articulating 29
  lighted 29–30, 108–109
  malleable 28–29
  optical see optical stylets
  removal of SGAs after intubation 119–120
  in video laryngoscopy 74, 79
subglottic cysts 190
subglottic hemangioma 191
subglottic stenosis 16, 133, 190, 197–200
succinylcholine 15, 95, 174, 179
suctioning
  bronchoscopy 97, 99–100, 114, 116
  extubation 163
  no port in optical stylets 103–105
  in trauma cases 171
sugammadex 95, 130
supraglottic airways (SGAs) 23, 38–51
  complications 13, 40–41, 122
  contraindications 121
  cuff volumes and pressures 39–41
  difficult placement 11
  extubation 164–166
  insertion 41–42
  intubation 44–49, 63
    using a fiberoptic bronchoscope 48–50, 101, 118–122
  in neonates 51, 194
  perilaryngeal sealers 38–47
  pharyngeal sealers 39, 47–48
  PPV 40, 51
  rescue airways 40–51
  spontaneous ventilation 51
Supreme LMA 43–44
Surch-Lite Stylet 29–30

TACA (transverse) ultrasound technique 148–154
teeth 2
  damage to 85, 114, 117
teratoma
  cervical 205, 208–209
  oropharyngeal 190, 205
thermal injuries 170, 173–176
thoracic trauma 169–172
three axes alignment theory (TAAT) 31
tongue 2

Index

macroglossia 186, 189
  pulling out of mouth 97
  on ultrasound 145
tonsils 3, 22
tooth guards 114
topical anesthesia
  flexible bronchoscopy 92, 94
  laryngoscopy 180
  rigid bronchoscopy 114
  SGA in awake infant 50, 121
trachea
  anatomy 3, 187
  long segment stenosis 191
  on ultrasound 146
    internal diameter 149–151
    tube placement 151–152
tracheobronchomalacia 197
tracheomalacia 191
tracheostomy 24, 133, 135, 137
  in neonates 192–193, 200–202
  one-lung ventilation 224
Trachway (Clarus videoscope) 107–108
training 61, 79, 85
  CICO 134
  DAC use 159
  ED personnel 178
transverse (TACA) ultrasound technique 148–154
trauma to the airways 169–176
  airway management (general) 171–173
  burns 170, 173–176
  iatrogenic 16, 170–171
trauma, facial 33–34, 169–170
traumatic brain injury 177, 180

Treacher Collins syndrome 4–5, 60
triple airway maneuver 22
Truflex stylet 29
TRUST (tracheal rapid ultrasound saline test) 152
Truview PCD video laryngoscope 61–62, 82

UESCOPE video laryngoscope 82–83
ultrasonography (US)
  appearance of airways and associated tissues 143–147
  equipment 143
  indications for use 145–153, 170, 172
Unique LMA 43
Univent Tube 223, 225
upper airway obstruction 2–5, 22–23, 132
  EXIT procedure 204–206
  failed extubation 161
  in neonates 186–191, 197–198, 204–206
  in trauma cases 171
upper respiratory tract infections 15
US *see* ultrasonography

vallecular cysts 189
vascular structures, on US 144
vasoconstricting agents 94
vecuronium 179
Ventrain oxygen ventilation device 62–65, 139
video-assisted laryngoscopy (VAL) 70, 82, 85
video laryngoscopy (VL) 69–85

  in burns cases 175
  complications 83–85
  efficacy 72, 75, 80, 82–83, 122
  equipment 73, 83
    Airtraq SP 83
    Bullard 61, 72–73
    GlideScope 69, 71, 73–78, 85, 122
    McGrath 80–82
    Pentax AWS 83
    Storz C-Mac 78–80
    Truview PCD 61–62, 82
    UEScope 82–83
  fiberoptic intubation (VLAFOI) 122–125
  history 69
  neonates 194–195
  oxygenation 61–62, 82
  problems
    insufficient view 70–72, 74–75, 79–80
    view-tube discrepancy 72, 75, 80
  techniques 69–72, 74–75, 79–80
    fiberoptic intubation 122–124
  as a training aid 61, 79, 85
VLAFOI (video laryngoscopy-assisted fiberoptic intubation) 122–125
vocal cords
  laryngospasm 14–15, 95, 130
  paralysis 190–191, 198

Wis-Hipple laryngoscopy blade 27–28
Wisconsin laryngoscopy blade 27–28